COMPLETE AROMATHERAPY *for* BEGINNERS

Everything You Need to Get Started with Essential Oils

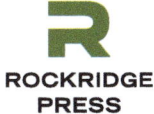

ROCKRIDGE PRESS

No book, including this one, can ever replace the diagnostic expertise and medical advice of a physician in providing information about your health. The information contained herein is not intended to replace medical advice. You should consult with your doctor before using the information in this or any health-related book.

As of press time, the URLs in this book link or refer to existing websites on the internet. Rockridge Press is not responsible for the outdated, inaccurate, or incomplete content available on these sites.

Copyright © 2015, 2016, 2018 by Rockridge Press

All rights reserved. No part of this publication may be reproduced, stored in a retrieval system, or transmitted in any form or by any means, electronic, mechanical, photocopying, recording, scanning, or otherwise, without the prior written permission of the Publisher. Requests to the Publisher for permission should be addressed to the Permissions Department, Rockridge Press, 1955 Broadway, Suite 400, Oakland, CA 94612.

First Rockridge Press trade paperback edition 2022

Rockridge Press and the Rockridge Press logo are trademarks or registered trademarks of Callisto Media Inc. and/or its affiliates in the United States and other countries and may not be used without written permission.

For general information on our other products and services, please contact our Customer Care Department within the United States at (866) 744-2665, or outside the United States at (510) 253-0500.

The content in this book was previously published in *DIY Aromatherapy* (9781623156442), *Aromatherapy for Natural Living* (9781623157494), and *Aromatherapy for Beginners* (9781939754608).

Paperback ISBN: 978-1-68539-493-6
eBook ISBN: 979-8-88608-977-6

Manufactured in the United States of America

Interior and Cover Designer: Heather Krakora
Art Producer: Hannah Dickerson
Editor: Olivia Bartz
Production Editor: Dylan Julian
Production Manager: Holly Haydash

Photography © Shannon Douglas, cover and pp. X, 8, 16; Trinette Reed/Stocksy, p. II; Nature Picture Library/Alamy Stock Photo, p. 73; All other photography used under license from Shutterstock.com and iStock.com. Illustrations used under license from iStock.com.

10 9 8 7 6 5 4 3 2 1 0

CONTENTS

Introduction xi

PART ONE: EVERYTHING YOU NEED TO KNOW ABOUT AROMATHERAPY 1

CHAPTER ONE: AROMATHERAPY BASICS 3

Benefits of Aromatherapy 4

How Essential Oils Work 5

CHAPTER TWO: THE SCIENCE BEHIND AROMATHERAPY 9

Behind the Scents 10

Producing Essential Oils 12

Chemistry 101 13

Moving Forward 14

CHAPTER THREE: WORKING WITH ESSENTIAL OILS 17

Determining Your Needs 18

Shopping for Essential Oils 18

All About Carrier Oils 21

Items to Have on Hand: Essential and Nice to Have 22

Store Your Oils Well 25

Using Essential Oils Safely 26

Your Starter Kit Essential Oil All-Stars 35

Dilution and Substitution 35

PART TWO: ESSENTIAL OIL PROFILES 41

PART THREE: RECIPES, REMEDIES, AND APPLICATIONS FOR HEALTH AND WELLNESS 129

CHAPTER FOUR: CHRONIC CONDITIONS, DISEASES, AND ILLNESSES 131

Asthma 132
Bronchitis 134
Canker Sores 136
Colds 138

Congestion 140
Fever 142
Fibromyalgia 144
Halitosis 146

Laryngitis and Sore Throat 148
Pinkeye 150
Sinusitis 152

CHAPTER FIVE: ACHES AND PAINS 155

Backache 156
Cuts and Scrapes 158
Hangover 160
Headache 162
Joint Pain 164
Motion Sickness 166
Muscle Cramps 168
Muscle Soreness 170
Neck Pain 172
Nosebleed 174
Sprain 176
Toothache 178

CHAPTER SIX: SKIN CONDITIONS AND CONCERNS 181

Blisters 182
Boils 184
Burns 186
Chapped Lips 188
Cold Sores 190
Diaper Rash
  (for Infants) 192
Eczema 194
Hives 196
Psoriasis 198
Stretch Marks 200
Warts 202

CHAPTER SEVEN: STRESS, WELL-BEING, AND SLEEP 205

Anxiety 206
Concentration 208
Exhaustion 210
Insomnia 212
Moodiness 214
Nervousness 216
Relaxation 218
Stress 220

CHAPTER EIGHT: GUT HEALTH 223

Bloating 224
Constipation 226
Diarrhea 228
Heartburn 230
Hemorrhoids 232
Indigestion 234
Nausea and
  Vomiting 236

CHAPTER NINE: SEXUAL HEALTH 239

Arousal 240
Menopause 242
Menstrual
  Symptoms 244
Urinary Tract Infection
  (UTI) 246
Vaginal Yeast Infection 248

PART FOUR: RECIPES, REMEDIES, AND APPLICATIONS FOR BEAUTY AND COSMETIC CARE 251

CHAPTER TEN: ACNE, WRINKLES, AND OTHER SKIN CARE 253

Acne 254
Age Spots 256
Body Odor 258
Cellulite 260
Dry Skin 262
Ingrown Hair 264
Oily Skin 266
Puffy Eyes 268
Razor Bumps 270
Rosacea 272
Wrinkles 274

CHAPTER ELEVEN: MOISTURIZERS AND TONERS 277

CHAPTER TWELVE: HEALTHY, STRONG HAIR 283

Dandruff 284
Dry Hair 286
Oily Hair 288
Split Ends 290

CHAPTER THIRTEEN: NURTURING THE HANDS AND FEET 293

Athlete's Foot 294
Brittle Nails 296
Bunions 298
Calluses 300
Cracked Heels 302
Dry Hands 304
Foot Odor 306
Ingrown Toenails 308

CHAPTER FOURTEEN: SCENTS AND PERFUMES 311

PART FIVE: RECIPES, REMEDIES, AND APPLICATIONS FOR THE HOME AND OUTDOORS 317

CHAPTER FIFTEEN: CLEANING AROUND THE HOME 319

Air Fresheners 320
Bathroom Cleansers 322
Floors 324
Glass and Mirrors 326
Kitchen Cleansers 328
Mold and Mildew 330
Refrigerator Cleansers 332
Stain Removers 334

CHAPTER SIXTEEN: PROTECTING PETS AND BANISHING PESTS 337

- Ant Repellent 338
- Fleas 340
- Mosquitoes 342
- Moths 344
- Spiders 346

CHAPTER SEVENTEEN: TENDING TO THE OUTDOORS AND TREATING OUTDOOR CONCERNS 349

- Hay Fever and Allergies 350
- Insect Bites and Bee Stings 352
- Lawn and Garden 354
- Poison Ivy 356
- Sunburn 358

Measurement Conversions 361

Glossary 362

Resources 364

Continuing Education 364

Ailments and Oils Quick Reference 365

References 366

Oils Index 375

General Index 391

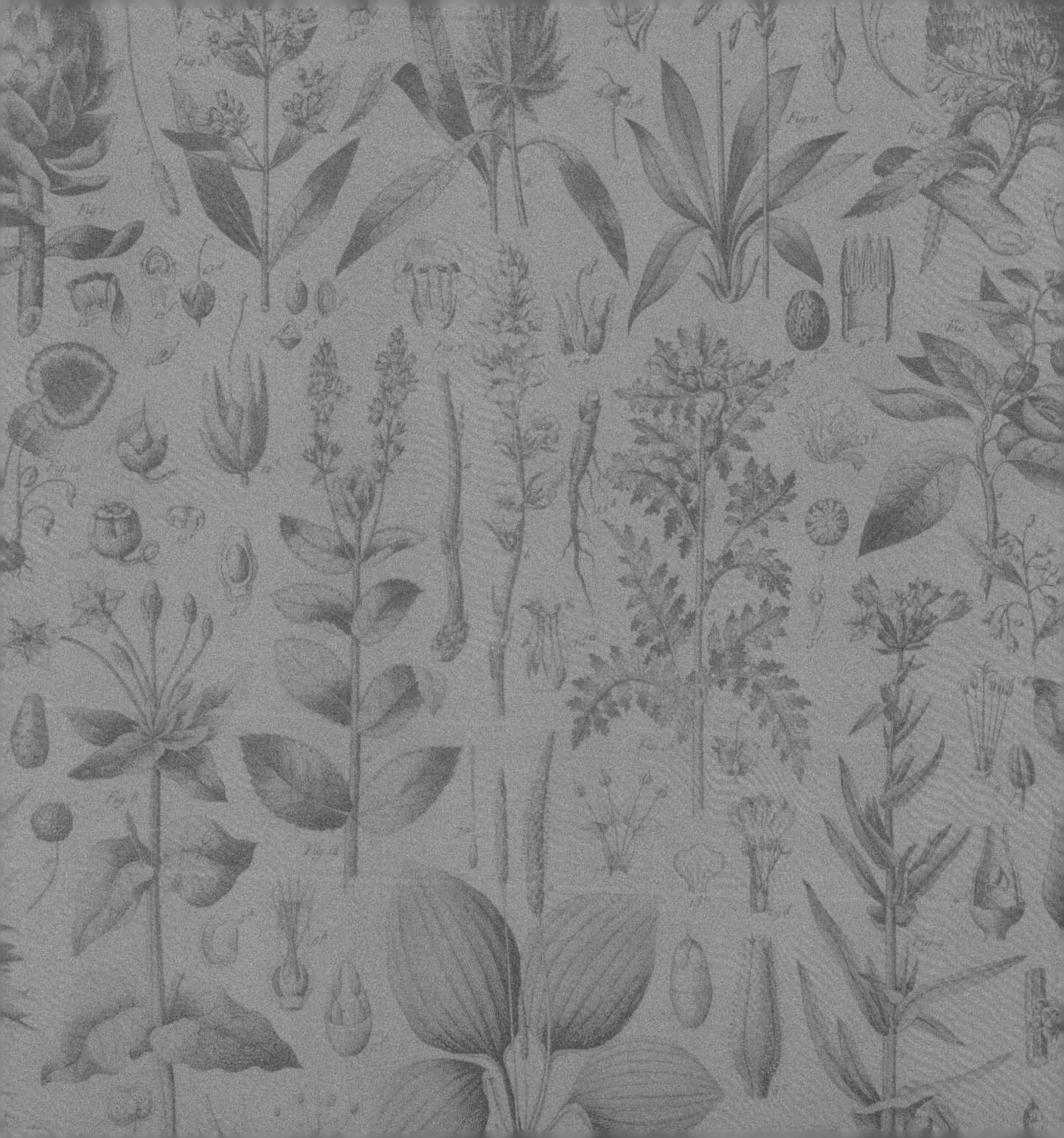

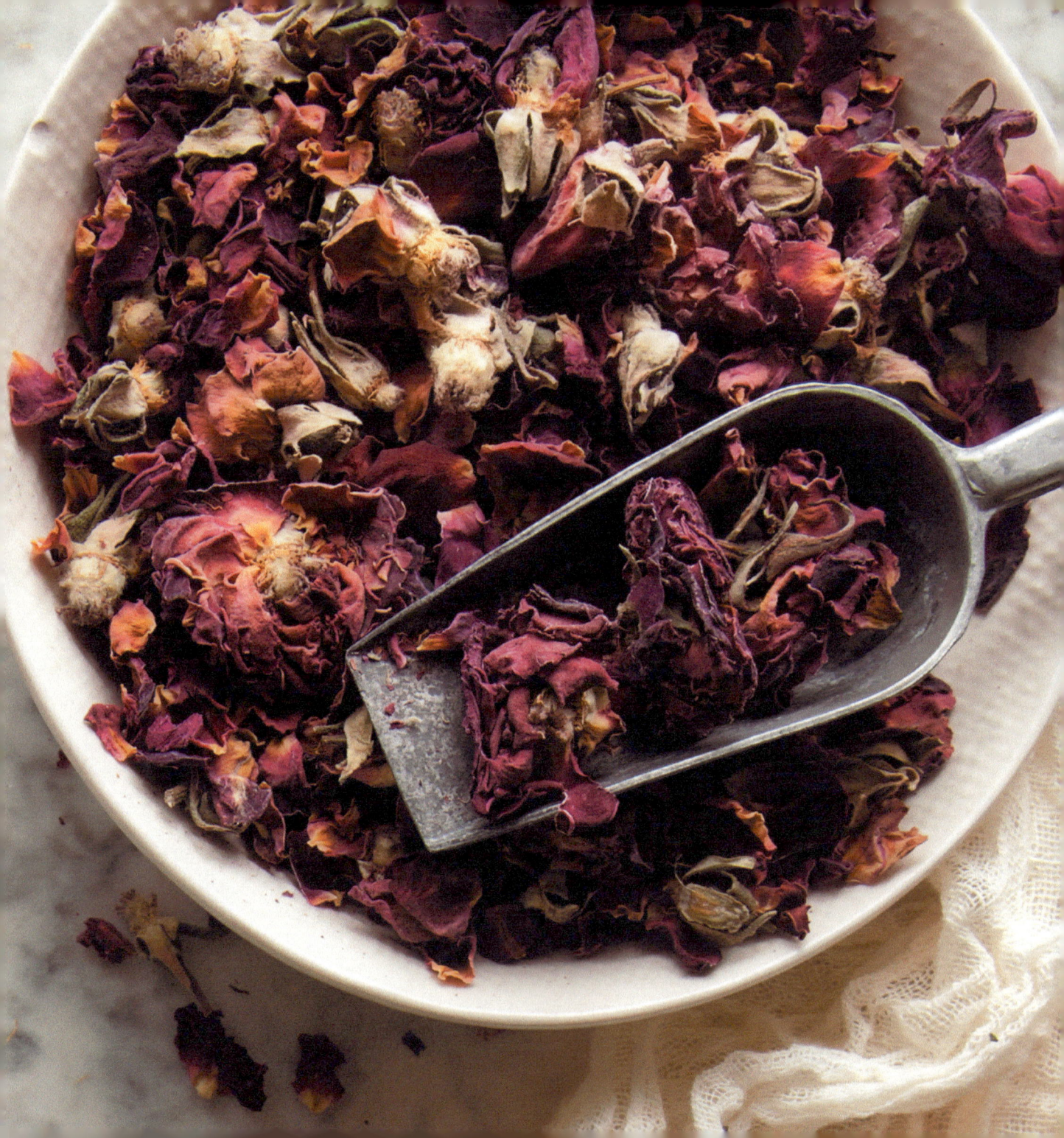

INTRODUCTION

The ancients knew the value of essential oils—aromatic distillations of plant parts they used for medicinal, cosmetic, and ritual purposes. Egyptians buried their dead with jars of fragrant ointment; Romans treated wounds with poultices of honey and basil; the New Testament speaks of the Magi bringing gifts of precious frankincense and myrrh to the newborn Christ child. In medieval times every monastery had a "physick" garden, and every housewife knew which plants could be used to cure a fever or induce childbirth or numb the pain of a sore tooth. Over the years, herb craft and plant lore faded into obscurity, but in recent years a new emphasis on organic food and purposeful living has brought attention back to the basics—the "essentials," one might say. Using essential oils will improve your health, increase your happiness, and raise your overall well-being; plus, it's a lot of fun playing with the scented oils and practicing a modern kind of alchemy.

These days, there are many essential oils and blends to choose from, and they are fairly easy to find. It's great to have so many options, but there is also a lot of marketing hype surrounding certain essential oils and brands. This can create some confusion for beginners. *Do I have the right oils? Do I have the best brand?* Relax! You don't need to buy every essential oil to reap the benefits of aromatherapy. Many people work with a small number of favorites; you can meet most of your everyday needs with a small number of versatile essential oils. Whether you've already purchased a starter kit that contains popular basics or are still deciding which essential oils to begin with, it's easy to put them to use with this book as your guide. These pages offer an introduction to the world of aromatherapy in a factual, friendly way, providing complete profiles of 86 top essential oils and more than 300 recipes, remedies, and applications. While anyone can buy essential oils and start diffusing them right away, this approach is different:

- You'll begin by learning easy steps to explore aromatherapy safely.
- You'll build a strong foundation of knowledge and gain the confidence to incorporate this wonderful practice into your everyday life.

Many of the oils are meant to complement Western medicine and promote natural wellness. Others are wonderful alternatives to toxic or expensive commercial products for body and home. Your knowledge of essential oils will grow and expand over time—no need to be in a hurry. Savor the process and discover the many ways in which aromatherapy can enhance your life. Soon, you'll be enjoying your favorite essential oils to their fragrant fullest.

PART ONE

Everything You Need to Know About Aromatherapy

You're about to embark on an exploration of aromatherapy. The first part of this book is designed to help you become comfortable with and knowledgeable about some basic concepts, and you'll learn common terminology. How do essential oils work? What are the most popular—and safest—ways to use these oils to enhance your daily life? What should you look for, and what's best to avoid? These are just a few of the questions answered here.

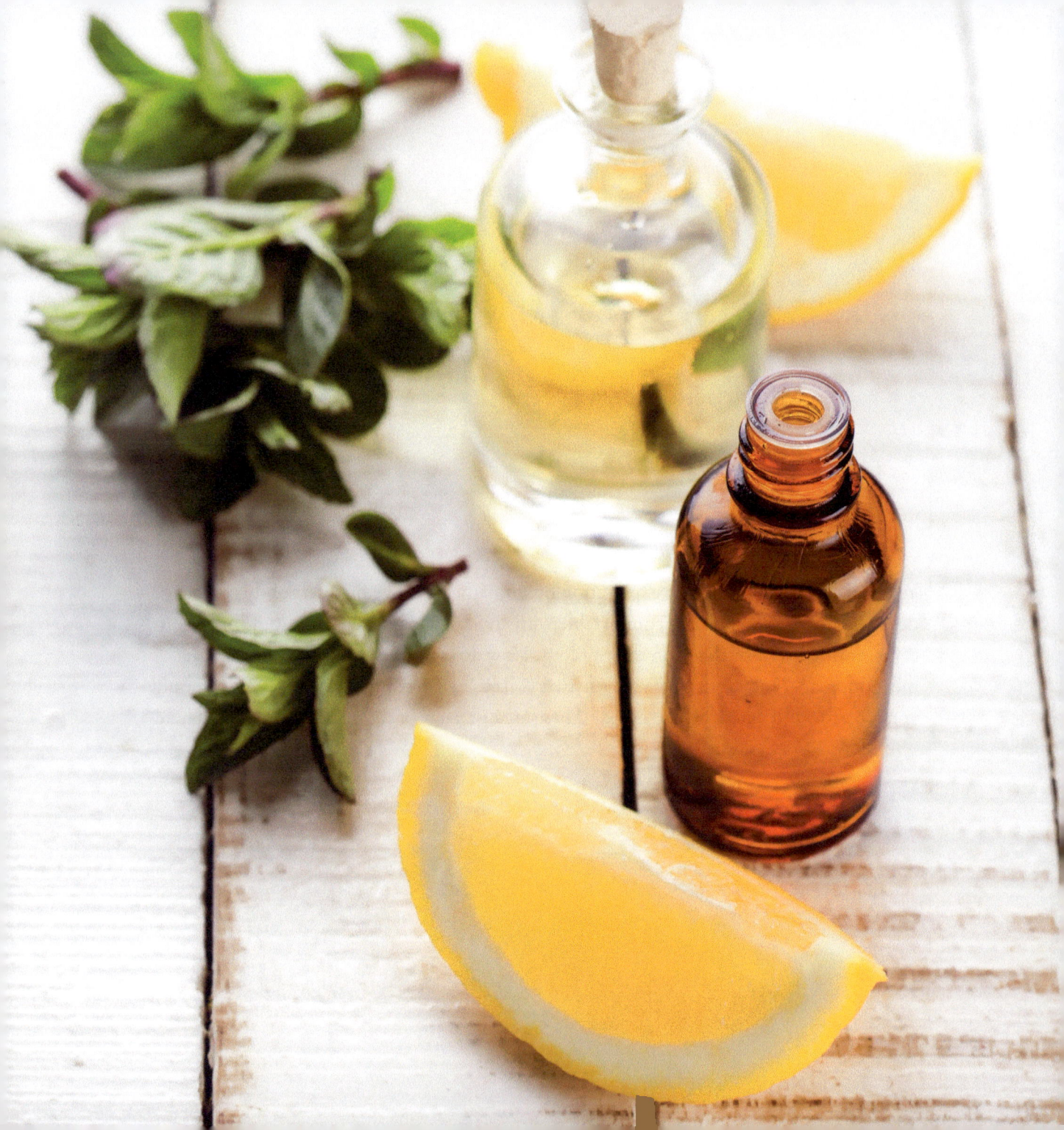

CHAPTER ONE

AROMATHERAPY BASICS

Your sense of smell is very powerful. Many species, including humans, rely partially on their sense of smell to survive. Scent can evoke memories, calm or invigorate the senses, help you wake up or fall asleep, and let you discern whether foods have gone bad, among many other functions. Many people think, and understandably so, given the name, that aromatherapy is purely about scents.

However, aromatherapy goes far beyond the practice of simply inhaling fragrant oils. The "aroma" part of the word tells you how this therapeutic practice works: When an essential oil's fragrance reaches your nose, you also inhale microscopic particles of the oil itself. These tiny droplets contain potent chemical components that can relieve common cold symptoms, ease tension, and more. Blended and applied topically, these same constituents can perform a variety of functions: Some provide natural pain relief, others help minor wounds heal faster, and still others discourage bugs from biting.

BENEFITS OF AROMATHERAPY

Aromatherapy provides many benefits, and as you'll learn in part 2, each essential oil offers different properties. The following list outlines some examples of the many ways you can use aromatherapy to enhance your well-being.

Boost energy levels Whether you're trying to cut back on caffeine or looking for a way to keep your energy level up during long workdays, you'll find that aromatherapy offers a variety of fragrant solutions. Many essential oils improve circulation, gently stimulating your body and mind without causing any unpleasant side effects. Peppermint, black pepper, and cinnamon leaf are some examples.

Change cognitive states Anxiety, nervousness, and other negative emotions are difficult to deal with, especially when they happen frequently. The essential oils used in aromatherapy have a direct impact on the brain's emotional center, and they can provide rapid relief from troublesome thought processes. Lavender and basil both address anxiety, and rose oil helps decrease stress.

Enhance memory Scents and memories are closely intertwined, and some essential oils have the ability to improve memory. Rosemary has been proven to increase cognitive learning and decrease the amount of time it takes students to answer test questions correctly.

Heighten immunity You may already know that good nutrition boosts your immune system; aromatherapy works in a similar way, by making cells strong and healthy so that they are better at fighting disease when needed. Bergamot, lavender, and tea tree are just a few examples of essential oils that stimulate the immune system.

Nourish skin Many aromatherapy recipes call for rich, moisturizing carrier oils and creams, and essential oils themselves help improve skin. Just like the plants they come from, essential oils like lavender and helichrysum contain vitamins and antioxidants, which nourish the skin on a cellular level.

Promote healing Many plants have the power to help the body heal faster: Because essential oils are highly concentrated, they can have an impressive healing effect. Helichrysum, for example, offers strong anti-inflammatory action, and it contains regenerative molecules that facilitate skin's ability to knit itself back together following an injury.

Provide stress relief Stress is a normal response to life's challenges, but that doesn't mean you have to live with it. Most aromatherapy treatments are a pleasure to use, and that alone can help you feel less stressed. Some essential oils have been studied for their ability to reduce stress; frankincense, for example, contains sesquiterpenes that cross the blood-brain barrier and stimulate the limbic system, immediately calming the mind and making it easier to deal with difficult emotions.

Relieve discomfort Aspirin and acetaminophen are two examples of analgesics—substances that stop pain. Many essential oils, such as tagetes and rosewood, also offer analgesic properties, and they often make suitable substitutes for over-the-counter medications. Sunburns, paper cuts, and minor sprains are just a few examples of painful problems that respond well to aromatherapy.

HOW ESSENTIAL OILS WORK

While some manufacturers market essential oils for internal use, *it's best to take a very cautious approach to assure your safety and ensure anything you take internally is labeled for dietary use.* This book does not discourage internal use, but it focuses on traditional aromatherapy methods that rely on inhalation and topical use, which allow beneficial molecules to enter the body and provide beneficial effects.

When inhaled: The fragrance from an essential oil carries molecules into the nose, where they stimulate smell receptors and interact with the body's nervous and limbic systems. The limbic system is a deep, primal portion of the brain responsible for controlling emotion.

At the same time, essential oil particles are delivered to the lungs with each breath. There, they enter the bloodstream and are carried throughout the entire body, where they act directly on the brain and other organs. A 2015 study published in the *Journal of Alternative and Complementary Medicine* showed impressive results. One group of subjects applied inhalation patches containing lavender essential oil to their chests each night. A second control group wore blank patches. The group using lavender enjoyed better sleep.

When applied topically: While the aroma enters your lungs and nostrils, even more molecules are absorbed into your skin. This often provides an immediate benefit: stopping the itch from a mosquito bite, soothing the pain from a sunburn, or taking some of the sting out of a minor wound.

Just one essential oil can provide a variety of benefits. Clove, for example, can repel mosquitoes and numb pain. At the same time, it is a powerful antifungal agent, as shown in a 2009 study published in the *Journal of Medical Microbiology*. It can destroy *Candida albicans*—the fungus that causes yeast infections—and other fungi, including some strains that resist the antifungal drug fluconazole. This backs up its traditional use as a remedy for common fungal infections such as athlete's foot.

FAQ: ESSENTIAL OILS, HYDROSOLS, AND FRAGRANCE OILS: WHAT'S THE DIFFERENCE?

Essential oils, hydrosols, and fragrance oils are aromatics. Because they are derived in different ways and have different chemical properties, they are used for different purposes.

Essential Oils are aromatic liquids derived from the various parts of a plant—from root to blossom to bark or berry. Depending on what part of the plant they come from, essential oils can have different properties and attributes. For example, cinnamon bark essential oil has a stronger scent than cinnamon leaf essential oil and is also roughly five times more expensive. Essential oils are safe for use on the body, although they are typically so powerful they need to be diluted with carrier oils (see page 21), to prevent side effects such as photosensitization (a strong reaction to sunlight) or sensitization (an allergylike reaction on the skin). While essential oils can be ingested, they are extremely potent and best used with the guidance of a trained practitioner. Use essential oils for aromatherapy and for the recipes and projects in this book.

Hydrosols (sometimes referred to as floral waters or flower waters) are the waters left behind from the process of distilling plant matter to extract essential oils. During the distillation process, manufacturers typically use steam or water. The resulting products are the essential oils and the water, both of which have extracted parts of the plants' essences. The essential oils contain the fat-soluble compounds while the hydrosols contain the water-soluble substances. Hydrosols have their own benefits, uses, and properties in aromatherapy, but they tend to be more fragile than essential oils, and therefore need to be kept in the refrigerator. They also tend to be less concentrated in both scent and power. Because they are weaker, hydrosols are usually gentler than essential oils. Therefore, hydrosols may work with someone in need of gentler therapies, such as infants or someone with a lot of chemical sensitivities. Chamomile hydrosol, for example, is an excellent and popular remedy for teething babies.

Fragrance Oils (also known as "perfume oils") are artificial scents that use synthetic chemicals to mimic the natural scents of essential oils. They are cheaper than essential oils and often used in candle and soapmaking, as well as in cosmetic blends. Unfortunately, while fragrance oils may successfully replicate the scent of an essential oil, they do not have the other properties that make the essential oil so valuable. They are used only for fragrance and not in health care or cooking applications. Do not use fragrance oils for the projects in this book.

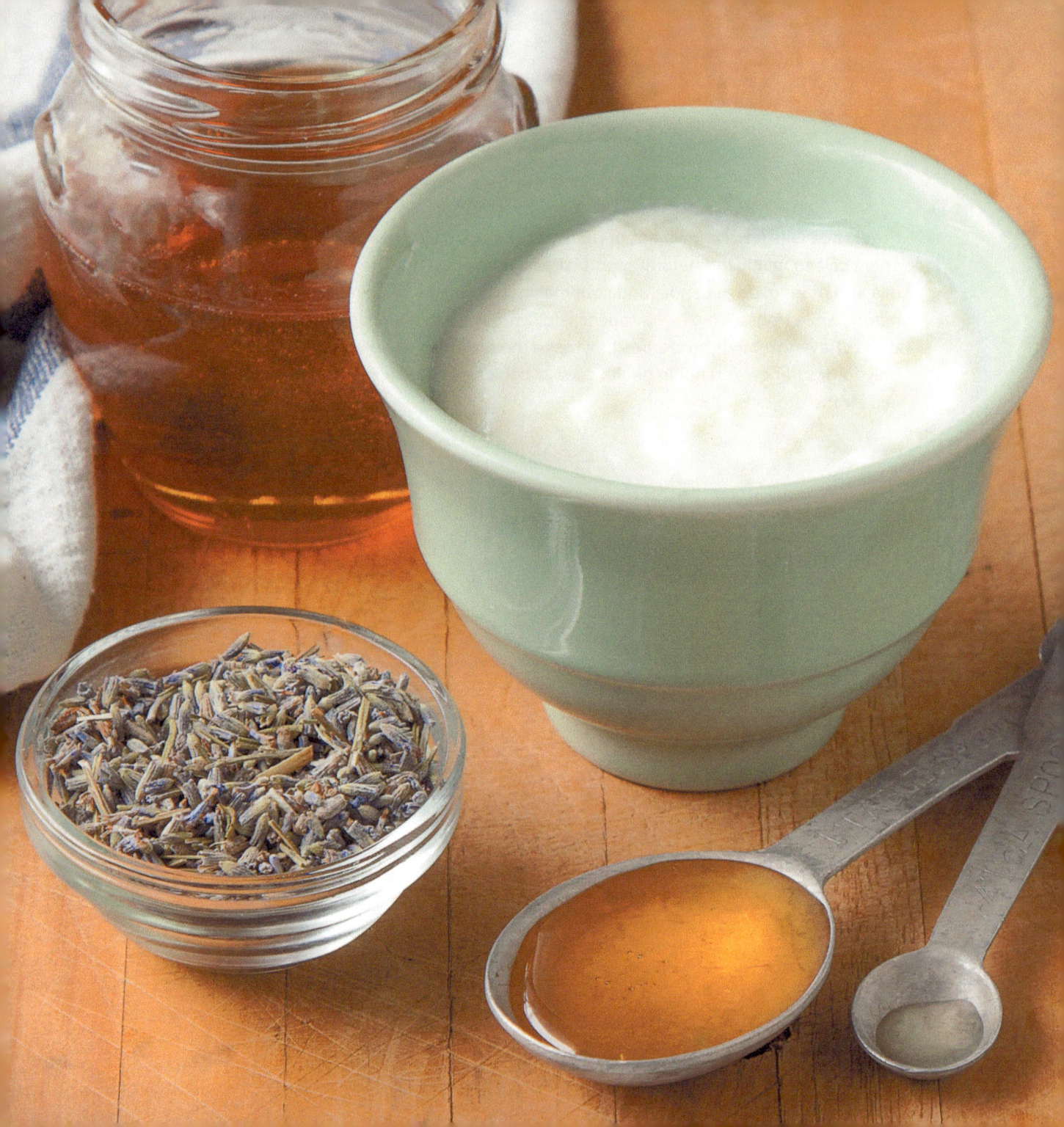

CHAPTER TWO

THE SCIENCE BEHIND AROMATHERAPY

A degree in chemistry certainly isn't necessary to use and enjoy the benefits of aromatherapy treatments. For the curious, however, there is a wealth of scientific evidence that supports treatments and provides insight into how and why aromatherapy works.

BEHIND THE SCENTS

So, how does aromatherapy actually work? All of the following are involved in the inner workings of aromatherapy:

It Begins with Your Nose

The nose serves as a direct link between the world around you and your brain; the knowledge of whether certain things smell good or bad is partly built in. For example, when you smell something burning unexpectedly, you may feel a sense of urgency. Alternatively, when you smell food cooking at mealtimes, the stomach responds with hungry growls. Other smells are directly connected to emotions. The crisp scent of freshly mowed grass, the clean tang of salty sea air, and the sweet aroma of holiday treats baking in the oven are examples of smells that can transport you back to times when you experienced some of life's most memorable moments.

The incredible sense of smell works when any substance with a scent emits molecules into the air. When the nose picks up those molecules, it transports them past the trigeminal nerve receptors, which are responsible for guarding the olfactory system by sensing irritants and triggering sneezes that eject the offending molecules. Molecules that make their way past these guard cells are taken up by nasal mucus, where they are dissolved before being transported through tiny olfactory receptor cells in the epithelium, the thin tissue that lines the outer layer of hollow body structures.

Once olfactory receptor cells are activated, they signal the olfactory bulb, which is the part of the brain's structure located above the nasal cavity, directly beneath the frontal lobe. Next, the receptor cells synapse with the second-order neurons that form the olfactory tract, and the scent's signal travels farther into the brain, where it synapses with cells in the amygdala and prepiriform cortex before traveling to the hypothalamus and other parts of the brain.

The sections of the brain that receive scent signals are directly involved in emotional control, memory recall, immune function, hormone production, basic drives, and more. Aromas can alter your heart rate, blood pressure, and breath rate. They can also stimulate the release of beta-endorphins, including endogenous opioids, which are the body's natural mood elevators and painkillers. These peptides are responsible for creating the euphoria, or "runner's high," following a great workout.

There is nothing—not even an advanced drug—you can take orally that affects your brain as quickly as scent will. And, if you inhale via both nose and mouth, the molecules will quickly enter your lungs and make their way into your bloodstream.

And Gets under Your Skin . . .

Aromatherapy isn't just about fragrance; it's also about the effect essential oils have when they come in contact with your skin. If you're familiar with transdermal patches, like those used to deliver nicotine to people trying to quit tobacco, then you already have a good idea how topical aromatherapy treatments work. Like those found in nicotine patches, the molecules in essential oils are capable of transdermal action, penetrating the skin and rapidly making their way through the entire body.

Then Impacts Your Cells . . .

Because they are made up of tiny molecules, essential oils are capable of passing through tissue and cell walls easily. These microscopic molecules are so minuscule that they're even able to pass through the blood-brain barrier, a filtering mechanism that blocks the passage of certain substances into the brain. No wonder they work so quickly!

Once an aromatherapy treatment's active essential oil molecules get into your cells, they perform some specific functions. Some treatments support the digestive, endocrine, circulatory, nervous, or reproductive systems, and some provide defense against bacteria and viruses.

Many essential oils are also powerful antioxidants with the ability to cleanse the cells of harmful free radicals that form as part of the natural metabolic process, as well as those that enter the body via external sources such as cigarette smoke, air pollution, or exposure to chemicals.

Because free radicals can damage cells, it's important to treat your body with plenty of antioxidants. Colorful vegetables and fruits are also a great source, so eating right and using aromatherapy in place of products laden with synthetic chemicals can be an important part of building a solid foundation for defense of your health.

PRODUCING ESSENTIAL OILS

The essential oils at the heart of aromatherapy treatments are produced via a few key methods. Some are centuries or even millennia old; others are new, highly technical procedures. The two most common are *steam distillation* and *CO_2 extraction*.

Steam distillation is the most common method for extracting essential oils. Vast quantities of aromatic plants are loaded into a machine and tightly compacted. Steam is then forced through the plant "filter," heating it up and releasing the oils as a gas. As the gas cools, it liquefies into oil and water, which are then separated. The fragrant water that's left behind by this process is a hydrosol (see page 6) and is valued in its own right.

CO_2 extraction is a process similar to steam distillation, but it uses carbon dioxide instead of water to extract the essential oil from the raw plant material. The CO_2 returns to its gaseous form when pressure is released, and only the essential oil remains. The finished product is usually more expensive than the same essential oil produced from traditional distillation.

Other extraction methods include:

Enfleurage is an ancient French technique that involves extracting the fragrance of flowers by exposing them to the sun until the essential oils leach into a fixed oil or fat. At that point, a separation process ensues that purifies the oil to make it ready for sale.

Expression (aka "cold pressing") is used mostly for extracting the essential oil from the peels of citrus fruit. In this method the fruit peels are pressed and then the oil is separated from the juice and pulp in a centrifuge. Expression is also the process used in winemaking and creating olive oil.

Maceration sounds like a process that would involve grinding or chewing up herbs, but it isn't. Plants are soaked in hot oil, which breaks down their cell walls to release the essential oils. The result is then filtered and bottled. The Egyptians used this method extensively in their perfume making.

Solvent extraction is used when flowers have too little volatile oil for other extraction methods. The essential oils are extracted with the help of chemical solvents such as methylene chloride, hexane, or benzene, and are called *absolutes*. Solvent extraction is an expensive, labor-intensive process that often involves several solvent treatments. Purists do not consider absolutes to be true essential oils owing to the solvent that is left behind.

The end result of these processes is a bottle of essential oil that can be used alone or in combination as part of a DIY medicine chest, cosmetic case, and home-care cabinet.

In order to create a safe and effective collection of essential oils, choose the purest and best essential oils. Price isn't always a determiner of quality. Research the various essential oil manufacturers to determine the processes they use to create the essential oils, as well as the purity of their oils, before purchasing the essential oils you want to include in your personal aromatherapy kit.

CHEMISTRY 101

What follows is a rundown of the chemical compounds that make up many of your favorite essential oils. While this is by no means an extensive lesson in organic chemistry, it will provide you with additional insight into the way aromatherapy works. *The Chemistry of Aromatherapeutic Oils* by E. Joy Bowles is one of the most comprehensive resources available for an in-depth study at the time of this writing.

Alcohols Highly preservative, with the ability to resist damage from oxidation. They offer strong antibacterial action, and are antifungal and antiviral as well. Geranium, lavender, and tea tree are some examples of essential oils with a high percentage of alcohol.

Esters An ester is the result of an alcohol combining with an acid. Essential oils that contain a high percentage of esters are often quite calming and relaxing. Examples include valerian, German chamomile, Roman chamomile, and citrus bergamot.

Ketones Carbon-based compounds that often possess calming or sedative properties. Essential oils with high ketone content are excellent for expelling mucus, and they stimulate cellular regeneration. Examples include rosemary, hyssop, and western red cedar.

Monoterpenes Also known as monoterpene alcohols, monoterpenes provide antiseptic, antifungal, and antiviral effects, usually without irritating skin. Citronella, lavender, and juniper are some examples of monoterpene-rich essential oils.

Oxides When other chemical compounds are oxidized, the result is an oxide. Oxides often come from terpenes, alcohols, and ketones. They are a good choice for expelling mucus that accompanies a cold or flu, and can be mildly stimulating. Examples include eucalyptus, ravensara leaf, and rosemary.

Phenols Oxygenated compounds, including carvacrol, eugenol, and thymol. Phenols are antiseptics, but they are strong enough to irritate skin and mucous membranes. Cinnamon, clove, and wintergreen are some examples of highly phenolic essential oils.

Sesquiterpenes Also known as sesquiterpene alcohols, sesquiterpenes are less common than many other essential oil components. Their anti-allergen and anti-inflammatory properties make them particularly valuable for dealing with hay fever, skin irritation, and minor wounds. Examples include myrrh, sandalwood, and patchouli.

MOVING FORWARD

Although this is a brief overview of essential oil chemistry, it can give you insight into what type of action you might be able to expect from aromatherapy treatments that contain oils that are high in certain constituents. It would take an entire book to provide an in-depth analysis of the hundreds of essential oils available, especially because each oil has more than one hundred components. Further, when you combine essential oils with one another, a synergistic effect is produced; in short, the therapeutic action of each oil can be increased. In the next chapter, you'll learn more about working with essential oils for aromatherapy.

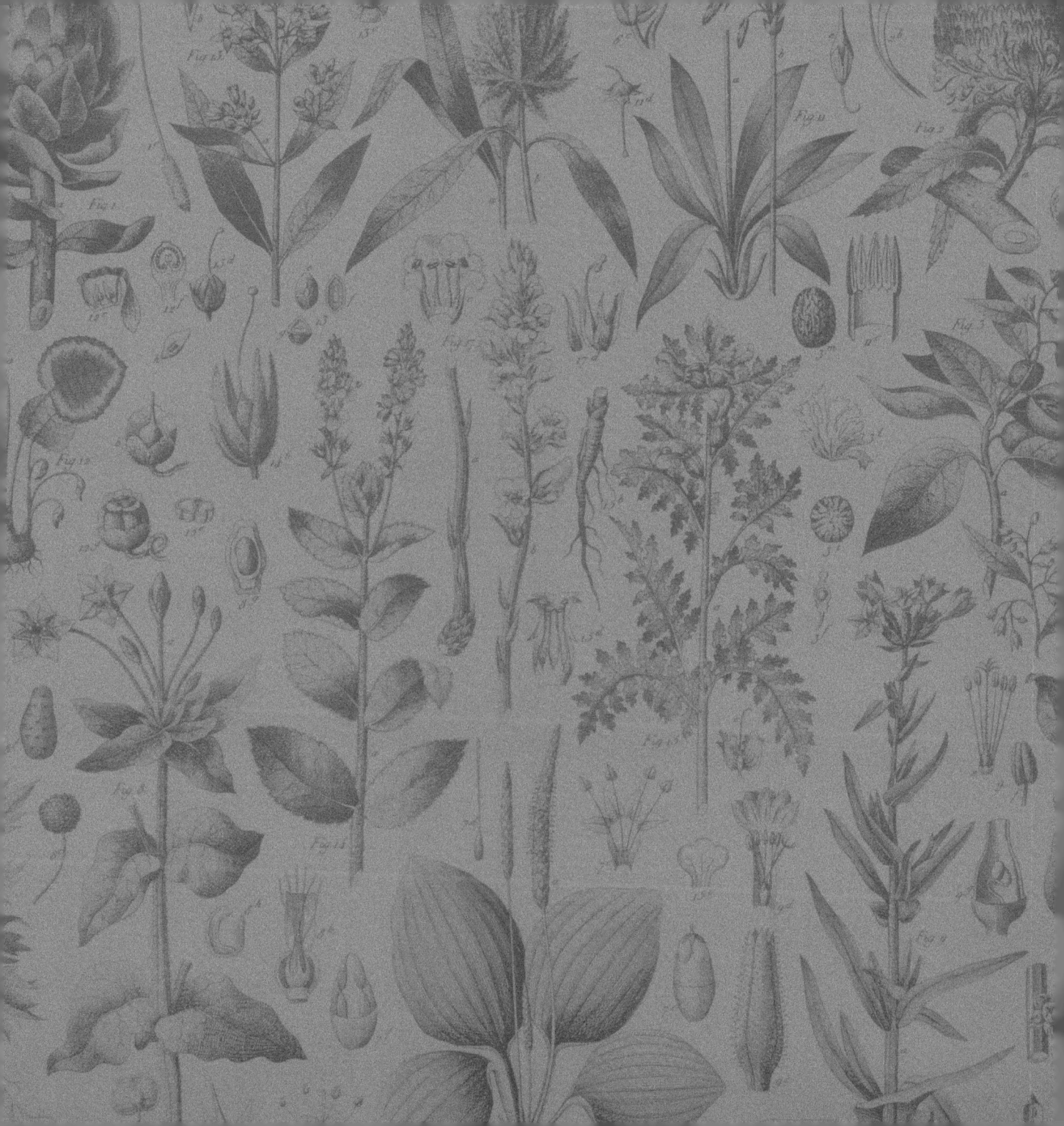

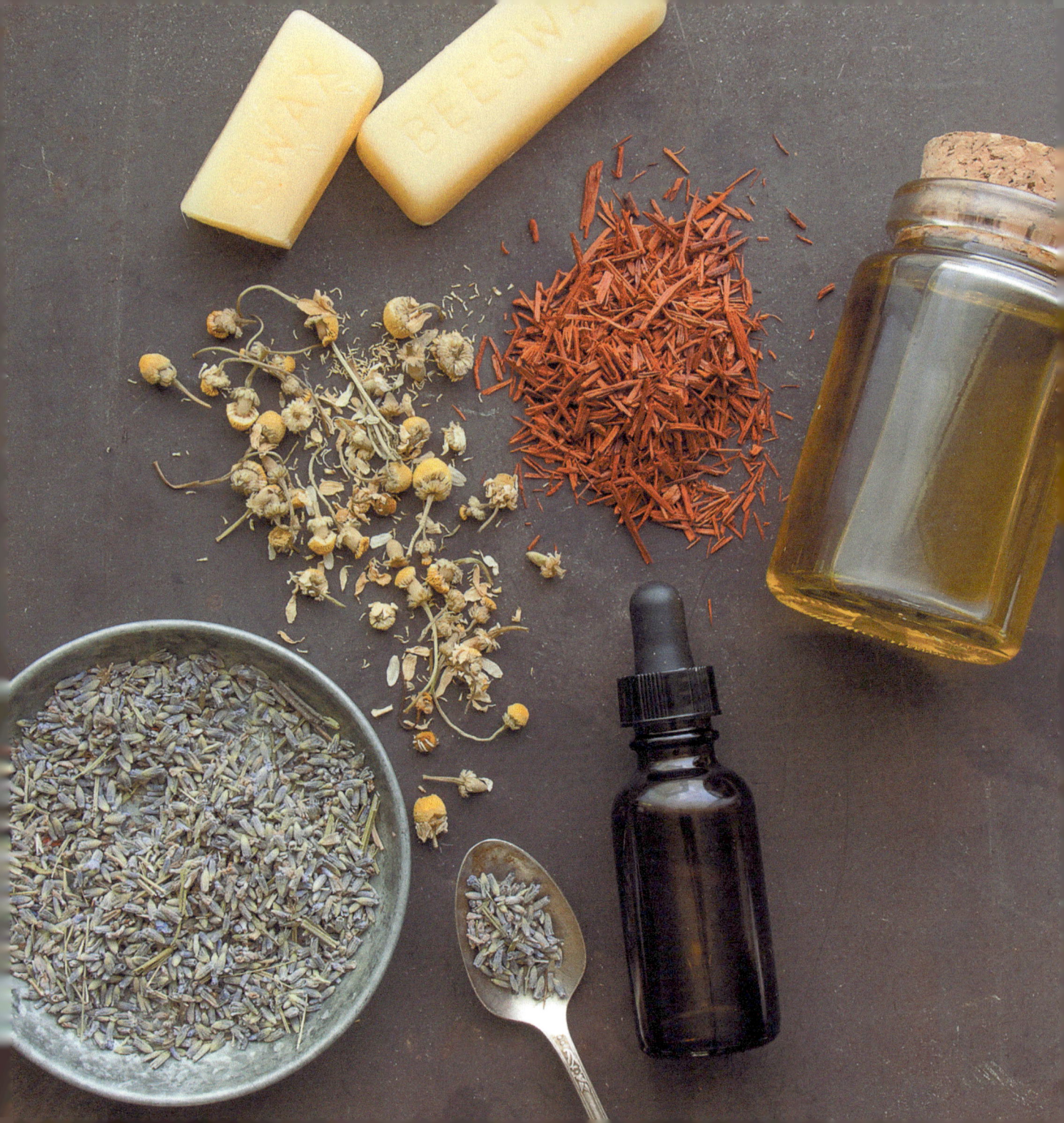

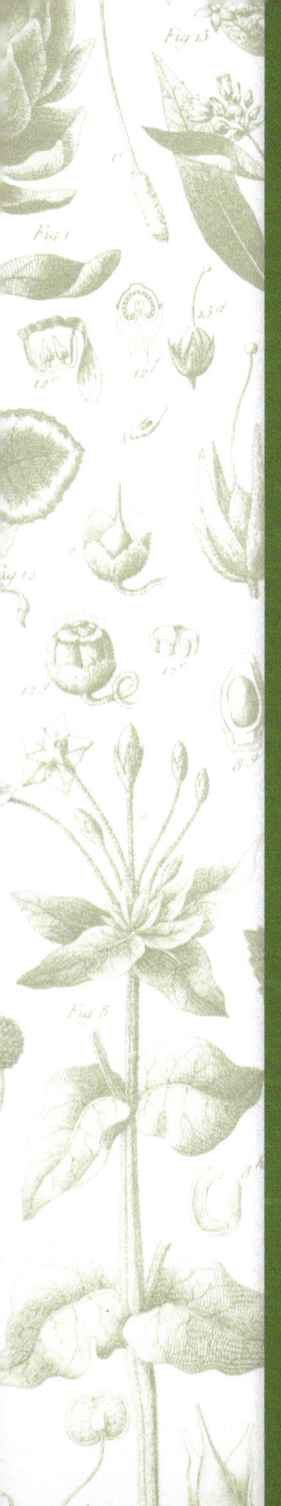

CHAPTER THREE

WORKING WITH ESSENTIAL OILS

There are so many wonderful ways to put your essential oils to work in your life. They lend themselves to a wide range of uses—from freshening the air, revitalizing foot soaks, improving oral hygiene, soothing sore muscles, promoting clearer thinking, to relieving a wide variety of mild health complaints. You'll love the personalized blends you can create for use in your own bath and body care products, and you can use your oils to create thoughtful, yet inexpensive gifts for others. The sky is the limit!

As you'll soon discover, there are many ways to use aromatherapy as part of a natural lifestyle. You'll find full essential oil profiles in part 2, but before you jump in, it's important to learn how to choose good essential oils and carriers, mix basic aromatherapy recipes, and use them safely.

DETERMINING YOUR NEEDS

What brings you to aromatherapy? What do you want to accomplish with your essential oils? These are two great questions to ask yourself to determine your needs, which will help you decide which essential oils to begin with. Some common reasons include:

- Treating common ailments naturally, instead of with over-the-counter remedies
- Saving money on high-quality bath and body products
- Reducing use of harsh household chemicals
- Interest in holistic health

If you're hoping to treat a specific ailment or two, you should research which essential oils are best for addressing your concerns. Whether you're looking for a way to increase energy naturally, enjoy better sleep, or get rid of tough headaches without reaching for pills, you'll find solutions in this book.

The same applies to other applications. Want a way to clean your home and do your laundry without worrying about potential problems listed on chemical warning labels? Look for essential oils that offer strong antibacterial properties and you'll be on your way to making effective, great-smelling household products.

For cosmetic concerns, research to see if an aromatherapy solution is available. The odds are high you'll find at least one that appeals to you—without the exorbitant price tags that typically accompany commercial preparations.

Once you've determined which issues you'd like to address, check the ingredients needed so you can buy your supplies before you get started. Once you know which oils you want to try first, and how little you actually need to get started, you're ready to take the next step.

SHOPPING FOR ESSENTIAL OILS

You may feel tempted to buy all the oils in this book, and you might opt to do that if cost isn't a concern. However, if you're on a budget, use your goals to decide which ones are the highest priorities. You can simply make a list of oils from the list of "Must Haves" presented later in this chapter (see page 35) to create a foundation for learning. If you aren't sure about your goals, or you just want to dip your toes into the water, try starting with just one essential oil. Of all those available, lavender is the most versatile, with excellent benefits for your mind and body, such as the ability to help you have a naturally clean home, fresh-smelling laundry, and a good night's sleep.

Once you've started, and as finances allow, you can decide how you'd like to expand your collection. When you begin shopping for essential oils—especially online—you'll notice there are many brands available, and each brand does its best to outshine its competitors. Take marketing claims with a grain of salt; it's easy to find high-quality essential oils online, in stores, and from private distributors. Use the following tips to determine which brands are likely to be best.

Avoid purchasing a product labeled *fragrance oil*. Other watchwords to avoid include *perfume oil* and *identical oil*. These are usually a combination of essential oil, carrier oil, and chemicals, usually offered for craft use. They are nice for making candles, but most aren't suitable for aromatherapy use.

Know the difference between absolutes and prediluted oil. Sometimes very expensive essential oils, such as rose and jasmine, are offered for sale prediluted in carrier oil. These are nice to have, and they cost much less than absolutes, but they cannot be substituted for absolutes, drop for drop, in aromatherapy recipes. Feel free to try these if you want to stretch your wings and experience some lovely, luxurious florals that might otherwise be outside your budget. If you purchase a prediluted oil, make sure the label contains the absolute's Latin name—for example, *Jasminum grandiflorum*, which is one of three jasmine varieties used to produce jasmine absolute.

Take note of the materials in the packaging. Most vendors offer essential oils in bottles of dark-colored glass or lined aluminum, which protects the oil from the oxidizing effect of light. Avoid essential oils packaged in clear glass containers, as well as plastic containers, even if those containers are dark colored. One exception is bulk purchasing; if you are making lots of personal-care products, you may find some reputable companies ship large quantities of essential oils in protective, BPA-free plastic bottles with instructions to transfer the essential oil to dark-colored glass containers as soon as possible. Skip essential oils packaged in bottles that come with rubber droppers on their lids. While they may look convenient, the droppers will break down and cause contamination over time.

Essential oil prices should vary widely within the same brand. Very common oils like lemon and mandarin shouldn't cost much, but absolutes like jasmine and rose will have prices that may give you sticker shock.

There should be plenty of other prices between the two extremes. If a vendor's oils all cost the same for the same amount, move on.

Look for the Latin name on the label. It's best to avoid essential oils with labels that fail to provide a Latin name for the plant from which the essential oil was obtained. There are many different varieties within species, and each variety has something different to offer.

Read reviews and do your research. A few companies sell their essential oils via multilevel marketing, a pyramid-type business practice in which individuals are compensated for the sales they generate and for sales made by the individuals they recruit. Protect yourself by reading reviews and independently verifying any unusual claims being made before investing in the company's essential oils.

There is no governing body that tests or regulates essential oils. Most companies make statements concerning the purity of their essential oils, and some take it a step further by mentioning that their products are "certified," "aromatherapy grade," or "therapeutic grade," but it's best to conduct research about the product in question. After all, anyone can make marketing claims.

If offered the option, consider choosing organic essential oil whenever possible. As long as an organic oil stands up to your scrutiny and falls within your budget, go for it. While nonorganic oils are certainly beneficial, organics are often superior. Of course, the choice is all yours.

Search for oils by aroma category. Essential oils have nine basic scent categories that can help you identify the type of fragrance you'll get with each essential oil. Because essential oils come tightly sealed, you can't open the lid to smell them in the store. Knowing the basic aroma category of the essential oil will, at least from a broad perspective, give you an understanding of how the essential oil will smell. Some essential oils fall into more than one of the nine categories:

- Citrus (orange, lemon, grapefruit, bergamot, mandarin, etc.)
- Earthy (sandalwood, cypress, patchouli, black pepper, etc.)
- Floral (rose, jasmine, lavender, chamomile, ylang-ylang, etc.)
- Herbaceous/Herbal (rosemary, clary sage, hyssop, basil, etc.)

- Medicinal (eucalyptus, cajuput, tea tree, etc.)
- Minty (peppermint, wintergreen, etc.)
- Spicy (cinnamon, ginger, clove, etc.)
- Woody (cedarwood, rosewood, pine, frankincense, etc.)

Don't be afraid to buy essential oils online. Shopping online gives you access to more variety than most local stores are able to provide, and all major essential oil companies maintain strong online presences, complete with knowledgeable customer-service representatives who are able to answer questions. Shopping online also gives you the ability to compare oils side by side with no pressure. As a bonus, many sources offer tools for making aromatherapy products, as well as high-quality packaging in which to store balms, lotions, sprays, and other remedies.

ALL ABOUT CARRIER OILS

With just a few exceptions, essential oils need to be diluted before they are applied to the skin or inhaled. Most commonly, they are combined with carrier oils, although you may also dilute them in alcohol, gels, and liquid soap, or add them to water for specific projects.

Carrier oils come in a wide variety of weights and prices. One of the most affordable and readily available carrier oils is olive oil, but its strong fragrance isn't ideal for use in formulas with delicate scents. Fortunately, plenty of other options exist, including plain old (inexpensive) safflower oil, which you can find near the salad dressing in any supermarket.

Six of the most affordable and versatile carrier oils are:

1. **Grapeseed oil is particularly good for those with sensitive skin because it's naturally nonallergenic.** Because it is so affordable, it is also great for use in large quantities, such as for massage therapy. Grapeseed oil has a shelf life of between six and twelve months. Refrigeration may make it last a bit longer.

2. **Sweet almond oil is practical for all skin types and has a light, nutty odor that does not conflict with most blends.** It works well as a massage blend, or in some cosmetic applications. It is extremely affordable and has a shelf life (unrefrigerated) of about twelve months.

3. **Rosehip oil is considered a dry oil because it is absorbed by the skin so quickly.** It's not great for massage, but is wonderful in cosmetic applications for dry and aging skin, though not for acne-prone skin. It is more expensive and more perishable than some of the other carrier oils. Rosehip oil needs to be refrigerated because of its propensity to rancidity, and it lasts about three months, so buy it in small quantities if you plan to use it. Don't use it if you have oily skin.

4. **Apricot kernel oil is reasonably affordable and great for dry or very dry skin.** It works well in cosmetic applications. It is high in essential fatty acids and contains vitamins A and E, which are wonderful antioxidants for mature skin. Because of its light peach color, it may stain clothing. It has a shelf life of about twelve months and doesn't require refrigeration.

5. **Jojoba oil is unique in that it remains shelf stable for a very long time—two or three years in most cases.** The skin also absorbs it very well, so it's great for cosmetic use.

6. **Coconut oil has its own, relatively strong coconut fragrance.** However, because it is a solid at room temperature, it's wonderful for creating salves. To use it with essential oils, you need to melt it and mix in the essential oils, and then allow it to return to a solid at room temperature. It is shelf stable for two or three years, and works well in cosmetic and alternative health applications.

ITEMS TO HAVE ON HAND: ESSENTIAL AND NICE TO HAVE

You can create many of the recipes in this book with basic kitchen tools such as mixing bowls, measuring spoons, and measuring cups (metal or glass is preferred). Some do call for special containers, such as glass sugar shakers, which are inexpensive when purchased at large home goods retailers and online. What else might you need? The list of essentials is surprisingly short.

Essentials

Dark glass containers These are essential for storing blends for long periods of time, because exposure to light shortens shelf life. There are many sizes and shapes available, ranging from glass bottles with misting spray tops or trigger spray tops to salve and cosmetics containers. Clear glass containers—even sanitized jam jars—will do in a pinch, as long as you keep your remedies in a dark place.

Diffuser If you want to scent your home naturally and enjoy the many psychotherapeutic benefits of aromatherapy, invest in at least one diffuser. There are a variety of sizes, colors, and styles available.

Funnels From tiny, purpose-built funnels that fit essential oil bottles to large, wide-mouth funnels that fit quart jars, these keep spills to a minimum when transferring finished products into storage containers.

Glass or metal bowls It's a good idea to get bowls in different sizes and to keep them separate from those used for food prep. Strong oils can damage plastic bowls and utensils; while they will do in a pinch, they're far from ideal. Whichever you choose, be sure to wash them well with soap and water after each use.

Labels These are a must for marking your blends. You can buy special labels that correspond with the containers you choose, or you can make your own with something as simple as masking tape.

Liquid measuring cups Get at least one liquid measuring cup to use for carrier oils. Most of the remedies in this book make 8 fluid ounces or less, so a 1-cup measure might serve your purposes perfectly for now.

Stainless steel pans These are good for warming carrier oils and very carefully melting waxes.

Travel-size containers If you plan to bring remedies along in a carry-on bag, travel-size containers are essential. They're available in glass or plastic; although plastic isn't ideal, it's okay for storing blends you plan to use within a week or two. You can justify the cost of glass ones by mixing up larger batches of your favorite portable remedies and then refilling your travel-size ones for continuous use on the go.

Nice to Have

Double boiler This is an excellent tool for melting waxes and crafting your own skin creams.

Glass droppers or disposable pipettes Droppers let you easily measure essential oils and other ingredients accurately. If you don't get droppers or pipettes, make sure that all of your essential oil bottles are fitted with orifice reducers, which are small discs that dispense one drop of liquid at a time.

Glass roller bottles Rollers make using homemade lip balms, perfumes, and portable aromatherapy remedies more convenient.

Massage chair or table If you really want to reap the rewards of aromatherapy, learn alongside a partner and use your blends in soothing massages. It's true that you can sit or lie anywhere to receive a massage, but massage chairs and tables make muscle groups accessible, and they are much more comfortable for both parties.

Metal measuring spoons Metal measuring spoons help you ensure accuracy when creating blends. Plastic will do in a pinch because you won't be using these for straight essential oils in most cases.

Oil-dispensing syringe This is a good tool to have for making blends when recipes use increments marked in milliliters (ml) rather than drops. They are typically available in 1-ml increments. Medical syringes such as those found at drugstores will work, too; just make sure that measurements are marked in milliliters.

Stirring utensils Special stirring utensils such as glass rods are nice to have, but not necessary. Although some recipes benefit from an electric hand mixer, a fork or whisk works nicely for most things; even a chopstick will do in a pinch. Avoid wood because it absorbs oil and wastes your products.

Storage bag or box An insulated bag or box offers the ideal solution for protecting your essential oils from heat and light.

Other Ingredients to Have on Hand

Many recipes in this book call for some ingredients you may need in addition to essential oils and the carrier oils of your choice. This is by no means an exhaustive list, but it will help you stock up before getting started. When shopping, be sure to check expiration dates if applicable, and buy only what you need. Some items, such as beeswax, don't come with expiration dates, making it easy to save some money by purchasing in bulk.

- **Creams, gels, and waxes.** Beeswax, shea butter, cocoa butter, and coconut oil make thick, creamy lotions, salves, and more. Unscented aloe vera gel dilutes essential oils beautifully, and gives body care products a light, fresh feel.

- **Dry ingredients.** Basics like baking soda, white and brown sugar, milk powder, and sea salt extend your repertoire, allowing you to make scented foot and body powders, bath salts, body scrubs, smelling salts, and other items. Diatomaceous earth (both regular and food grade) also comes in handy for several recipes. Epsom salts are the perfect medium for a soothing aromatherapy bath without leaving a messy ring behind.

- **Liquids.** Vinegar, hydrogen peroxide, and alcohol-free witch hazel lend themselves to a variety of uses. Foot soaks, toners, and first-aid treatments are some of the recipes that call for these ingredients.

- **Natural body supplies.** Unscented all-natural body supplies such as shampoo, conditioner, and body wash offer convenience, allowing you to add essential oils that suit your needs. Liquid or bar castile soap is another staple to have on hand, particularly if you want to try your hand at formulating complicated body care recipes from scratch.

It's often fine to substitute similar ingredients for one another. For example, if a recipe calls for cocoa butter and you only have shea butter, feel free to use it.

STORE YOUR OILS WELL

Storing essential oils properly preserves their therapeutic properties. While essential oils don't go rancid the same way carrier oils can, they are subject to oxidization when exposed to heat and light. Citrus oils start to lose their potency about six months after opening, so make use of them when they're at their freshest. The good news is, when properly stored, most essential oils have a shelf life of at least one year, and many will stay fresh for two years or longer. Some, such as patchouli, actually improve with age.

The best way to store your essential oils is to keep them in a cool, dark area with a stable temperature. An insulated case is ideal, and a padded cooler can do the trick. Never store your essential oils in direct sunlight, as this causes rapid deterioration.

Once blended, most remedies keep for about six months, depending on the ingredients and the storage conditions. Make small batches to avoid waste or share your products with others. Refrigeration can greatly extend shelf life, too.

It's time to replace your oils and blends when their scents weaken or start to smell a bit off. Your nose is an excellent tool for detecting oils that are no longer suitable for aromatherapy.

USING ESSENTIAL OILS SAFELY

Essential oils are powerful substances. Although they're all-natural, it's very important to follow these simple safety guidelines. There are safety issues to consider when you use them. If you have children or pets in your home, there are essential oils you'll want to avoid using around them. Pregnant people need to use caution, as there are some essential oils known to cause harm to a growing baby when misused. Some essential oils can elicit bad reactions if applied topically and the skin is exposed to the sun.

There is no reason to fear any of the essential oils in this book as long as you use them appropriately. Essential oil safety isn't complicated, so by taking just a few simple precautions, you can enjoy their many benefits without worry or overexposure.

Less Is Truly More

It takes an enormous amount of plant matter to make just one drop of essential oil. For example, it takes about sixty roses to make a single drop of pure rose essential oil—no wonder it's expensive! Cost isn't the only reason to approach essential oil use with a judicious hand; every drop of essential oil contains the concentrated chemical components from all the plants that went into it, so there is a risk of overuse. Using too much essential oil can cause adverse effects, just like using too much medicine.

Even though these are natural remedies and are generally safe, improper or excessive use can be dangerous. It's important to approach aromatherapy mindfully and respect these natural medicines the same way you respect prescription and drugstore remedies. By using only the amount required, you'll receive the benefits you need, you'll save money, and you won't risk injury, irritation, or illness.

Essential Oils to Avoid

The following oils are highly toxic, extremely irritating to skin or lungs, or even lethal if ingested. Some of these essential oils are used in perfumery, and some are described as safe by certain resources. It's always best to be safe and to avoid the following essential oils despite reports of their potential benefits.

- **Bitter almond** Toxic; contains cyanide; small quantities can be lethal
- **Boldo leaf** Toxic; can produce convulsions
- **Horseradish** Caustic; can cause severe pain and inflammation
- **Mugwort** Toxic; can cause miscarriage; neurotoxin
- **Mustard** Caustic; burns skin; causes respiratory distress
- **Pennyroyal** Toxic; causes liver damage; causes lung damage; can cause death if ingested
- **Rue** Toxic; irritates lungs and mucous membranes; neurotoxin; can burn skin
- **Sassafras** Carcinogenic; small quantities can be lethal
- **Savin** Toxic; small quantities can be lethal
- **Tansy** Toxic; can produce convulsions; can cause uterine bleeding; small quantities can be lethal (Note: This is not the same oil as blue tansy.)
- **Tea Tree** (black) Black tea tree is different from the more common tea tree that is safe for use in pregnancy. When in doubt, check the Latin name. Black tea tree is known as *Melaleuca bracteata*. The common and safe tea tree bears the Latin name *Melaleuca alternifolia*.
- **Thuja** Toxic; can cause severe gastrointestinal distress; can cause convulsions; neurotoxin
- **Wintergreen** Extremely toxic; even tiny quantities can be lethal
- **Wormseed** Explosive; can explode when heated or combined with an acid; toxic to liver and kidneys; small quantities can be lethal; can cause deafness and vision loss
- **Wormwood** Toxic; can cause addiction and brain damage; neurotoxin

Patch Test

Because it's difficult to predict how a specific essential oil will affect your skin, it's best to conduct a patch test before use, even if you are not normally sensitive. Take extra care with patch testing whenever an essential oil is listed as having the potential to cause sensitive skin.

To conduct a patch test, combine one drop of the essential oil in question with 1 teaspoon of carrier oil. Apply a single drop of this blend to your inner elbow, and leave it alone for twenty-four hours.

Do not wash the area during the test period unless irritation develops.

If, after the twenty-four-hour test period passes, you have no sign of redness, itching, or swelling, then it should be safe for you to use the essential oil you're considering.

Because carrier oils can cause sensitive skin, too, it's best to perform a patch test using one drop of each new carrier oil before using it on larger areas of skin or combining it with essential oils for patch testing.

Safety for Everyone

Everyone should observe the following safety precautions:

- Because it is possible to develop sensitivities you haven't experienced before, if it's been a while since you've used a blend or oil, perform the patch test again.

- Avoid using oils around the eyes because they can cause pain and damage.

- Avoid putting oils near flames, as they are flammable.

- Always use a carrier oil for topical application, because the oils may irritate skin or cause a reaction.

- Follow the ratios for blends and recipes in this book exactly.

- Give yourself a break from oils from time to time. Don't use the same oils or blends day after day, or you may build sensitivity. A good rule of thumb for frequently used oils is to use them on a five-day-on, two-day-off schedule.

- If you've ever experienced a sensitization reaction to any essential oil (may appear as skin breakouts, hives, sensitivity, itchiness, and redness), do not use that oil again.

- Keep oils out of reach of children and pets.

- Some essential oils cause photosensitization, meaning they can increase your risk of sunburn. If you use an essential oil with a photosensitization warning, avoid sun exposure and tanning beds for six to twenty-four hours after application, depending on the individual essential oil and the warning that accompanies it.

- Think about your needs, and then decide which oils will meet them. Assure their safety by checking for contraindications, and check with your doctor if you take any prescription medicines. For example, grapefruit essential oil acts much like grapefruit, interacting with certain medications.

- When making your own essential oil blends, try to keep the essential oils between 1.5 percent and 3 percent of the solution, or about three drops of essential oil per two teaspoons of carrier oil.

Safety for People with Allergies

True allergies are triggered by protein molecules. While essential oils do not contain proteins (they are removed during distillation), they can combine with proteins in the skin to cause an allergic reaction. However, even if you have an allergy to an essential oil used topically, you may not have one with inhalation of the scent, because there is no protein with which the plant molecules can combine. Therefore, if you have allergic reactions to certain essential oils, inhalation of the aroma may be another option.

If you have allergies, always perform a patch test. If you react to the patch test, do not try using that oil again. Avoid using essential oils that correspond with any allergies you have. For example, if you are allergic to ragweed, you should avoid using chamomile essential oil on the skin.

Safety in Pregnancy

Many essential oils are emmenagogues, meaning that they promote menstruation. While those oils can be useful for treating painful periods, they should be avoided during pregnancy. Note that some emmenagogues, particularly jasmine and clary sage, are also parturient, meaning that they can assist with labor and delivery. If you'd like to use essential oils in the delivery room, ensure that you do so with the help of an experienced aromatherapist, doula, or midwife.

Many of the recipes used in this book call for one or a combination of the oils listed next, so keep substitution oils on hand. For pregnant people, lavender (*Lavandula angustifolia*) and spearmint are two of the best substitution oils, and they mix well in most recipes.

If you are pregnant and considering a specific oil, conduct some research beforehand to ensure that use of any of the following is safe.

- Angelica
- Anise (also known as aniseed)
- Basil
- Bay laurel
- Birch
- Black pepper
- Calendula
- Camphor
- Caraway seed
- Carrot seed
- Cedarwood
- Chamomile (German and Roman)
- Cinnamon leaf
- Clary sage
- Clove
- Copaiba
- Cypress
- Davana
- Elemi
- Eucalyptus
- Fennel seed
- Frankincense
- Geranium
- Ginger
- Hops flower
- Hyssop
- Jasmine
- Juniper
- Lavandin
- Marjoram
- Myrrh
- Myrtle
- Oakmoss
- Oregano
- Parsley
- Peppermint
- Ravintsara
- Rose
- Rosemary
- Rue
- Spanish sage
- Spanish lavender
- Spike lavender
- Tagetes
- Tarragon
- Vitex berry

Safety for Children

As mentioned previously, always keep essential oils out of reach of children. If you do plan to make preparations specifically for use with children, keep these points in mind:

- You will see that many oils are described as "safe for children and babies," but they are safe only when used in specific ways. Follow recipes as written.

- With the exception of recipes formulated specifically for babies or children, assume all other recipes are formulated for adults. Adapt these recipes at half-strength for children twelve and under.

- Always use caution to avoid burns when administering steam inhalation treatments to children.

Safety for Seniors

Just as children are more sensitive to essential oils than average adults, seniors—particularly, elderly and frail individuals—have heightened levels of sensitivity. Take extra care when preparing treatments intended for seniors. It's a good idea to make formulations at half-strength to prevent skin irritation or sensitization. Adjustments can be made only if there is no negative reaction after a few applications of the preparation.

Using Oils with Care

It's important to be careful with all essential oils, but some do come with particular warnings. When an essential oil has the potential to cause sensitive skin, dilute it with at least twice as much carrier oil. In other words, use at least two drops of carrier oil for every one drop of essential oil.

Be aware that different resources provide contradictory information, and err on the side of safety rather than taking chances.

- **Allspice** May cause sensitive skin
- **Anise** Also known as aniseed; avoid if diagnosed with any form of cancer
- **Basil** Avoid if diagnosed with any form of cancer; may cause sensitive skin
- **Bay** Avoid if diagnosed with any form of cancer; may cause sensitive skin
- **Benzoin** May cause sensitive skin; avoid if driving or operating machinery
- **Bergamot** Avoid if diagnosed with melanoma or skin cancer; may cause sensitive skin
- **Birch** May cause sensitive skin
- **Black pepper** May cause sensitive skin
- **Camphor** Avoid if diagnosed with epilepsy
- **Carnation** Avoid if driving or operating machinery
- **Cassia** May cause sensitive skin
- **Cedarwood** May cause sensitive skin
- **Chamomile** (German and Roman) Avoid if driving or operating machinery
- **Cinnamon** Avoid both cinnamon leaf and cinnamon bark if diagnosed with any form of cancer; may cause sensitive skin
- **Citronella** Avoid if diagnosed with estrogen-dependent cancer; may cause sensitive skin
- **Clove bud** Avoid if diagnosed with any form of cancer; may cause sensitive skin
- **Costus** May cause sensitive skin
- **Cumin** May cause sensitive skin
- **Elecampane** May cause sensitive skin
- **Eucalyptus** Avoid all species if diagnosed with estrogen-dependent cancer; *Eucalyptus globulus* may cause sensitive skin
- **Fennel seed** Avoid if diagnosed with any form of cancer; may cause sensitive skin
- **Fir needle** May cause sensitive skin
- **Geranium** Avoid if driving or operating machinery
- **Ginger** May cause sensitive skin
- **Grapefruit** Avoid if diagnosed with melanoma or skin cancer

- **Helichrysum** May cause sensitive skin
- **Ho leaf** Avoid if diagnosed with any form of cancer
- **Hops** Avoid if driving or operating machinery
- **Hyacinth** Avoid if driving or operating machinery
- **Hyssop** Avoid if diagnosed with epilepsy; avoid if diagnosed with high blood pressure
- **Juniper** May cause sensitive skin
- **Laurel** Avoid if diagnosed with any form of cancer
- **Lavender** Avoid if driving or operating machinery
- **Lemon verbena** May cause sensitive skin
- **Lemon** Avoid if diagnosed with melanoma or skin cancer; may cause sensitive skin
- **Lemongrass** Avoid if diagnosed with estrogen-dependent cancer; may cause sensitive skin
- **Lime** Avoid if diagnosed with melanoma or skin cancer
- **Linden blossom** Avoid if driving or operating machinery
- **Mace** Avoid if driving or operating machinery
- **Mandarin** Avoid if diagnosed with melanoma or skin cancer
- **Marjoram** Avoid if driving or operating machinery
- **Melissa** May cause sensitive skin
- **Neroli** Avoid if driving or operating machinery
- **Oakmoss** May cause sensitive skin
- **Oregano** May cause sensitive skin
- **Ormenis flower** Avoid if driving or operating machinery
- **Parsley seed** May cause sensitive skin
- **Peppermint** Avoid if diagnosed with heart problems; may cause sensitive skin
- **Petitgrain** Avoid if driving or operating machinery
- **Pine** May cause sensitive skin
- **Rosemary** Avoid if diagnosed with epilepsy or high blood pressure
- **Sage** Avoid if diagnosed with epilepsy or high blood pressure
- **Sandalwood** Avoid if driving or operating machinery
- **Spike lavender** Avoid if diagnosed with epilepsy

- **Spikenard** Avoid if driving or operating machinery

- **Star anise** Avoid if diagnosed with estrogen-dependent cancer

- **Sweet orange** Avoid if diagnosed with melanoma or skin cancer; may cause sensitive skin

- **Tagetes** May cause sensitive skin

- **Tangerine** Avoid if diagnosed with melanoma or skin cancer

- **Thyme** May cause sensitive skin; avoid if diagnosed with high blood pressure

- **Valerian** Avoid if driving or operating machinery

- **Verbena** Avoid if diagnosed with estrogen-dependent cancer

- **Vetiver** Avoid if driving or operating machinery

- **Ylang-ylang** Avoid if driving or operating machinery

Additional Safety Q&A

Q: How often can I diffuse?
A: It's fine to diffuse essential oils daily, but it's a good idea to rotate oils throughout the week to avoid sensitization.

Q: Can I use different essential oils for different needs all at the same time?
A: You can use multiple essential oils throughout the day, but pace yourself. You should give each oil enough time to do its job. If you're using heavily diluted essential oils in bath and beauty products, it's fine to enjoy them one after another as you would normally do with other body products.

Q: Is it possible to use too much essential oil?
A: Yes: Unless you're treating an acute condition over a period of several days, you should use no more than 3 to 4 drops of each essential oil over the course of a given day, and you shouldn't use strong topical solutions unless necessary. Overuse can lead to allergies and hypersensitivity. If this happens, you'll get an unpleasant reaction each time you use the oil in the future.

Q: Should I take a break from my essential oils?
A: It's fine to use highly diluted oils daily—for example, in soaps and shampoos. If you've been using stronger remedies, give your body a one-week break for every two weeks of topical essential oil use.

Q: Should I switch application sites to avoid sensitization?
A: Yes, if you tend to use the same oil over and over again, and particularly if you use oils neat. Overuse can cause rashes, and in some cases serious skin irritation can develop.

YOUR STARTER KIT ESSENTIAL OIL ALL-STARS

There are countless essential oils available, so how did just a handful make it onto this list? The criteria were simple. The 15 oils at the heart of this book were selected because they are versatile, affordable, and easy to find. Many come in starter kits from top essential oil companies, and all are fantastic for blending with a few others on the list.

Nine Must-Have Essential Oils

Clove	Lavender	Peppermint
Eucalyptus	Lemon	Rosemary
Geranium	Lemongrass	Tea tree

Six Great-to-Have Essential Oils

Clary sage	Grapefruit	Roman chamomile
Frankincense	Patchouli	Thyme

DILUTION AND SUBSTITUTION

Because essential oils are so powerful, it's important to understand how they should be diluted and substituted for one another. Here are the basics.

Using Oils Neat and in Dilutions

There are different opinions on how best to dilute essential oils, and whether it is ever safe to apply essential oils neat—that is, without diluting them first. Just like the subject of taking oils internally, neat application is a controversial topic with opinions that vary from one practitioner to the next. It is up to you to determine how best to apply your essential oils safely. Neat peppermint oil that some people use to stop headaches isn't appropriate for everyone; in someone with highly sensitive skin, it would probably cause some irritation.

The best way to avoid skin irritation or sensitization is to dilute your oils before using them. When you blend essential oils with anything—a carrier oil, aloe vera gel, your bathwater, or an unscented soap or lotion base for example—you're diluting it. Most topical treatments in this book are heavily diluted, but there are exceptions for certain first-aid applications, as well as other remedies. Certain acute conditions can respond best to undiluted essential oils. A drop of undiluted lavender essential oil, for example, is an excellent treatment for a minor cut or scrape, while a drop of undiluted tea tree essential oil makes an outstanding treatment for foot fungus. These are just two of many instances when neat application can be highly beneficial. Certain oils are often used neat on acupressure points, too. In almost all cases though, the total amount is just 1 or 2 drops.

If you have sensitive skin, or want to treat an elder or a child under twelve with essential oils, it's a good idea to dilute even the oils generally considered safe for neat use before applying them. The same logic applies to people who are pregnant, people with serious illnesses, and anyone with a compromised immune system. Don't worry—the essential oil will still do its job; the carrier "carries" the essential oil into the skin, while acting as a buffer.

Remember, even when heavily diluted, certain oils are not safe for everyone. Check for contraindications before using an essential oil on anyone—especially if that person falls into one of the categories mentioned previously, such as a young child or elderly person.

General Dilution Guide: Create New Recipes Safely

Essential oil dilution isn't an exact science: Drop sizes differ depending on the essential oil's viscosity and the type of dropper used. Additionally, some essential oils are far stronger or "hotter" than others and can require higher dilution rates—the percentage of essential oil relative to the percentage of carrier—for safety reasons as well as to ensure the scents aren't overpowering. Recipes often fall into gray areas, too. For example, a blend might contain between 1.5 and 2 percent essential oil to provide a balanced, pleasing scent, while offering a high level of safety.

For beginners ready to create new blends for topical use, the following basic dilution guidelines represent a road map. You can follow them exactly, or you can calculate how many drops of essential oil to use with a simple equation. Imagine you'd like to make just 1 teaspoon of a remedy that calls for 3 percent dilution. The following chart shows that a 3 percent dilution with 2 tablespoons (1 fluid ounce) of carrier oil calls for 24 drops of essential oil. Basic measurement guidelines tell you that 1 teaspoon is one-sixth of a fluid ounce: So, 24 divided by 6 is 4, meaning that 1 teaspoon of your remedy should contain 4 drops of essential oil.

Whenever you use a new essential oil, you'll find it helpful to conduct some research on recommended dilution rates. Since opinions about dilution tend to vary widely, it's often best to check a few sources before deciding how to proceed.

Essential oils are never safe for premature infants.

Dilution Guide

This chart shows the number of drops of essential oil required for different dilution rates in varying amounts of carrier oils. If you need the carrier oil amount specified in ounces, see the measurement conversions chart on page 361.

Dilution Rate	0.25%	0.5%	1%	1.5%	2%	2.5%	3%	4%	5%	10%
1 tablespoon carrier	1 drop	2 drops	4 drops	6 drops	8 drops	10 drops	12 drops	16 drops	20 drops	40 drops
2 tablespoons carrier	2 drops	4 drops	8 drops	12 drops	16 drops	20 drops	24 drops	32 drops	40 drops	80 drops
¼ cup carrier	4 drops	8 drops	16 drops	24 drops	32 drops	40 drops	48 drops	64 drops	80 drops	160 drops
½ cup carrier	8 drops	16 drops	32 drops	48 drops	64 drops	80 drops	96 drops	128 drops	160 drops	320 drops
¾ cup carrier	12 drops	24 drops	48 drops	72 drops	96 drops	120 drops	144 drops	192 drops	240 drops	480 drops
1 cup carrier	16 drops	32 drops	64 drops	96 drops	128 drops	160 drops	192 drops	256 drops	320 drops	640 drops

USING STARTER ESSENTIAL OILS AS SUBSTITUTES

Dig deeper into the world of aromatherapy and you'll notice that many essential oils offer similar benefits to one another, and others have similar scents. In many cases, it's possible to use one essential oil in place of another—which is especially nice when a recipe calls for something expensive and you'd rather save your money. Listed here are 17 of the world's most expensive essential oils, plus some possible substitutions you can try.

You'll notice some of these costly oils have scents that can't be re-created by substituting another oil; these fragrances are uniquely complex. Many of the most expensive oils are primarily used in perfumery, even though they often come with psychotherapeutic effects.

GERMAN (BLUE) CHAMOMILE
Scent: Roman chamomile shares a similar scent profile; the two are not identical but can easily stand in for each other.
Action: Try clove for a similar pain relief effect. Try Roman chamomile for a similar relaxing effect.

HELICHRYSUM
Scent: Try blending a drop of lavender with a drop of clary sage for a similar fresh, herbaceous scent.
Action: Try lavender, frankincense, or patchouli for a similar healing effect.

HYSSOP
Scent: Try blending a drop of clary sage and a drop of peppermint or rosemary to replicate hyssop's very light, fresh, herbal fragrance.
Action: Try lavender, patchouli, or tea tree for a similar antiviral effect.

JASMINE
Scent: No substitute.
Action: Try lavender or geranium for a similar skin-soothing effect. Try clary sage for similar relief from menstrual and menopausal symptoms.

MELISSA
Scent: Try blending a drop of peppermint or clary sage with 2 drops of lemon for a similar fresh, lemony fragrance.
Action: Try clary sage or lavender for a similar relaxing effect. Try rosemary for similar relief from respiratory discomfort.

MYRRH
Scent: Try frankincense for a fragrance that shares a similar richness and warmth.
Action: Try frankincense, lavender, or geranium for similar skin-healing effects.

PALO SANTO
Scent: Try frankincense; the two are close relatives and their scents share some similar qualities.
Action: Try frankincense for similar anti-inflammatory and pain-relieving effects.

ROSE
Scent: No substitute, but preblended rose oil is an inexpensive option worth exploring.
Action: Try geranium for similar skin-soothing effects.

SANDALWOOD
Scent: No substitute.
Action: Try frankincense for similar skin-soothing effects.

SPIKENARD
Scent: Try clary sage as a stand-in for spikenard's strong, earthy fragrance.
Action: Try clary sage for similar relief from menstrual symptoms. Use lavender, clary sage, or patchouli for similar relief from stress and anxiety.

VETIVER
Scent: No substitute.
Action: Try lavender or clary sage for a similar soothing, relaxing effect. Topically, try tea tree or lavender for minor cuts and scrapes.

VITEX BERRY
Scent: Try blending 1 drop of lavender or geranium with 2 or 3 drops of clary sage for a somewhat similar herbal, earthy, slightly floral fragrance.
Action: Try clary sage for similar relief from menstrual and menopausal symptoms.

YUZU
Scent: Try grapefruit, lemon, or a combination of the two.
Action: Try grapefruit or lemon for a similarly uplifting sensation. Grapefruit and lemon readily stand in for other applications, such as increasing focus, reducing stress, and easing cold symptoms.

PART TWO

Essential Oil Profiles

Essential oils are the backbone of aromatherapy, and it's vital you learn the basics of each before using it on your skin or in your home. Each of the eighty-six short profiles included here covers important safety information and interesting facts about some of the most versatile and useful essential oils available, along with a list of medicinal properties, ideas for use, and inspiration for creating blends.

The botanical name is listed with each entry, along with a basic price estimate. Please note that prices can vary widely and are subject to change depending on market conditions.

There are hundreds of essential oils and blends available, but discovering which one suits your needs can take a little research. If you're interested in making your own nontoxic baby lotions, for example, you need to know which oils are safe for infants (lavender and dill, for instance) and, more importantly, which are not (rosemary or eucalyptus).

Just as you wouldn't treat a headache with a spoonful of cough syrup, it makes sense to focus on the oils that fit the specific requirement of your project—whether it's making an antiseptic salve, a nourishing eye cream, or a disinfectant spray to remove pet odors.

$	$15 and under
$$	$16–$34
$$$	$35–$50
$$$$	more than $50

ALLSPICE
Pimenta dioica

SPICY SCENT
COST: $

Also known as pimenta or pimento berry oil, allspice essential oil is made from the leaves and/or fruit of an evergreen tree that grows primarily in South America and the West Indies. Its warm, pleasant fragrance helps with stress and mild depression, and is similar to the aroma of cloves. Allspice contains a high level of eugenol, which fights bacteria, numbs pain, and inhibits fungal growth, among other tasks. Eugenol is found in a variety of commercial products, including mouthwash and toothpaste.

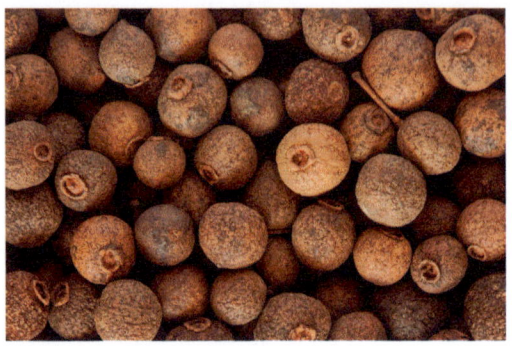

MEDICINAL PROPERTIES
Analgesic, anesthetic, antiseptic, carminative, muscle relaxant, rubefacient, stimulant

USES
Effective in treating bronchitis and sore muscles; ideal for making personal fragrances

BLENDS WELL WITH
Bergamot, clove bud, geranium, ginger, jasmine, lavender, lemon, patchouli, sweet orange, ylang-ylang

PRECAUTIONS
Do not use during pregnancy. Allspice can cause skin irritation if applied neat. Because it can irritate mucous membranes, it should not be inhaled directly.

ANISE
Pimpinella anisum

LICORICE SCENT
COST: $

With a rich, sweet aroma reminiscent of authentic black licorice, anise has a long history of culinary and medicinal applications. Traditional liqueurs including arak, ouzo, Pernod, and raki rely on the herb for their signature flavors. Anise is often sold as anise seed or aniseed essential oil. Be careful not to confuse it with star anise, or *Illicium verum*, because it offers different properties.

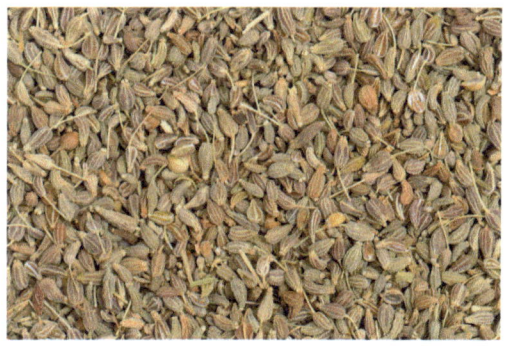

MEDICINAL PROPERTIES
Antibacterial, antifungal, antiseptic, antispasmodic, aperient, aphrodisiac, carminative, cordial, decongestant, digestive, expectorant, insecticide, sedative, vermifuge

USES
Effective in treating bronchitis, cold, and flu; ideal for treating ailments that include digestive discomfort

BLENDS WELL WITH
Bay laurel, black pepper, fir needle, ginger, lavender, lime, pine, rose, spruce, sweet orange

PRECAUTIONS
Do not use during pregnancy or if breastfeeding. Avoid if diagnosed with endometriosis or an estrogen-dependent form of cancer. Not recommended for children under five years old. Anise can irritate sensitive skin. Heavy doses have a narcotic effect, causing heartbeat and respiration to slow. Avoid if you are allergic to carrots, celery, or pollen. Use caution around pets; anise is toxic to birds and rodents.

ATLAS CEDARWOOD
Cedrus atlantica

WOODY SCENT
COST: $

Atlas cedarwood has a long, storied history of use in architecture and furniture making, and these beautiful evergreen trees are popular with landscapers. Its woody, balsamic fragrance makes it a favorite in perfumery and incense making. Because both Atlas cedarwood and cedarwood essential oil from the *Cedrus deodara* species offer similar scents and medicinal properties, they are often interchangeable.

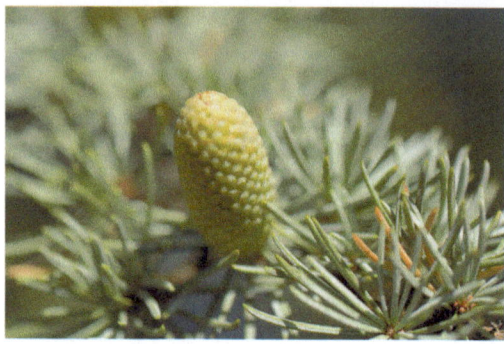

MEDICINAL PROPERTIES
Antibacterial, antifungal, anti-inflammatory, antiseptic, antispasmodic, aphrodisiac, astringent, diuretic, expectorant, insect repellent, insecticide, sedative, vulnerary

USES
Effective in treating acne, dandruff, and oily hair; ideal for making insect repellents

BLENDS WELL WITH
Bergamot, clary sage, cypress, frankincense, German chamomile, jasmine, juniper berry, lavender, neroli, palmarosa, petitgrain, Roman chamomile, rosemary, vetiver

PRECAUTIONS
Do not use during pregnancy. Atlas cedarwood can cause skin irritation if applied neat.

BALSAM OF PERU
Myroxylon balsamum

SWEET VANILLA SCENT
COST: $

A wonderful essential oil for skin care, balsam of Peru also soothes feelings of minor depression, reduces stress, and promotes peaceful sleep. Its fragrance is strongly reminiscent of vanilla, with undertones of chocolate, making it a favorite with perfumeries and soap makers. It is considered an inexpensive substitute for costly vanilla essential oil.

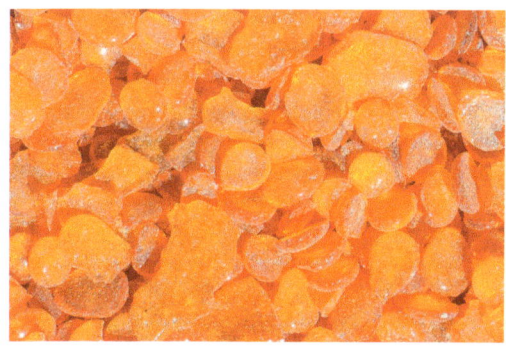

MEDICINAL PROPERTIES
Antibacterial, anti-inflammatory, antioxidant, antiseptic, cicatrizant, deodorant, diuretic, expectorant

USES
Effective in treating dry, chapped skin; ideal for making bath and body products

BLENDS WELL WITH
Atlas cedarwood, cardamom, cedarwood, cinnamon leaf, clove bud, ginger, lavender, lemon, lime, mandarin, marjoram, peppermint, rosemary, sweet orange, thyme

PRECAUTIONS
Balsam of Peru can cause skin sensitivity, especially in the elderly and children under two years old.

BASIL
Ocimum basilicum

SWEET, HERBACEOUS SCENT
COST: $

Basil essential oil comes from the common culinary herb, which gets its name from the Greek word *basileum*, meaning "king." A fantastic skin tonic for acne, it also relieves menstrual cramps, rheumatism, gout, and sore muscles. Basil should be avoided during pregnancy. However, when nursing, its use promotes greater milk production. In Italy, new moms traditionally eat basil leaves to stimulate lactation.

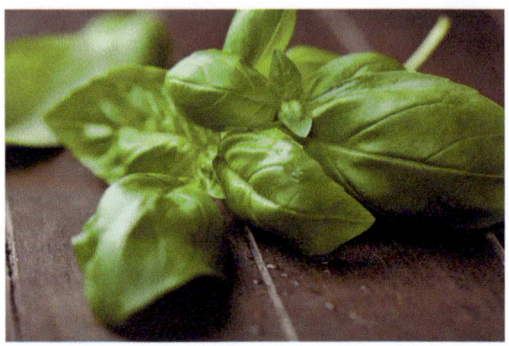

MEDICINAL PROPERTIES
Antibacterial, antidepressant, antiseptic, antispasmodic, digestive, expectorant, restorative, stomachic

USES
Effective in treating headaches, eliminating anxiety, and soothing insect bites

BLENDS WELL WITH
Bay laurel, black pepper, citronella, lemon, lemongrass, lime, marjoram, melissa, oregano, peppermint, ravintsara, spearmint, vetiver, yuzu

PRECAUTIONS
Do not use during pregnancy.

BAY LAUREL
Laurus nobilis

SPICY, SWEET SCENT
COST: $

Also known as sweet bay or laurel leaf, bay laurel essential oil offers an uplifting fragrance, with hints of camphor and spice. Sourced from the same plant as the bay leaves used for culinary purposes, this essential oil is ideal for diffusing when you have a cold or the flu. You can also diffuse it when you're feeling stressed and on the edge of illness; it supports a healthy immune system while promoting clarity and peace of mind.

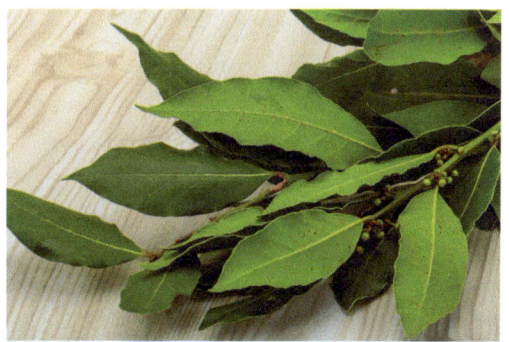

MEDICINAL PROPERTIES
Analgesic, antibacterial, antiseptic, antispasmodic, antiviral, astringent, cholagogue, emmenagogue, expectorant, febrifuge, insecticide, sedative, stomachic, sudorific

USES
Effective in treating cold and flu; ideal for supporting digestive health

BLENDS WELL WITH
Bergamot, clary sage, cypress, eucalyptus, frankincense, ginger, juniper berry, lavender, lemon, myrtle, patchouli, pine, ravensara leaf, ravintsara, rosemary, Spanish sage, sweet orange, ylang-ylang

PRECAUTIONS
Do not use during pregnancy. Bay laurel can cause skin irritation.

BENZOIN
Styrax benzoin, S. tonkinensis

WARM, SWEET SCENT
COST: $$

With a pleasant aroma that carries a strong hint of vanilla, benzoin essential oil is very popular with perfumeries and incense makers. Historically used in India and Asia, it was also quite popular with ancient Egyptians. It is no surprise, then, that this beautiful oil is ideal for alleviating stress and creating a sense of euphoria.

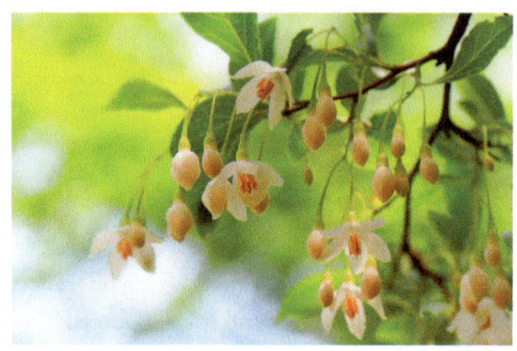

MEDICINAL PROPERTIES
Antidepressant, anti-inflammatory, antiseptic, astringent, carminative, cordial, deodorant, diuretic, expectorant, sedative, vulnerary

USES
Effective in treating arthritis, rheumatism, body aches, and joint pains; ideal for relieving chapped, dry skin

BLENDS WELL WITH
Bergamot, black pepper, cinnamon leaf, coriander, cypress, frankincense, ginger, jasmine, juniper berry, lavender, lemon, marjoram, myrrh, petitgrain, rose, rosemary, sandalwood, sweet orange

PRECAUTIONS
Avoid use before driving or undertaking important tasks.

BERGAMOT
Citrus bergamia

SPICY, CITRUS SCENT
COST: $$

A valuable essential oil for treating oily skin, abscesses, and boils, bergamot is also a good choice for dealing with stress and exhaustion. If you suffer from seasonal depression, you may find that diffusing bergamot is a good way to lift your mood and give you the inspiration you need to get up and go. Choose bergamot FCF, which stands for furocoumarin free, if possible; it has had the bergaptene (furocoumarin) removed and is far less phototoxic than standard bergamot.

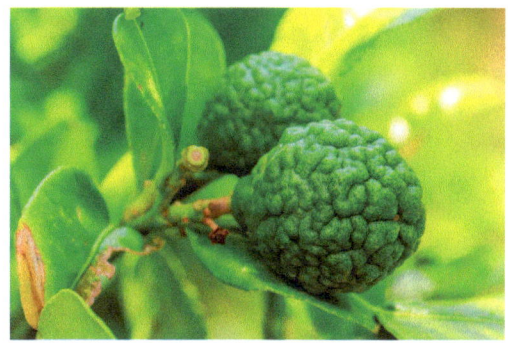

MEDICINAL PROPERTIES
Analgesic, antidepressant, antiseptic, antispasmodic, calmative, cicatrizant, deodorant, digestive, febrifuge, stomachic, vermifuge, vulnerary

USES
Effective in treating acne, oily skin, psoriasis, and eczema; ideal for making bath and body products

BLENDS WELL WITH
Basil, clary sage, coriander, cypress, geranium, German chamomile, ginger, hops flower, jasmine, juniper berry, palo santo, Roman chamomile, rose, sandalwood, vetiver

PRECAUTIONS
Phototoxic if not labeled "bergamot FCF"; do not apply to skin that will be exposed to direct sunlight. Bergamot can cause sensitive skin.

BLACK PEPPER
Piper nigrum

WARM, SPICY SCENT
COST: $

Offering a crisp, spicy scent with hints of green and the slightest touch of flowers, black pepper essential oil smells a little bit like freshly ground peppercorns. It stimulates the mind and promotes alertness. Its ability to facilitate circulation while providing a deep, warming effect makes it a good choice in blends designed to ease muscle pain and aching joints.

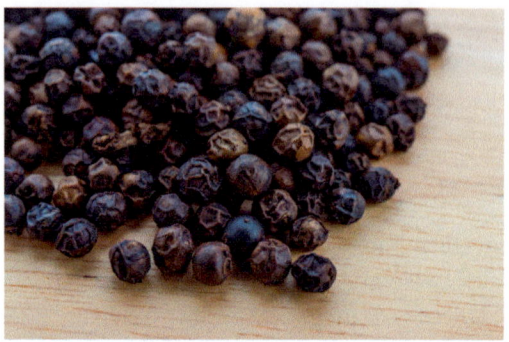

MEDICINAL PROPERTIES
Analgesic, antiseptic, antispasmodic, aphrodisiac, diaphoretic, digestive, diuretic, febrifuge, laxative, rubefacient

USES
Effective in treating digestive problems, arthritis, flu, and colds; ideal for use in blends designed to provide emotional motivation

BLENDS WELL WITH
Bergamot, clary sage, clove bud, coriander, fennel seed, frankincense, geranium, ginger, grapefruit, juniper berry, lavender, lemon, lime, mandarin, sandalwood, Spanish sage, rosewood, ylang-ylang

PRECAUTIONS
Avoid topical use during pregnancy due to increased risk of skin sensitization. Black pepper can cause sensitive skin.

CAJUPUT
Melaleuca leucadendron, M. minor

SWEET, CAMPHOROUS SCENT
COST: $

Also known as cajeput, or *Melaleuca minor*, cajuput essential oil relieves cold and flu symptoms, including congestion and sore throat. A close relative of tea tree, it is also suitable for treating asthma and bronchitis, muscle aches, and oily skin. Its sweet, lightly camphorous aroma promotes a clear, alert state of mind, and makes it an excellent choice for use in natural insect repellents.

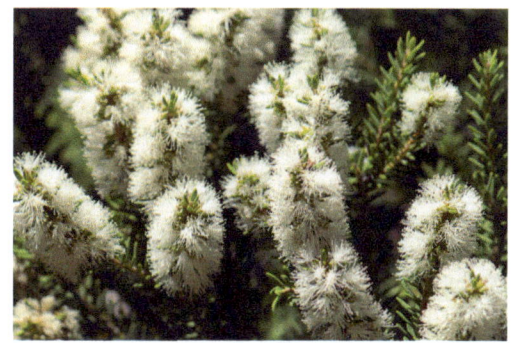

MEDICINAL PROPERTIES
Analgesic, antiseptic, antispasmodic, carminative, decongestant, expectorant, febrifuge, insect repellent, insecticide, stimulant, sudorific, vermifuge

USES
Effective in treating skin conditions such as acne, eczema, and psoriasis; ideal for making insect repellents

BLENDS WELL WITH
Bergamot, citronella, clary sage, clove bud, geranium, lavender, lemongrass, rosemary, thyme, vetiver

PRECAUTIONS
Avoid topical use during pregnancy due to increased risk of skin sensitization. Cajuput can cause skin irritation when used at high concentrations.

CALENDULA
Calendula officinalis

FLORAL SCENT
COST: $

Also known as the pot marigold, calendula is one of the few flowers that produces an essential oil and not an absolute. The flower has a long history of being associated with sacred rituals and was used to adorn Hindu temples, and was revered by the Egyptians for its regenerative properties. Calendula ointments have long been used to treat conjunctivitis (pinkeye) and as a gentle lotion for diaper rash.

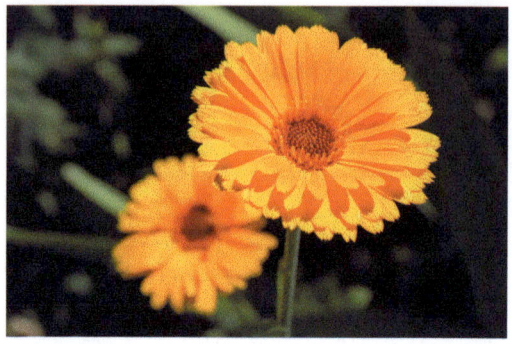

MEDICINAL PROPERTIES
Anti-inflammatory, antispasmodic, sedative, skin care, soporific, tonic

USES
Effective in easing acne, anxiety, burns, cold sores, menstrual issues, psoriasis, and skin irritations

BLENDS WELL WITH
Orange, lemon, neroli, lavender, chamomile, cypress, pine, cedarwood

PRECAUTIONS
Avoid use if pregnant or breastfeeding.

CARAWAY SEED
Carum carvi

SWEET, SPICY SCENT
COST: $

A wonderfully energizing essential oil, caraway seed offers an aroma that has variously been described as spicy and sweet, fruity, peppery, and herbaceous. It makes an intriguing addition to personal scents and when diffused, it proves useful in easing laryngitis, bronchitis, and cold symptoms.

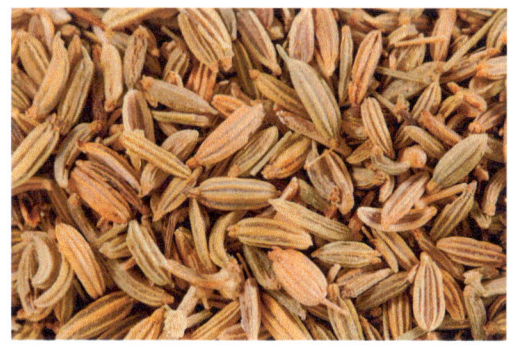

MEDICINAL PROPERTIES
Antihistaminic, antiseptic, antispasmodic, aperitive, astringent, carminative, digestive, disinfectant, diuretic, emmenagogue, expectorant, galactagogue, stimulant, stomachic, vermifuge

USES
Effective in treating digestive ailments and gastric spasms; ideal for soothing mental fatigue

BLENDS WELL WITH
Basil, coriander, frankincense, German chamomile, ginger, lavender, Roman chamomile, sweet orange

PRECAUTIONS
Do not use during pregnancy. Caraway seed can cause skin irritation when used at high concentrations.

CARDAMOM
Elettaria cardamomum

SWEET, SPICY SCENT
COST: $$

You might recognize cardamom as one of the spices that gives chai its irresistible flavor. Cardamom essential oil comes from the seeds of a perennial herb with a reedlike structure. Highly prized by Egyptians for perfumery and incense, these seeds were also chewed as tooth whiteners, and the Romans nibbled on them to ease indigestion.

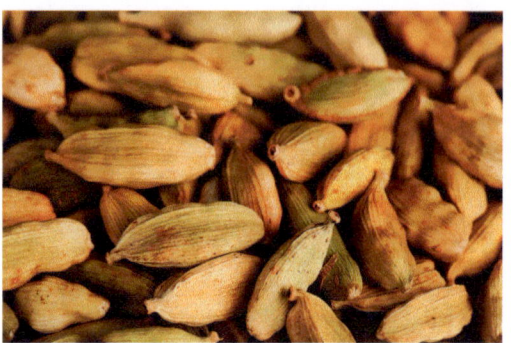

MEDICINAL PROPERTIES
Antiseptic, antispasmodic, carminative, digestive, diuretic, expectorant, stimulant, stomachic

USES
Effective in treating nausea and indigestion; ideal for making refreshing bath and body products

BLENDS WELL WITH
Bergamot, caraway seed, cedarwood, cinnamon leaf, clove bud, hops flower, lime, mandarin, rose, spikenard, sweet orange, tangerine

PRECAUTIONS
Generally regarded as safe.

CARROT SEED
Daucus carota

EARTHY, HERBACEOUS SCENT
COST: $$

Primarily obtained from European wild carrots, carrot seed essential oil is sometimes confused with inexpensive carrot oil, which is a macerated infusion of domestic carrots and carrier oil. Carrot seed essential oil contains high levels of carotene and vitamin A. Its ability to stimulate and rejuvenate skin makes it a valuable addition to bath and body products, while combining it with complementary essential oils such as geranium and rose is an excellent tactic for naturally reducing the appearance of wrinkles.

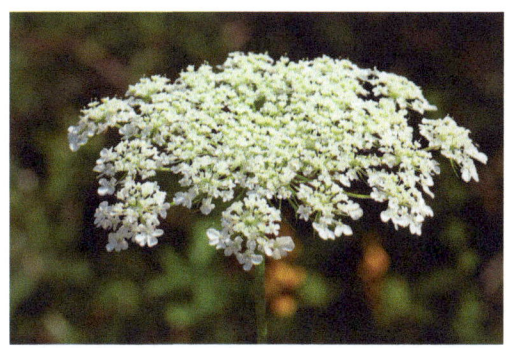

MEDICINAL PROPERTIES
Antiseptic, carminative, cytophylactic, depurative, diuretic, emmenagogue, stimulant, vermifuge

USES
Effective in treating dermatitis, rashes, and eczema; ideal for making rejuvenating bath and body products

BLENDS WELL WITH
Atlas cedarwood, bergamot, caraway seed, cardamom, cedarwood, cinnamon leaf, clove bud, geranium, ginger, juniper berry, lavender, lemon, lime, mandarin, rose, rose geranium, sweet orange

PRECAUTIONS
Do not use during pregnancy.

CEDARWOOD
Juniperus virginiana

SOFT, WOODY SCENT
COST: $

Sometimes confused with Atlas cedarwood, this essential oil comes from Virginian red cedar trees, which are also known as eastern red, Bedford, or southern red cedars. Prized by American Indigenous Peoples, the oldest examples of these trees are estimated to have sprouted more than nine hundred years ago. Like many other products made with this beautiful red wood, cedarwood essential oil deters insect activity. Meanwhile, its soft fragrance helps soothe nervous tension and ease anxiety.

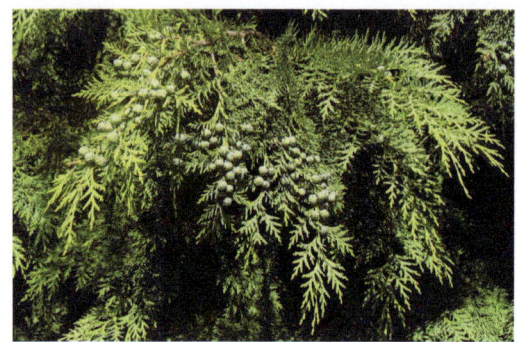

MEDICINAL PROPERTIES
Antiseborrheic, antiseptic, antispasmodic, astringent, diuretic, emmenagogue, expectorant, fungicide, insect repellent, insecticide, sedative

USES
Effective in treating arthritis, respiratory illnesses, and urinary tract infections (UTIs); ideal for making products to combat oily skin and hair

BLENDS WELL WITH
Benzoin, bergamot, cinnamon leaf, citronella, cypress, frankincense, helichrysum, jasmine, juniper berry, lavender, lemon, lime, neroli, rose, rose geranium, rosemary

PRECAUTIONS
Do not use during pregnancy. Cedarwood can cause skin irritation when used at high concentrations.

CINNAMON LEAF
Cinnamomum zeylanicum, C. verum

WARM, SPICY SCENT
COST: $

While cinnamon leaf essential oil comes from the same trees as cinnamon bark oil does, it has a higher eugenol content that increases its value as a topical analgesic. As a spice, cinnamon finds its way into sweet and savory dishes that span cultures worldwide. The essential oil was historically used for a variety of purposes, ranging from temple incense to massaging sore feet.

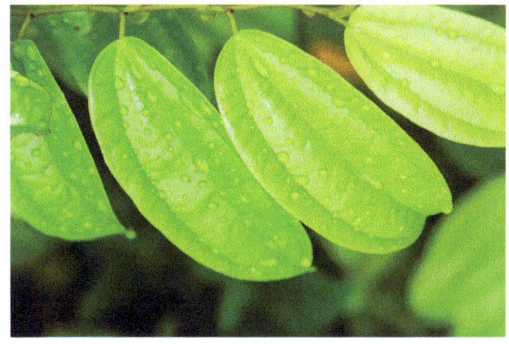

MEDICINAL PROPERTIES
Analgesic, antibiotic, antiseptic, antispasmodic, aphrodisiac, astringent, carminative, emmenagogue, insecticide, stimulant, stomachic, vermifuge

USES
Effective in treating joint and muscle pain, cramps, and painful periods; ideal in aromatherapy blends for respiratory ailments and depression

BLENDS WELL WITH
Balsam of Peru, benzoin, cardamom, clove bud, coriander, frankincense, ginger, grapefruit, lavender, lemon, mandarin, petitgrain, rosemary, sweet orange, tangerine, thyme, ylang-ylang

PRECAUTIONS
Do not use during pregnancy. Cinnamon leaf can cause severe skin irritation and mucous membrane irritation when used at high concentrations.

CITRONELLA
Cymbopogon nardus,
Andropogon nardus

SWEET, CITRUS SCENT
COST: $

Citronella essential oil comes from a fragrant tropical grass that has been employed in culinary and medicinal roles for thousands of years. Popular throughout China, Africa, and Southeast Asia, it is used for a wide range of ailments that include fevers, headaches, and menstrual problems, along with digestive illnesses. In the Western world, its greatest value lies in its efficacy as an insect repellent.

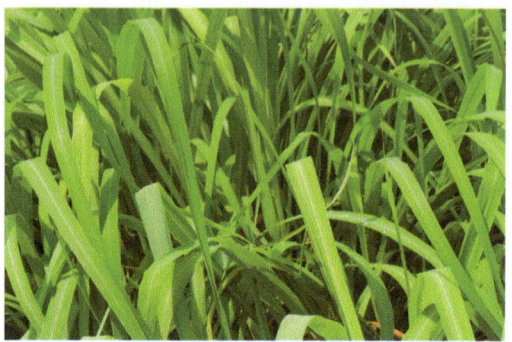

MEDICINAL PROPERTIES
Antiseptic, antiviral, bactericidal, deodorant, diaphoretic, febrifuge, insect repellent, insecticide, stimulant

USES
Effective in treating cold, fever, and flu; ideal for use in refreshing bath and body products that double as insect repellents

BLENDS WELL WITH
Atlas cedarwood, bergamot, cedarwood, cypress, fir needle, frankincense, geranium, lavender, lemon, lemon eucalyptus, lemongrass, pine, sandalwood, vetiver

PRECAUTIONS
Citronella can cause sensitive skin.

CLARY SAGE
Salvia sclarea

HERBACEOUS, SLIGHTLY FRUITY SCENT
COST: $$

Clary sage is an excellent essential oil for relaxation, and when used in bedtime blends, it can lull you gently to sleep. It is most popular, though, for its value in treating PMS, painful periods, and menopause symptoms. It contains sclareol, a constituent with an estrogen-like structure that helps bring hormones into balance. When diffused or worn in personal fragrance blends, clary sage can promote a calm feeling of self-confidence.

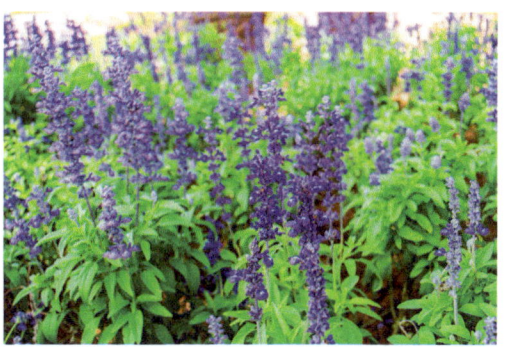

MEDICINAL PROPERTIES
Antidepressant, anti-inflammatory, antiseptic, antispasmodic, aphrodisiac, astringent, bactericidal, carminative, deodorant, digestive, emmenagogue, euphoriant, hypotensive, nervine, parturient, sedative, stomachic

USES
Effective in treating depression and postnatal depression; ideal for making relaxing bath and body products

BLENDS WELL WITH
Bergamot, cedarwood, frankincense, geranium, juniper berry, lavender, lemon, sandalwood, sweet orange, vitex berry

PRECAUTIONS
Do not use during pregnancy. Do not use before driving or operating machinery.

CLOVE BUD
Eugenia caryophyllata,
Syzygium aromaticum

SWEET, SPICY SCENT
COST: $

The irresistible aroma of clove bud essential oil stimulates the mind and helps lift depression; however, its greatest value lies in its ability to aid digestion and ease physical discomfort. An excellent remedy for dental pain, it is also ideal for soothing stiff, aching muscles and joints. Placed on a cotton ball, a few drops of clove bud essential oil will make any linen cabinet fragrant while keeping insects away.

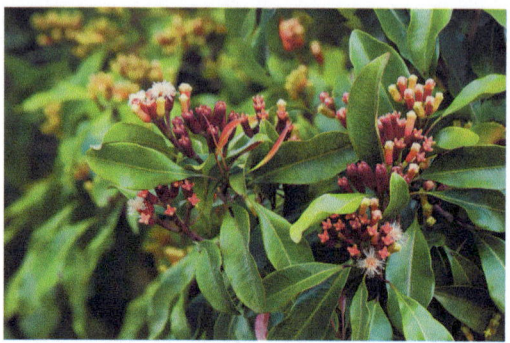

MEDICINAL PROPERTIES
Analgesic, antifungal, antiseptic, antispasmodic, carminative, disinfectant, insecticide, stimulant, stomachic

USES
Effective in treating athlete's foot, toothache, and digestive complaints; ideal for making warming massage blends to ease muscle pain, cramping, and spasms

BLENDS WELL WITH
Allspice, basil, benzoin, bergamot, cinnamon leaf, clary sage, ginger, helichrysum, hops flower, lavender, lemon, lime, myrtle, sandalwood, sweet orange, yuzu

PRECAUTIONS
Do not use during pregnancy. Do not use if diagnosed with liver or kidney disease. Clove bud can cause skin irritation and mucous membrane irritation when used at high concentrations.

COPAIBA
Copaifera reticulata

MILD, WOODY SCENT
COST: $ TO $$$

Traditionally used by Indigenous Peoples of Brazil to heal skin, copaiba has a very mild, almost wet-smelling wood aroma that blends very well with almost all other fragrances. It's advisable to use a little at a time because the scent gets stronger when exposed to air or placed on skin.

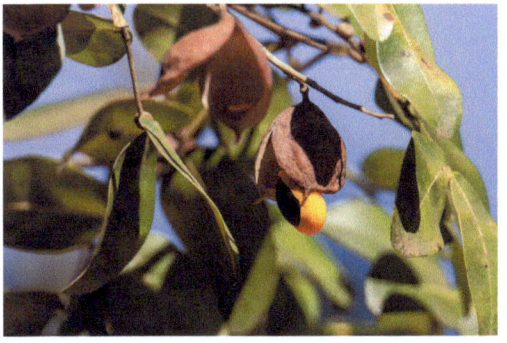

MEDICINAL PROPERTIES
Antibacterial, anti-inflammatory, decongestant, disinfectant, diuretic, expectorant, stimulant

USES
Effective in treating intestinal issues, including diarrhea; ideal for making antianxiety blends and blends that increase concentration while alleviating stress

BLENDS WELL WITH
Atlas cedarwood, bay laurel, bergamot, carrot seed, cedarwood, cinnamon leaf, clary sage, frankincense, lavender, mandarin, palmarosa

PRECAUTIONS
Do not use during pregnancy. Undiluted copaiba can cause sensitive skin.

CORIANDER
Coriandrum sativum

SWEET, SPICY SCENT
COST: $$

If coriander's name sounds familiar to you, it's probably because of its use as a culinary spice. Ancient Greeks and Romans used coriander to lend more depth to the flavor of wine; it is also a flavoring component in Benedictine and Chartreuse liqueurs. Beyond its use as a flavoring agent, coriander eases indigestion, diarrhea, and nausea, and its warming action has a therapeutic effect on muscle pain.

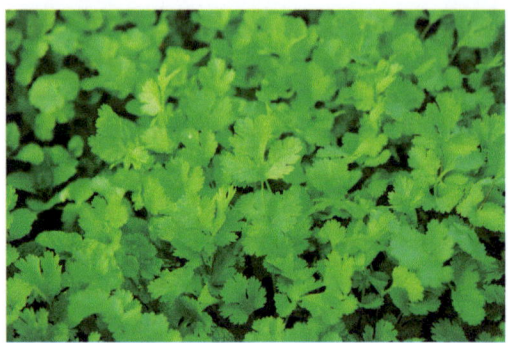

MEDICINAL PROPERTIES
Analgesic, antispasmodic, aphrodisiac, carminative, deodorant, depurative, digestive, fungicidal, stimulant, stomachic

USES
Effective in treating coughs, headaches, and mental fatigue; ideal for making warming massage blends

BLENDS WELL WITH
Bergamot, cajuput, cinnamon leaf, eucalyptus (all types), ginger, grapefruit, lavender, lemon, lemongrass, lime, may chang, neroli, sandalwood, spikenard, sweet orange

PRECAUTIONS
Generally regarded as safe.

CUCUMBER SEED
Cucumis sativus

SWEET, REFRESHING SCENT
COST: $

Cucumbers are enjoyed worldwide for their refreshing flavor, and they have a long history of use in face masks and rejuvenating skin treatments. Cucumber seed essential oil has a bright, uplifting fragrance and, thanks to its high level of vitamin C and omega-6 fatty acid, it makes a marvelous addition to cleansers, facial toners, and moisturizers.

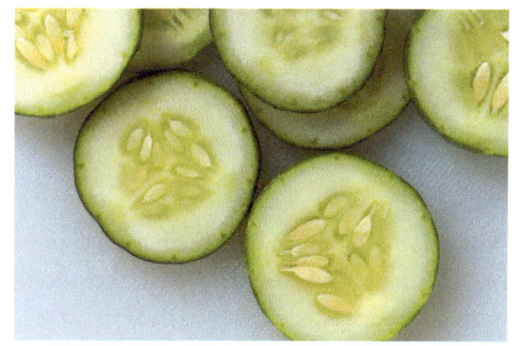

MEDICINAL PROPERTIES
Anti-inflammatory, antioxidant, antiseptic, diuretic

USES
Effective in treating psoriasis, acne, sunburn, and stretch marks; ideal for making nourishing hair and body products

BLENDS WELL WITH
Bergamot, carrot seed, geranium, grapefruit, lavender, lemon, lime, mandarin, neroli, sweet orange, ylang-ylang

PRECAUTIONS
Generally regarded as safe.

CYPRESS
Cupressus sempervirens

WOODY, SLIGHTLY SPICY SCENT
COST: $

Besides offering a versatile essential oil, cypress has a fascinating history. Thanks to the wood's durability and resilience, it was used to carve Egyptian sarcophagi, while the ancient Greeks often used it to carve statues of their gods. Because of its association with cemeteries and grave goods, cypress is nicknamed the "tree of death," but its botanical name alludes to its long life. Cypress essential oil has a long litany of uses, benefiting ailments as varied as hemorrhoids, muscle cramps, and stress.

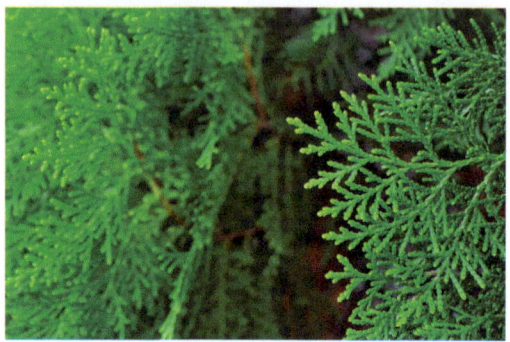

MEDICINAL PROPERTIES
Antiseptic, antispasmodic, astringent, calmative, deodorant, diuretic, hemostatic, insect repellent, insecticide, sedative, styptic, sudorific, vasoconstrictor

USES
Effective in treating varicose veins, asthma, bronchitis, and flu; ideal for making massage blends for muscle aches and cramping

BLENDS WELL WITH
Bergamot, clary sage, copaiba, frankincense, helichrysum, juniper berry, lavender, marjoram, myrtle, pine, ravensara leaf, rosemary, sandalwood, sweet orange, yuzu

PRECAUTIONS
Avoid topical use during pregnancy owing to increased risk of skin sensitization. Cypress essential oil gets stronger with age, so the older the oil, the less you'll need.

DAVANA
Artemisia pallens

GREEN, HERBAL SCENT
COST: $$$

While davana is expensive, it makes a fascinating addition to bath and body blends, as its aroma smells different on every wearer. If you are interested in making your own perfumes, then davana should be on your list of must-haves. Beyond its usefulness in perfumery, davana essential oil is a strong antidepressant, and its antiviral and antiseptic properties make it useful in treating a variety of illnesses.

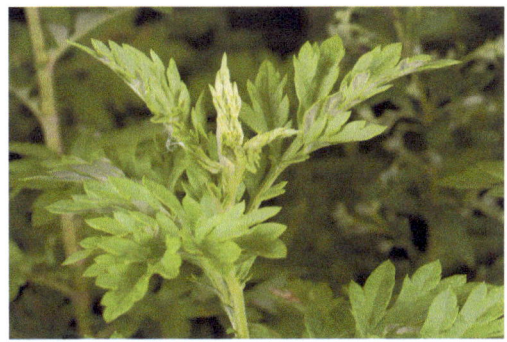

MEDICINAL PROPERTIES
Antiviral, disinfectant, emmenagogue, expectorant, relaxant, vulnerary

USES
Effective in treating minor wounds, muscle cramps, and headaches; ideal for making delightful personalized perfumes

BLENDS WELL WITH
Allspice, Atlas cedarwood, bergamot, cedarwood, cypress, geranium, grapefruit, mandarin, neroli, palo santo, rose, rose geranium, rosewood, sweet orange, tangerine, ylang-ylang, yuzu

PRECAUTIONS
Do not use during pregnancy. Davana can cause sensitive skin.

DILL SEED
Anethum graveolens

FRESH, HERBACEOUS SCENT
COST: $$

While dill seed is commonly put to culinary use, and its aroma might automatically remind you of homemade pickles, its usefulness extends far beyond the kitchen. It is an effective treatment for nausea and indigestion, and is gentle enough for use on young children.

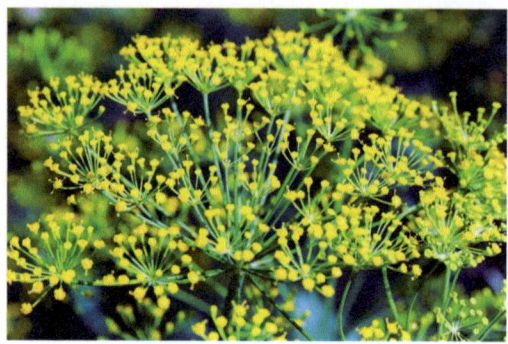

MEDICINAL PROPERTIES
Antibacterial, antioxidant, antiseptic, antispasmodic, aperitive, carminative, digestive, disinfectant, diuretic, emmenagogue, galactagogue, laxative, sedative, stomachic

USES
Effective in treating a wide range of digestive complaints

BLENDS WELL WITH
Bergamot, caraway, coriander, lemon, lime

PRECAUTIONS
Do not use during pregnancy. Dill seed can be very relaxing and may slow your reflexes; be mindful of how it affects you before driving or operating machinery.

ELEMI
Canarium luzonicum

FRESH, CITRUS-LIKE SCENT
COST: $

The elemi tree is in the same family as frankincense and myrrh. Not only did ancient Egyptians use it in embalming, but they also valued it for its usefulness in skin care, medicinal salves, incense, and more. In the Middle East, elemi was used as an antiseptic and healing agent. Today, it remains an excellent choice for skin care, and it makes a valuable addition to your cold and flu arsenal.

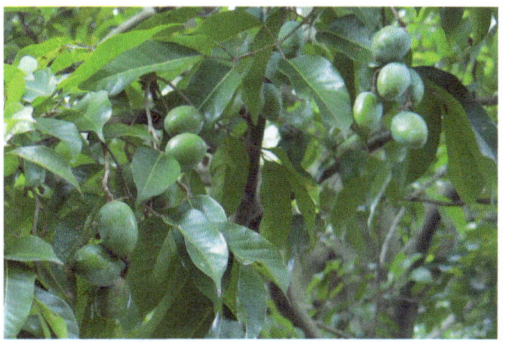

MEDICINAL PROPERTIES
Analgesic, antiseptic, expectorant, stimulant

USES
Effective in treating respiratory ailments, excess mucus, and minor wounds; ideal for making rejuvenating bath and body products

BLENDS WELL WITH
Cardamom, carrot seed, cinnamon leaf, clary sage, clove bud, cucumber seed, frankincense, geranium, helichrysum, lavender, myrrh, rose, rose geranium, rosemary, Spanish sage

PRECAUTIONS
Elemi can cause sensitive skin.

EUCALYPTUS GLOBULUS
Eucalyptus globulus

CRISP, CAMPHOROUS SCENT
COST: $

Of the many types of eucalyptus essential oil commonly offered for sale, *Eucalyptus globulus* is among the most popular. It offers a variety of medicinal actions, and its ability to reduce swelling of the mucous membranes makes it a valuable ally during cold and flu season. Topically, it eases inflammation and muscle soreness.

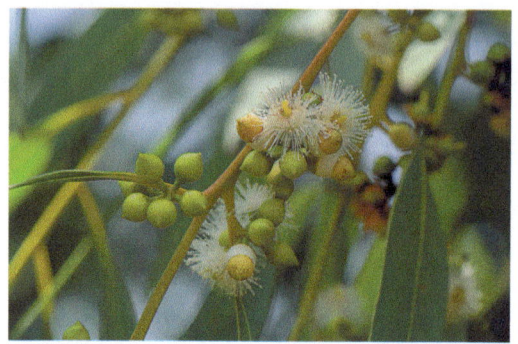

MEDICINAL PROPERTIES
Analgesic, antibacterial, anti-inflammatory, antiseptic, antispasmodic, antiviral, astringent, cicatrizant, decongestant, deodorant, depurative, diuretic, expectorant, febrifuge, rubefacient, stimulant, vermifuge, vulnerary

USES
Effective in treating headaches, asthma, sinusitis, and congestion; ideal for making healing salves for burns, blisters, insect bites, and minor wounds

BLENDS WELL WITH
Benzoin, cajuput, lavender, lemongrass, lemon, pine, rosemary, tea tree, thyme

PRECAUTIONS
Do not use on children under six years old. Avoid if diagnosed with epilepsy or high blood pressure. Excessive use of eucalyptus can cause headaches.

EUCALYPTUS RADIATA
Eucalyptus radiata

SOFT, CAMPHOROUS SCENT
COST: $

Offering a softer fragrance than its close cousin, *Eucalyptus globulus, E. radiata* is a milder choice for treating upper respiratory issues, particularly in children and the elderly. Diffuse or vaporize it to clear a stuffy nose or blend it into a soothing massage oil to ease the pain of arthritis or rheumatism.

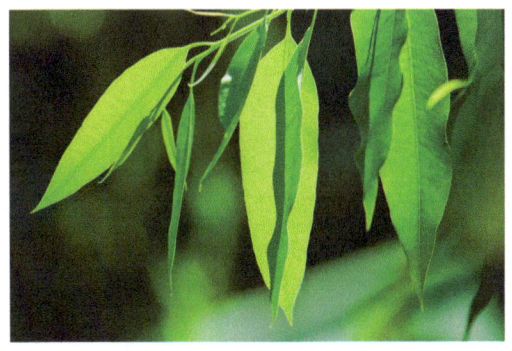

MEDICINAL PROPERTIES
Antibacterial, antifungal, anti-inflammatory, antiviral, insect repellent, stimulant

USES
Effective in treating minor cuts and scrapes; ideal for diffusing during cold and flu season

BLENDS WELL WITH
Bergamot, black pepper, cajuput, German chamomile, ginger, marjoram, peppermint, pine, Roman chamomile, spearmint, spruce

PRECAUTIONS
Do not use on children less than three years old. Avoid if diagnosed with diabetes, as it can raise blood sugar in diabetics. Asthmatics sometimes react to *Eucalyptus radiata*; proceed with caution if you have asthma.

FENNEL SEED
Foeniculum vulgare

SWEET, PEPPERY SCENT
COST: $

Also known as sweet fennel, this intriguing essential oil is excellent for addressing digestive issues. Besides helping with nausea, vomiting, flatulence, and hiccups, fennel seed can help with appetite control. Roman soldiers ate the seeds to keep hunger pangs at bay while on long marches, and early Christians chewed fennel seed to stave off hunger during periods of fasting.

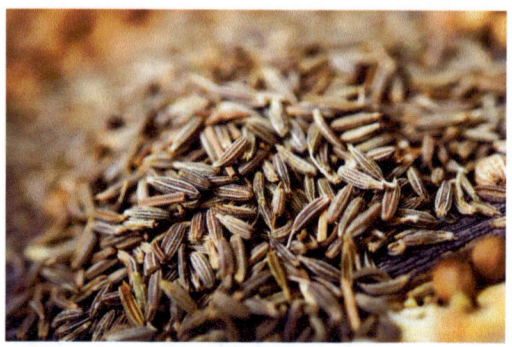

MEDICINAL PROPERTIES
Antiseptic, antispasmodic, carminative, depurative, diuretic, emmenagogue, expectorant, galactagogue, laxative, stimulant, stomachic, vermifuge

USES
Effective in treating bloating, constipation, and indigestion; ideal for making skin-care products to sort out oily skin, fight wrinkles, and smooth cellulite

BLENDS WELL WITH
Bergamot, black pepper, cardamom, cypress, dill seed, fir needle, geranium, ginger, grapefruit, hops flower, juniper berry, lavender, lemon, mandarin, marjoram, niaouli, orange, pine, ravensara leaf, rose, rose geranium, rosemary, tangerine, ylang-ylang

PRECAUTIONS
Do not use during pregnancy. Avoid if diagnosed with epilepsy or an estrogen-dependent form of cancer.

FIR NEEDLE
Abies balsamea

FRESH CONIFER SCENT
COST: $

Also known as European silver fir, white spruce, or white fir, the tree that produces this fragrant essential oil was historically used for a variety of health purposes. Its buds and bark were used in antiseptics, and its resin, bark, and needles were used for conditions ranging from muscle pain to fever. Like the tree, fir needle essential oil offers a variety of aromatherapy benefits, and its beautiful, green, forest fragrance makes it a pleasure to use.

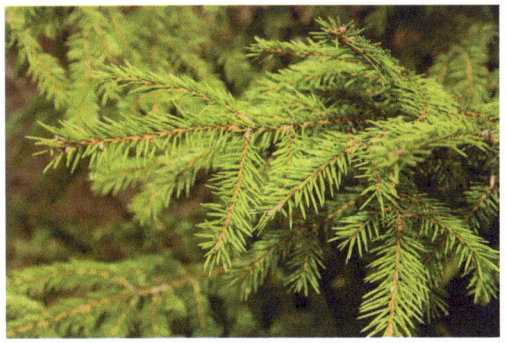

MEDICINAL PROPERTIES
Analgesic, antiseptic, astringent, decongestant, deodorant, diuretic, expectorant, rubefacient, stimulant, vasoconstrictor, vulnerary

USES
Effective in treating upper respiratory illnesses; ideal for making balms, salves, and compresses for pain relief

BLENDS WELL WITH
Atlas cedarwood, benzoin, cedarwood, copaiba, cypress, davana, juniper berry, lavender, lemon, marjoram, oregano, peppermint, pine, rosemary, spearmint, spruce, sweet orange

PRECAUTIONS
Fir needle can cause sensitive skin.

FRANKINCENSE
Boswellia carterii

SPICY, WOODY SCENT
COST: $$

Frankincense has been used in incense for thousands of years, and it is also used to treat a variety of skin ailments. Its ability to calm the mind and create inner peace makes it a valuable oil to diffuse during meditation, and its mild sedative property encourages deep, slow breathing. Combined with its expectorant and antiseptic properties, this makes it ideal for treating respiratory illnesses.

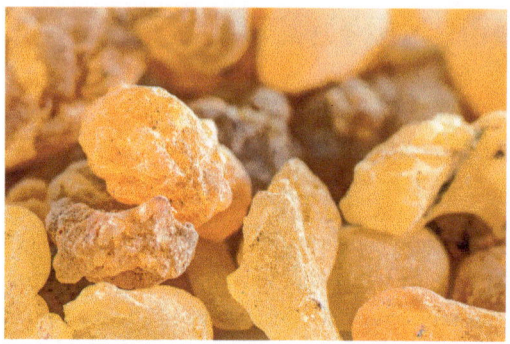

MEDICINAL PROPERTIES
Antiseptic, astringent, carminative, cicatrizant, cytophylactic, digestive, diuretic, emmenagogue, expectorant, sedative, vulnerary

USES
Effective in treating asthma, bronchitis, cough, colds, and laryngitis; ideal for making healing balms and salves for wounds, scars, aging skin, and inflammation

BLENDS WELL WITH
Bergamot, black pepper, cinnamon leaf, cypress, geranium, grapefruit, helichrysum, lavender, lemon, mandarin, neroli, orange, palmarosa, patchouli, pine, rose, rose geranium, sandalwood, vetiver, ylang-ylang

PRECAUTIONS
Do not use during pregnancy.

GALBANUM
Ferula galbaniflua

GREEN, WOODY SCENT
COST: $$

Ancient Romans and Greeks burned galbanum resin as incense or mixed the fragrant oil into their baths and used it to formulate healing balms and decadent perfumes. Galbanum essential oil is a wonderful tonic for weary minds as it stimulates circulation, eases inflammation, and helps wounds heal faster while diminishing the appearance of scars.

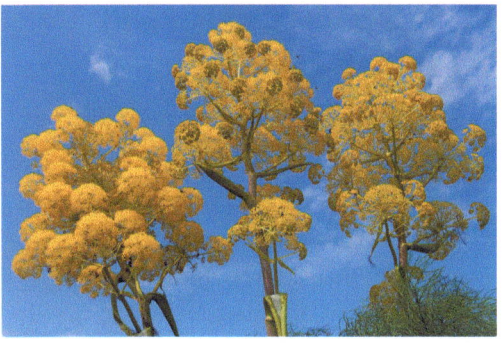

MEDICINAL PROPERTIES
Antispasmodic, cicatrizant, decongestant, detoxifier, emollient, insect repellent, insecticide, vermifuge, vulnerary

USES
Effective in treating arthritis, rheumatism, and gout; ideal for diffusion and vapor treatments for treating upper respiratory issues

BLENDS WELL WITH
Allspice, benzoin, cardamom, elemi, fir needle, frankincense, geranium, ginger, lavender, palmarosa, palo santo, pine, rose geranium, sweet orange

PRECAUTIONS
Generally regarded as safe.

GERANIUM
Pelargonium odoratissimum

FRESH, FAINTLY FLORAL SCENT
COST: $

Offering an irresistible, intriguing fragrance, geranium is a versatile essential oil useful for making insect repellent, creating comforting skin-care products to deal with dry or aging skin, and distilling for clean, fresh-smelling indoor air. This beautiful oil also offers relief from physical discomfort; its hormone-balancing qualities make it a good choice for treating PMS, painful periods, breast engorgement, and menopause symptoms.

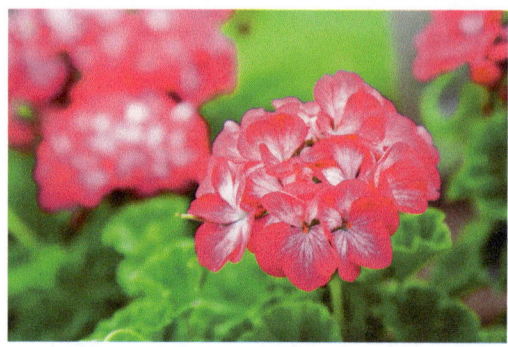

MEDICINAL PROPERTIES
Antiseptic, astringent, cicatrizant, cytophylactic, deodorant, diuretic, hemostatic, styptic, tonic, vermifuge, vulnerary

USES
Effective in treating sunburn and eczema; ideal for easing stress, anxiety, and tension

BLENDS WELL WITH
Atlas cedarwood, bergamot, carrot seed, cedarwood, clary sage, cucumber seed, grapefruit, helichrysum, jasmine, juniper berry, lavender, lime, melissa, neroli, petitgrain, ravensara leaf, rose, rosemary, sandalwood, sweet orange

PRECAUTIONS
Not recommended for use during pregnancy owing to geranium's hormone-balancing effect. Not recommended if diagnosed with diabetes, as geranium can reduce blood sugar.

GERMAN CHAMOMILE
Matricaria recutita

**STRONG, SWEET, HERBACEOUS SCENT
COST: $$$**

If you have ever spent time relaxing with a cup of hot chamomile tea, you have probably felt the wonderfully relaxing quality of German chamomile at work. Besides offering gentle sedation, particularly at bedtime or when suffering from a nasty cold, German chamomile contains levomenol, which helps heal compromised skin. Also known as blue chamomile, German chamomile essential oil gets its vivid color from azulene, which imparts a potent anti-inflammatory effect.

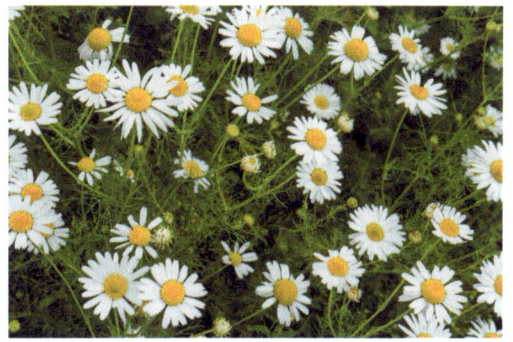

MEDICINAL PROPERTIES

Analgesic, anti-allergenic, antibiotic, anti-inflammatory, antispasmodic, bactericidal, carminative, cholagogue, cicatrizant, digestive, emmenagogue, sedative, stomachic, vasoconstrictor, vermifuge, vulnerary

USES

Effective in treating inflamed skin, psoriasis, and eczema

BLENDS WELL WITH

Benzoin, bergamot, clary sage, frankincense, geranium, grapefruit, helichrysum, jasmine, lavender, lemon, lime, mandarin, marjoram, neroli, patchouli, ravensara, rose, rosemary, sweet orange, tea tree, ylang-ylang

PRECAUTIONS

Do not use during pregnancy.

GINGER
Zingiber officinale

WARM, SPICY SCENT
COST: $

Ginger is a tropical perennial herb that bears fragrant flowers and a crown of narrow, spear-shaped leaves. While it is prized for its aboveground beauty and aroma, the spice and essential oil come from its swollen roots, which are thick, spreading rhizomes. Ginger has been used medicinally for millennia, with mentions in Chinese and Sanskrit texts as well as in ancient Roman, Greek, and Arabian literature. The plant's name is derived from India's Gingee district, where ginger tea is used to comfort upset stomachs.

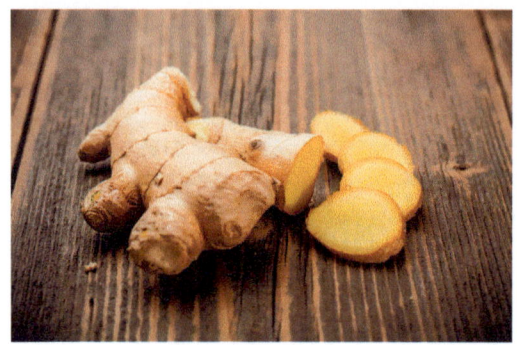

MEDICINAL PROPERTIES
Analgesic, anti-emetic, antiseptic, antispasmodic, bactericidal, carminative, expectorant, febrifuge, laxative, rubefacient, stimulant, stomachic, sudorific

USES
Effective in treating nausea, vomiting, hangovers, and travel sickness; ideal for making pain-relieving salves for sore joints and muscles

BLENDS WELL WITH
Allspice, anise, Atlas cedarwood, bergamot, cedarwood, clove bud, coriander, eucalyptus (all species), frankincense, galbanum, geranium, grapefruit, jasmine, juniper berry, lemon, lime, mandarin, neroli, palmarosa, patchouli, rose, sweet orange, vetiver, ylang-ylang, yuzu

PRECAUTIONS
Not recommended for use during pregnancy owing to increased risk of skin sensitization. Ginger can cause skin irritation and can be phototoxic; do not apply to skin that will be exposed to direct sunlight.

GRAPEFRUIT
Citrus paradisi, C. racemosa, C. maxima var. *racemosa*

SWEET, CITRUS SCENT
COST: $

Offering a sweet, tangy, refreshing smell, grapefruit essential oil comes from fresh grapefruit peels. High in vitamin C and valuable to the body's immune system, it offers some protection during cold and flu season. Its diuretic properties make it a valuable ally in the battle against cellulite, and its uplifting scent provides relief from mental fatigue, depression, and headache.

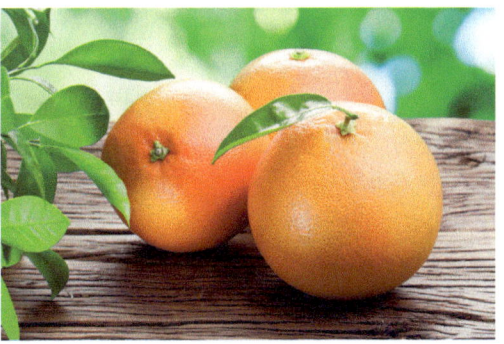

MEDICINAL PROPERTIES
Antibacterial, antidepressant, antiseptic, aperitive, astringent, digestive, disinfectant, diuretic, lymphatic stimulant, tonic

USES
Effective in treating water retention

BLENDS WELL WITH
Bergamot, cardamom, cedarwood, cinnamon leaf, coriander, cypress, davana, ginger, juniper berry, lemon, neroli, palmarosa, peppermint, ravensara leaf, Roman chamomile, rose, sweet orange

PRECAUTIONS
Phototoxic; do not apply to skin that will be exposed to direct sunlight. Grapefruit can cause sensitive skin. Do not use if taking medications that interact with grapefruit.

HELICHRYSUM
Helichrysum italicum

STRONG, HERBAL SCENT
COST: $$$

Helichrysum essential oil isn't cheap, but it is a powerful addition to your aromatherapy arsenal. Sourced from an aromatic evergreen, it is also known as *immortelle*, or everlasting. Traditional uses for this Mediterranean plant include treatments for allergies, colds and coughs, wound healing, indigestion, and much more.

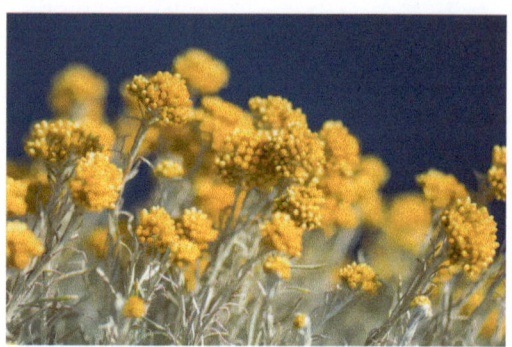

MEDICINAL PROPERTIES
Analgesic, anti-allergenic, antibacterial, antidepressant, antifungal, anti-inflammatory, antiseptic, antispasmodic, antitussive, antiviral, astringent, cholagogue, cytophylactic, diuretic, emollient, expectorant, nervine, sedative, skin regenerator

USES
Effective in treating chronic skin conditions, bruises, acne, and arthritis; ideal for making first-aid salves and stretch mark balms

BLENDS WELL WITH
Bergamot, black pepper, clary sage, clove bud, cypress, frankincense, galbanum, geranium, German chamomile, lavender, mandarin, oregano, Roman chamomile, rosewood, sweet orange, tea tree, vetiver, yuzu

PRECAUTIONS
Generally regarded as safe.

HOPS FLOWER
Humulus lupulus

SPICY, FLORAL SCENT
COST: $$$

Hops flowers impart flavor to beers and ales, and are a staple in herbal medicine, where they are revered for their sedative action. Besides helping with insomnia, hops flower essential oil is valuable for easing asthma symptoms and soothing coughs. Applied externally, it is useful for eczema, dandruff, and dry skin.

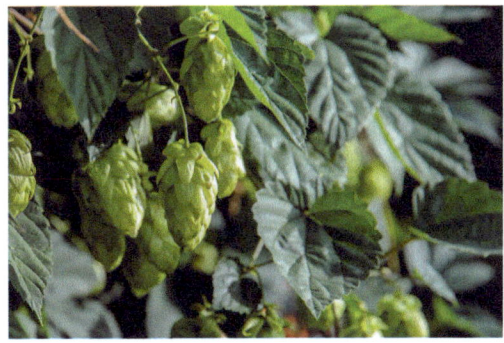

MEDICINAL PROPERTIES
Analgesic, anti-inflammatory, antispasmodic, antiviral, aphrodisiac, decongestant, relaxant, sedative

USES
Effective in treating stress, tension, and headaches; ideal for making relaxing bath and body products that nourish skin and hair

BLENDS WELL WITH
Anise, bergamot, bay laurel, caraway seed, cardamom, cinnamon leaf, clove bud, copaiba, fennel seed, fir needle, ginger, grapefruit, juniper berry, lemon, lime, mandarin, pine, sweet orange, tangerine, yuzu

PRECAUTIONS
Do not use if clinically depressed. Hops flower can irritate skin.

HYSSOP
Hyssopus officinalis

SWEET, MINTY, HERBAL SCENT
COST: $$

Hyssop was once nicknamed the "herb of protection" and was used to defend individuals and their homes from malicious influences. In England, it was added to remedies for easing sore muscles and joints. In gardens, its beautiful spikes of violet-blue flowers attract honeybees and other pollinators.

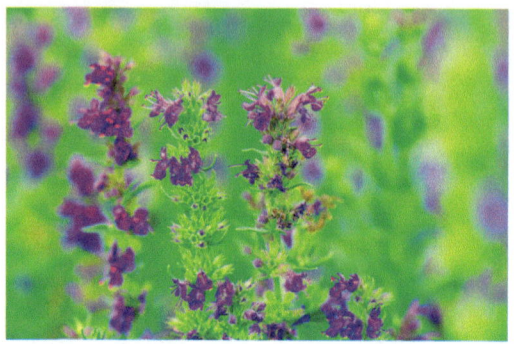

MEDICINAL PROPERTIES
Antibacterial, antiseptic, antispasmodic, astringent, carminative, cicatrizant, digestive, diuretic, emmenagogue, expectorant, febrifuge, hypertensive, nervine, tonic, vermifuge, vulnerary

USES
Effective in treating flu and cold symptoms; ideal for making pain-relieving salves for bruises, arthritis, rheumatism, and muscle aches

BLENDS WELL WITH
Bay laurel, clary sage, geranium, grapefruit, hops flower, lemon, lime, mandarin, melissa, myrtle, rosemary, spearmint, Spanish sage, sweet orange

PRECAUTIONS
Do not use during pregnancy. Do not use on children less than three years old. Do not use if diagnosed with asthma or epilepsy. Hyssop can cause sensitive skin.

JASMINE
Jasminum officinale, J. grandiflorum

RICH, FLORAL SCENT
COST: $$$$

Jasmine absolute is among the most expensive of oils, but a tiny drop goes an incredibly long way. Sourced from the star-shaped flowers of a climbing evergreen shrub of two varieties, jasmine oil begins its journey as a concrete that contains the power of about one thousand blossoms per pound. From there, absolute is solvent-extracted, and essential oil is steam-distilled from the absolute. You can experience the exquisite beauty of jasmine for less by purchasing a blend; many top companies carry prediluted jasmine, often with sweet almond oil.

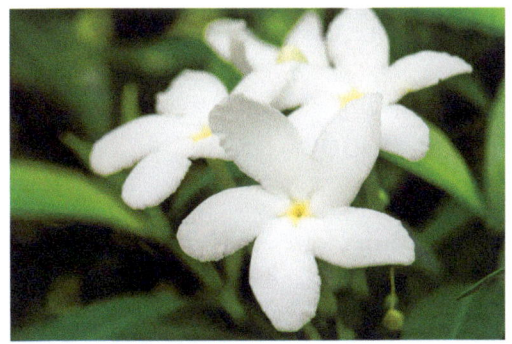

MEDICINAL PROPERTIES
Analgesic, antidepressant, anti-inflammatory, antiseptic, antispasmodic, aphrodisiac, calmative, carminative, cicatrizant, decongestant, expectorant, galactagogue, parturient, sedative

USES
Effective in treating impotence, anxiety, depression, and exhaustion; ideal for making personal fragrances and beautifully scented bath and body products

BLENDS WELL WITH
Clary sage, cypress, frankincense, geranium, lemon, lime, mandarin, rose, rose geranium, rosewood, sandalwood, sweet orange, tangerine, yuzu

PRECAUTIONS
Do not use during pregnancy. Overuse can cause a headache.

JUNIPER BERRY
Juniperus communis

FRESH, WOODY SCENT
COST: $

Juniper berries, leaves, and branches have been used for purifying and cleansing the mind, body, and spirit since ancient times, when the trees were believed to ward off illness and negativity while thwarting evil spirits. Native Americans put juniper to good use by making tonics to treat cold, flu, muscle aches, and other ailments, including UTIs.

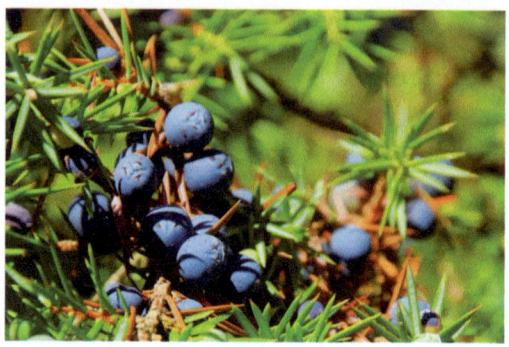

MEDICINAL PROPERTIES
Antiseptic, antispasmodic, astringent, carminative, depurative, diuretic, rubefacient, stomachic, sudorific, tonic, vulnerary

USES
Effective in treating enlarged prostate, painful periods, gout, arthritis, and rheumatism; ideal for making salves and lotions for treating acne, eczema, psoriasis, oily skin, and dandruff

BLENDS WELL WITH
Atlas cedarwood, bergamot, cedarwood, clary sage, cypress, geranium, grapefruit, lavandin, lavender, lemon, lemongrass, lime, vetiver

PRECAUTIONS
Generally regarded as safe.

LAVANDIN
Lavandula Hybrida

CLEAN, FLORAL SCENT
COST: $

Lavandin is an interesting hybrid plant that was developed in 1900 for use in the perfume and soapmaking industries. A cross between true lavender and spike lavender, lavandin is a larger, more productive plant that tolerates colder temperatures than its popular cousin. It is good for easing joint and muscle pain, and it clears lungs and sinuses; like lavender, lavandin is suitable for treating wounds and dermatitis.

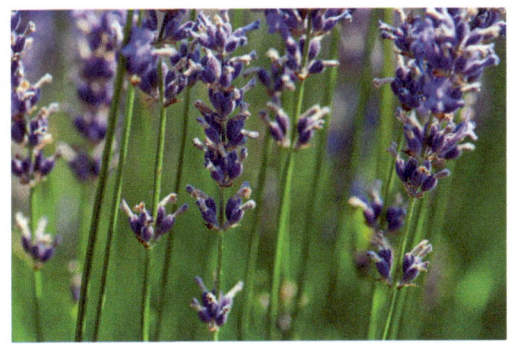

MEDICINAL PROPERTIES
Analgesic, antidepressant, antiseptic, antispasmodic, cicatrizant, deodorant, diuretic, emmenagogue, expectorant, nervine, sedative, vulnerary

USES
Effective in treating cold symptoms and muscle aches; ideal for making fragrant bath and body products

BLENDS WELL WITH
Bay laurel, bergamot, cinnamon leaf, clary sage, clove bud, lemongrass, lime, patchouli, pine, rosemary, tangerine, thyme

PRECAUTIONS
Do not use during pregnancy.

LAVENDER
Lavandula angustifolia

HERBACEOUS, FLORAL SCENT
COST: $

Lavender is among the most versatile of all essential oils, thanks to its ability to soothe pain, help wounds heal faster, and ease you into deep, relaxing sleep. Lavender gets its name from the Latin word *lavare*, meaning "to wash," and Romans used it extensively in bathing. It was the Romans who introduced lavender to England, where it remains a favorite today.

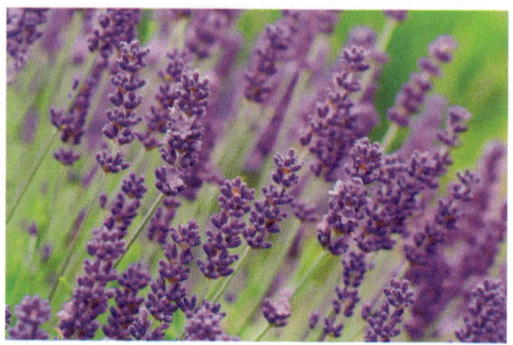

MEDICINAL PROPERTIES
Analgesic, antidepressant, anti-inflammatory, antiseptic, antispasmodic, antiviral, bactericide, carminative, cholagogue, cicatrizant, cordial, cytophylactic, decongestant, deodorant, diuretic, hypotensive, nervine, rubefacient, sedative, sudorific, vulnerary

USES
Effective in treating minor burns, cuts, and bruises; ideal for making soothing bedtime bath salts, lotions, and linen sprays

BLENDS WELL WITH
Atlas cedarwood, cedarwood, clary sage, cypress, galbanum, geranium, juniper berry, lemongrass, melissa, peppermint, pine, rosemary, spearmint, tagetes

PRECAUTIONS
Generally regarded as safe. Allergic reactions can develop with overuse; discontinue if irritation occurs.

LEMON
Citrus limonum

SHARP, CITRUS SCENT
COST: $

In Japan, lemon essential oil is often diffused in banks and other businesses where sharp attention to detail is required, because its crisp aroma helps promote alertness. Sourced from the same tree that provides the tangy, vitamin-rich citrus fruit that goes into popular beverages, candies, and culinary treats, lemon essential oil is a pleasant and useful addition to your aromatherapy kit.

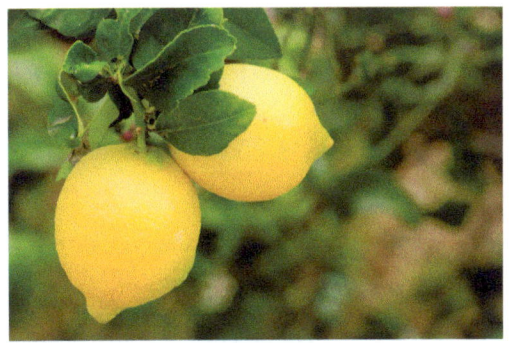

MEDICINAL PROPERTIES
Antiseptic, bactericidal, carminative, cicatrizant, depurative, diaphoretic, diuretic, febrifuge, hemostatic, hypotensive, insecticidal, rubefacient, tonic, vermifuge

USES
Effective in treating bronchitis, asthma, and respiratory infections; ideal for making bath and body products, as well as cleaning products

BLENDS WELL WITH
Allspice, benzoin, caraway seed, cardamom, eucalyptus (all types), fennel seed, geranium, juniper berry, neroli, ravensara leaf, ravintsara, rose, rose geranium, rosewood, tagetes

PRECAUTIONS
Phototoxic; do not apply to skin that will be exposed to direct sunlight. Lemon can cause sensitive skin.

LEMON EUCALYPTUS
Eucalyptus citriodora

CLEAN, CITRUS SCENT
COST: $

While it offers many of the same properties as other eucalyptus varieties, *Eucalyptus citriodora* has a crisp, lemon scent that some people prefer. Although less potent than *E. globulus* and *E. radiata*, it is an excellent choice for antiseptic and antifungal use, and its disinfectant qualities make it ideal for use in household cleaners.

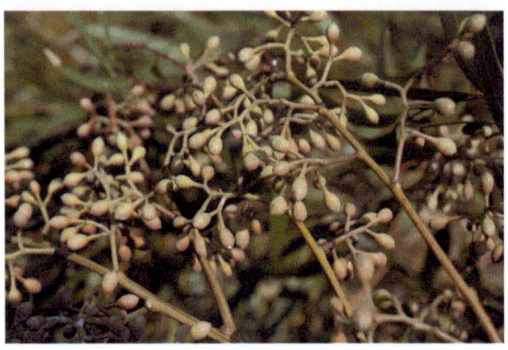

MEDICINAL PROPERTIES
Antibacterial, antidepressant, antifungal, anti-inflammatory, antiseptic, antiviral, expectorant, febrifuge, insect repellent

USES
Effective in treating congestion, insect bites, and dandruff; ideal for making insect repellent and household cleaners

BLENDS WELL WITH
Atlas cedarwood, bergamot, cedarwood, cucumber seed, ginger, lavandin, lavender, lemon, lime, marjoram, peppermint, pine, ravensara leaf, rosemary, tea tree

PRECAUTIONS
Lemon eucalyptus can cause skin irritation.

LEMON VERBENA
Lippia citriodora

WOODY, CITRUS SCENT
COST: $$

Offering a gorgeous aroma filled with bright lemon, sensual wood, and fruity, floral undertones, lemon verbena essential oil creates a cheerful atmosphere when diffused in your home or office. It calms tension while boosting your spirits, and it offers comfort during periods of digestive distress. Lemon verbena is a potent liver detoxifier, and is useful for dealing with hangovers and overindulgence in rich, fatty foods.

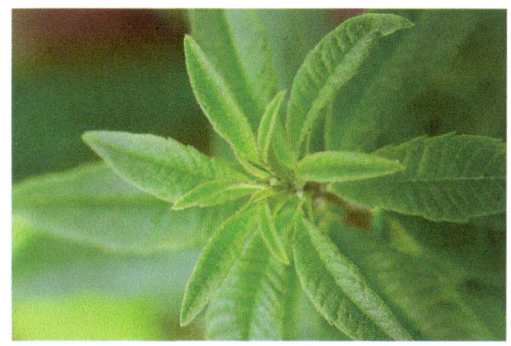

MEDICINAL PROPERTIES
Antiseptic, antispasmodic, aphrodisiac, digestive, emollient, febrifuge, insecticide, sedative, stomachic

USES
Effective in treating acne, bronchitis, and sinusitis; ideal for making compresses to deal with puffy eyes

BLENDS WELL WITH
Allspice, davana, elemi, lemon, lime, ginger, mandarin, melissa, palmarosa, yuzu

PRECAUTIONS
Phototoxic; do not apply to skin that will be exposed to direct sunlight. Lemon verbena can cause sensitive skin.

LEMONGRASS
Cymbopogon citratus, C. flexuosus

GREEN, CITRUS SCENT
COST: $

Lemongrass is a popular ingredient in Asian cuisine, and the essential oil often makes its way into natural insect repellents. This aromatic grass is a native of India, where it grows wild and reaches a height of about three feet. There, it is used in Ayurvedic medicine, where it is prized for its ability to treat infections and reduce fevers.

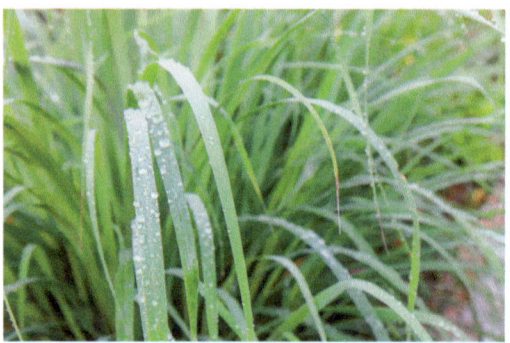

MEDICINAL PROPERTIES
Analgesic, antidepressant, antimicrobial, antiseptic, astringent, bactericidal, carminative, deodorant, diuretic, febrifuge, fungicidal, galactagogue, insect repellent, insecticidal, nervine

USES
Effective in treating jet lag, headaches, and stress; ideal for making insect repellent and antifungal bath and body products

BLENDS WELL WITH
Basil, cajuput, coriander, geranium, jasmine, lavandin, lavender, palmarosa, patchouli, tea tree, vetiver

PRECAUTIONS
Do not use on children less than two years old. Lemongrass can irritate diseased, damaged, or hypersensitive skin.

LIME
Citrus aurantifolia

CRISP, CITRUS SCENT
COST: $

Originally cultivated in Asia, lime is a delicious citrus fruit that makes its way into beverages, desserts, and more. In the days when sailing ships took months to transport goods from one continent to another, British sailors ate limes to prevent scurvy (a condition caused by a severe lack of vitamin C), thus earning the nickname "limeys." Lime essential oil offers a delightful fragrance that adds interest to a variety of aromatherapy blends.

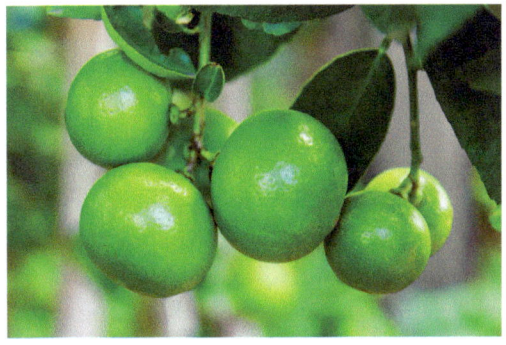

MEDICINAL PROPERTIES
Antiseptic, antiviral, aperitive, astringent, bactericidal, disinfectant, febrifuge, hemostatic

USES
Effective in treating painful joints and muscles, respiratory ailments, and acne; ideal for making bath and body products to combat cellulite

BLENDS WELL WITH
Bergamot, clary sage, juniper berry, lavandin, lavender, lemon, lemon eucalyptus, lemon verbena, lemongrass, neroli, tagetes, ylang-ylang

PRECAUTIONS
Phototoxic; do not apply to skin that will be exposed to direct sunlight. Lime can cause sensitive skin.

MANDARIN
Citrus reticulata

SWEET, CITRUS SCENT
COST: $

If you are a parent, mandarin is one of the best essential oils to add to your collection. Safe for children and ideal for soothing temper tantrums, it is beautifully uplifting and makes your home smell fantastic. Sometimes *Citrus reticulata* essential oil is labeled "tangerine." Although the two trees are very closely related, these are two different essential oils. They're quite alike though, so feel free to use them interchangeably.

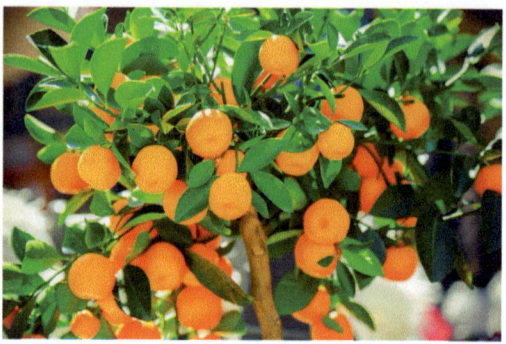

MEDICINAL PROPERTIES
Antiseptic, antispasmodic, cytophylactic, depurative, sedative, stomachic, tonic

USES
Effective in treating upset stomachs, temper tantrums, and hyperactivity; ideal for making delightfully uplifting bath and body products

BLENDS WELL WITH
Allspice, bergamot, clary sage, clove bud, elemi, frankincense, neroli, palo santo, ravensara leaf, tagetes, ylang-ylang

PRECAUTIONS
Generally regarded as safe.

MARJORAM
Origanum majorana

SWEET, SPICY SCENT
COST: $

Also known as sweet marjoram or knotted marjoram, *Origanum majorana* originated in North Africa and the Mediterranean and reached Egypt sometime around 2000 BCE. The herb was dedicated to Osiris, the Egyptian god of the underworld, and it was used in funerary preparations, as well as in love potions and medicines. Marjoram is a very relaxing essential oil, and it's a good choice for colds, flu, and digestive ailments.

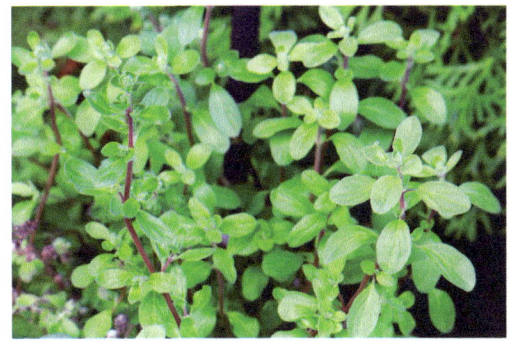

MEDICINAL PROPERTIES
Analgesic, antiseptic, antispasmodic, antiviral, bactericidal, carminative, cordial, diaphoretic, digestive, diuretic, emmenagogue, expectorant, fungicidal, hypotensive, laxative, nervine, sedative, stomachic, vasodilator, vulnerary

USES
Effective in treating congestion and sinusitis; ideal for use in warming blends to ease muscle pain

BLENDS WELL WITH
Atlas cedarwood, bergamot, black pepper, cedarwood, clary sage, cypress, German chamomile, lavender, lemon, lime, myrtle, ravensara leaf, Roman chamomile, rosemary, sweet orange

PRECAUTIONS
Do not use during pregnancy.

MAY CHANG
Litsea cubeba

TROPICAL, FRUITY SCENT
COST: $

Also sold under its botanical name or abbreviated as litsea, may chang essential oil offers a delightfully intriguing scent that might make it one of your favorites. This wonderful fragrance comes from a small tree native to China. It has a long history of use in treating ailments ranging from asthma to back pain. Its uplifting fragrance makes it an excellent choice for treating anxiety, fatigue, and depression.

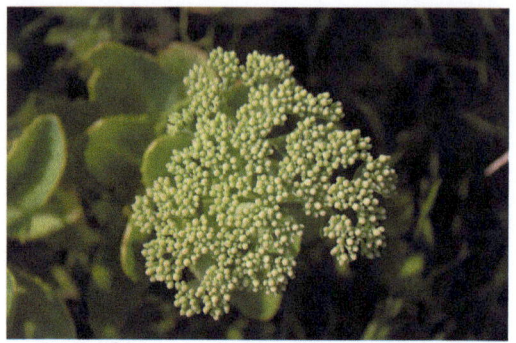

MEDICINAL PROPERTIES
Antibacterial, antidepressant, anti-inflammatory, antifungal, antiseptic, astringent, deodorant, disinfectant, diuretic, expectorant, insecticide, stimulant, tonic

USES
Effective in treating chest congestion and indigestion; ideal for making air fresheners, bath and body products, and cleaning products

BLENDS WELL WITH
Basil, bay laurel, black pepper, cardamom, cedarwood, clary sage, coriander, cypress, davana, eucalyptus (any species), frankincense, geranium, ginger, grapefruit, juniper berry, marjoram, neroli, palmarosa, patchouli, petitgrain, rose, rosemary, rosewood, sandalwood, sweet orange, tea tree, thyme, vetiver, ylang-ylang

PRECAUTIONS
Not recommended for use during pregnancy due to its ability to increase lactation. May chang can cause skin irritation.

MELISSA
Melissa officinalis

SWEET, HERBAL SCENT
COST: $$$

Melissa essential oil comes from a medicinal herb often referred to as lemon balm and nicknamed "the elixir of life." A marvelous choice for dealing with stress and tension, melissa reduces blood pressure and settles your nerves. It works wonders for headaches and can help regulate menstruation while easing associated discomfort.

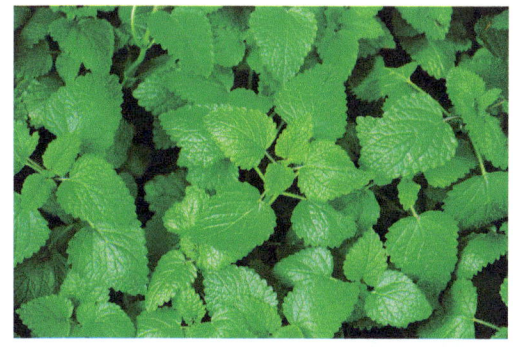

MEDICINAL PROPERTIES
Antidepressant, antifungal, antihistaminic, antispasmodic, antiviral, bactericidal, diaphoretic, febrifuge, hypertensive, insect repellent, nervine, sedative, stomachic, sudorific, vermifuge

USES
Effective in treating cold sores, cramping, and allergies; ideal for diffusing during times of stress and emotional upset

BLENDS WELL WITH
Basil, frankincense, galbanum, geranium, lavender, myrrh, myrtle, peppermint, Roman chamomile, rose, rose geranium, spearmint, ylang-ylang

PRECAUTIONS
Melissa can cause skin irritation.

MYRRH
Commiphora myrrha

WARM, WOODY SCENT
COST: $$

Renowned as one of the precious gifts presented to the Christ child by the Magi, myrrh essential oil comes from a small tree native to the Middle East and Somalia. Egyptians not only used it as medicine but also employed it in mummification and worship. Myrrh is a wonderful essential oil for skin care, cold and flu season, and diffusing to increase spiritual awareness.

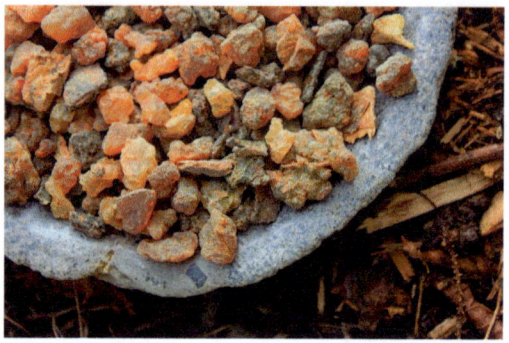

MEDICINAL PROPERTIES
Anti-inflammatory, antimicrobial, antiseptic, astringent, carminative, cicatrizant, digestive, emmenagogue, expectorant, fungicidal, sedative, stomachic, vulnerary

USES
Effective in treating sore throats, boils, and chapped skin; ideal for making soothing bath and body products

BLENDS WELL WITH
Benzoin, bergamot, clove bud, cypress, frankincense, geranium, German chamomile, grapefruit, jasmine, juniper berry, lavender, lemon, lemon eucalyptus, neroli, palmarosa, palo santo, patchouli, pine, Roman chamomile, rose, rosemary, rosewood, sandalwood, tea tree, vetiver, ylang-ylang

PRECAUTIONS
Do not use during pregnancy.

MYRTLE
Myrtus communis

LIGHT, FRESH SCENT
COST: $$

Myrtle has long been a representative of peace, love, and harmony; in Britain, it often finds its way into bridal bouquets. Ancient Romans and Greeks valued it for its ability to treat a litany of digestive complaints. Myrtle essential oil addresses a wide range of ailments, yet it is mild enough for young children and seniors.

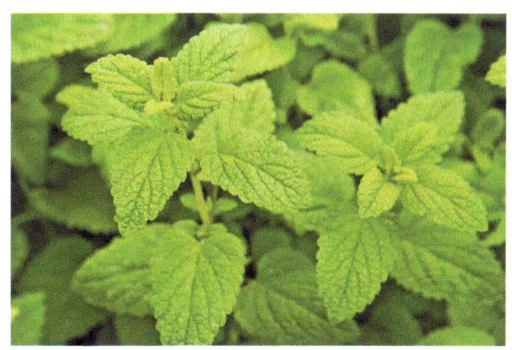

MEDICINAL PROPERTIES
Antibacterial, antifungal, anti-inflammatory, antimicrobial, antioxidant, antiseptic, antispasmodic, astringent, decongestant, deodorant, digestive, diuretic, emmenagogue, expectorant, laxative, nervine, sedative

USES
Effective in treating coughs, cold and flu symptoms, and abdominal issues; ideal for making skin-care products to sort out acne, psoriasis, and irritation

BLENDS WELL WITH
Allspice, bay laurel, bergamot, cinnamon leaf, clary sage, clove bud, cypress, ginger, hyssop, lime, melissa, neroli, rosemary

PRECAUTIONS
Do not use during pregnancy.

NEROLI
Citrus aurantium

SWEET, LINGERING FLORAL
COST: $$$$

Also known as orange blossom, neroli is extracted from the tiny, white flowers of the bitter orange tree. This extremely relaxing essential oil works well in bedtime blends, and it offers relief from depression, anxiety, and stress. Neroli is an excellent addition to skin-care products, as it regenerates skin cells and helps prevent scar tissue. If you find the cost prohibitive but want to enjoy neroli's fragrance, you'll find it is available in fairly inexpensive blends.

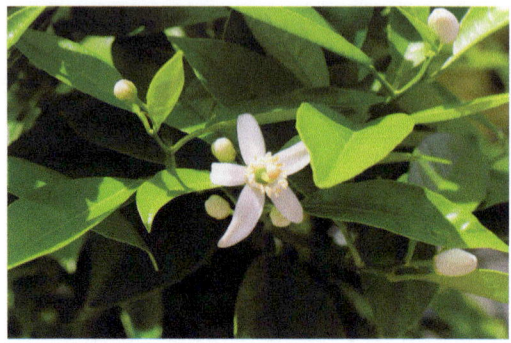

MEDICINAL PROPERTIES
Antidepressant, antiseptic, antispasmodic, aphrodisiac, bactericidal, carminative, cicatrizant, cordial, cytophylactic, deodorant, digestive, emollient, sedative

USES
Effective in treating insomnia, headaches, and depression; ideal for making lotions to combat stretch marks and scars

BLENDS WELL WITH
Benzoin, copaiba, cucumber seed, elemi, frankincense, geranium, grapefruit, lavender, lemon, lime, jasmine, mandarin, palo santo, petitgrain, rosemary, rosewood, sandalwood, spikenard, yuzu

PRECAUTIONS
Neroli can be very relaxing; be aware of how it affects you before driving or undertaking important tasks.

NIAOULI
Melaleuca quinquenervia, var. *cineole*

FRESH, SWEET SCENT
COST: $

Niaouli is closely related to tea tree, and although it is milder, it shares many of the same characteristics. A native of Australia, the niaouli tree's leaves were historically made into poultices for treating fevers, aching joints, and headaches. Niaouli essential oil has the ability to enhance the body's immune response, and is an excellent choice for respiratory illnesses.

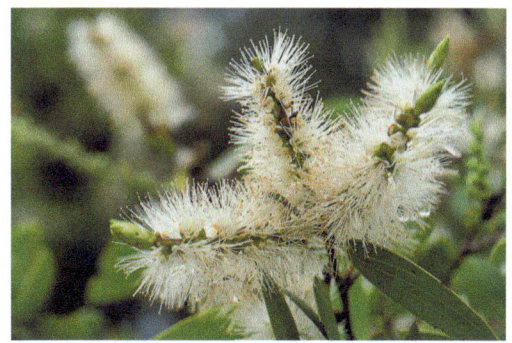

MEDICINAL PROPERTIES
Analgesic, antibacterial, antiseptic, antispasmodic, decongestant, expectorant, febrifuge, insecticide, vermifuge, vulnerary

USES
Effective in treating bronchitis, asthma, sinusitis, and laryngitis; ideal for making first-aid salves to treat minor cuts, burns, and insect bites

BLENDS WELL WITH
Clary sage, clove bud, coriander, eucalyptus (any species), fennel seed, juniper berry, lavender, lime, peppermint, pine, rosemary, spearmint

PRECAUTIONS
Generally regarded as safe.

ORANGE FAMILY:
Citrus aurantium (Neroli or Bitter orange) *C. sinesis* (Sweet orange) *C. reticulata* (Mandarin)

CITRUS SCENT
COST: $

With similar scents, the essential oils in the orange family also have similar properties and can typically be substituted for one another in both health and scent formulations. Orange is used as a flavoring and also as a solvent. It is used in Ayurvedic medicine to treat gout, digestive disorders, and anxiety. See also individual entries for Neroli, Sweet Orange, and Mandarin.

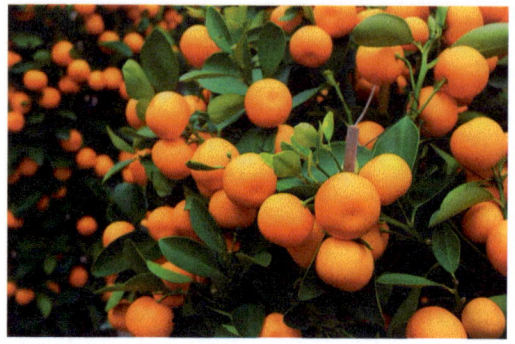

MEDICINAL PROPERTIES
Antidepressant, antifungal, digestive tonic, sedative, skin tonic, stimulant

USES
Effective in treating acne, anxiety, athlete's foot, colds and flu, depression, fungal infections, skin problems

BLENDS WELL WITH
Grapefruit, lemon, lime, bergamot, lavender, black pepper, ginger

PRECAUTIONS
Bitter orange (neroli) is phototoxic.

OREGANO
Origanum vulgare

SPICY, HERBACEOUS SCENT
COST: $$

While some sources decry oregano as too powerful an oil to use in aromatherapy, it offers a number of medicinal properties, and can be of great benefit when used with a careful hand. The herb itself is potent; ancient Greeks used oregano leaves on sore, aching muscles and wounds, and early European herbalists recommended it as a digestive aid.

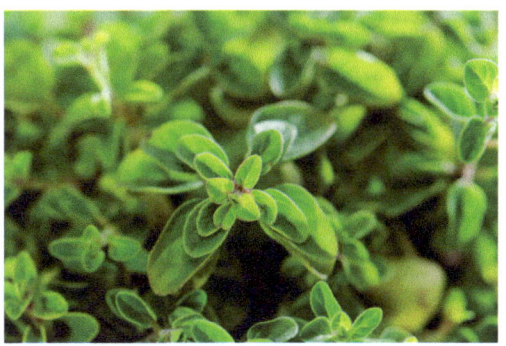

MEDICINAL PROPERTIES
Analgesic, anthelmintic, antibacterial, antifungal, anti-inflammatory, antiseptic, antispasmodic, anti-toxic, antiviral, carminative, disinfectant, diuretic, emmenagogue, expectorant

USES
Effective in treating warts and sinus infections; ideal for use in insect repellents

BLENDS WELL WITH
Cypress, German chamomile, lavender, marjoram, pine, Roman chamomile, rosemary

PRECAUTIONS
Do not use during pregnancy. Do not use on children less than ten years old. Oregano can cause severe skin irritation.

PALMAROSA
Cymbopogon martinii

SWEET, FLORAL SCENT
COST: $

While palmarosa is sometimes referred to as Turkish or East Indian geranium, it comes from a wild grass with straw-colored leaves and flowering tops. Despite its floral scent, the herb is harvested before the flowers appear. Palmarosa essential oil is used commercially to scent tobacco, soaps, cosmetics, and perfumes.

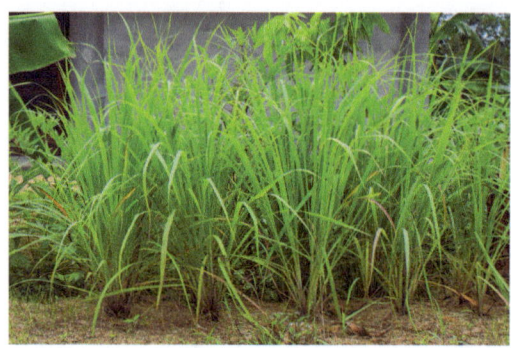

MEDICINAL PROPERTIES
Analgesic, antiseptic, antiviral, bactericide, cicatrizant, cytophylactic, digestive, febrifuge

USES
Effective in treating digestive issues, colds, and flu; ideal for making nourishing skin-care blends that address acne and dermatitis while regenerating skin

BLENDS WELL WITH
Bergamot, geranium, lemon, lime, mandarin, melissa, neroli, patchouli, petitgrain, ravensara leaf, rose, rose geranium, rosemary, rosewood, sweet orange, tangerine, ylang-ylang, yuzu

PRECAUTIONS
Generally regarded as safe.

PALO SANTO
Bursera graveolens

SWEET, WOODY SCENT
COST: $$

If you like frankincense, you're likely to appreciate palo santo. This essential oil offers a calming, grounding presence that eases anxiety, depression, and emotional upset, and a tiny drop goes a long way. In Ecuador and Peru, where this "holy wood" is grown, the smoke is used to keep flying insects at bay and to treat respiratory ailments.

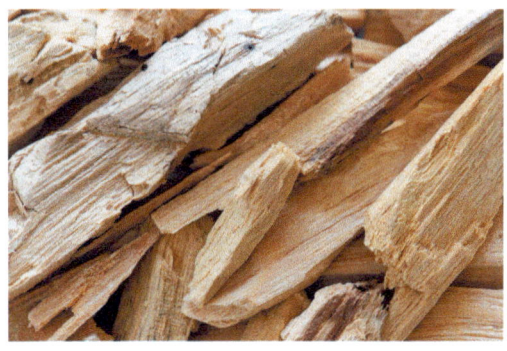

MEDICINAL PROPERTIES
Antidepressant, anti-inflammatory, calmative, deodorant, insect repellent, relaxant

USES
Effective in treating irritated skin and joint soreness; ideal for creating a peaceful, meditative atmosphere in your home

BLENDS WELL WITH
Atlas cedarwood, bergamot, cedarwood, davana, frankincense, helichrysum, mandarin, myrrh, neroli, patchouli, rose, rosewood, sandalwood, vetiver, ylang-ylang

PRECAUTIONS
Generally regarded as safe.

PATCHOULI
Pogostemon cablin

SWEET, SPICY, WOODY SCENT
COST: $$

Arguably one of the most intriguing of scents, patchouli became popular when textile companies began using it to repel lice and fleas in the fabric used to make clothing and bedding. It was also used to give India ink its signature smell. Patchouli essential oil has a long history of masking unpleasant odors and serving as a base note in perfumes; despite its popularity in aromatic applications, it offers a wide range of medicinal properties.

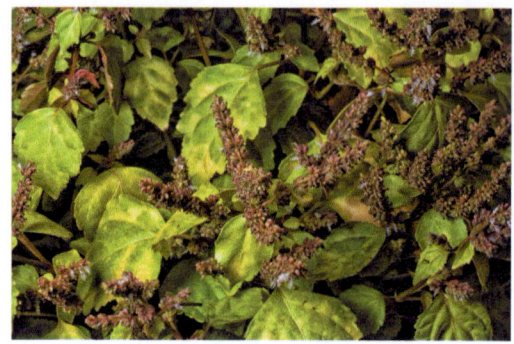

MEDICINAL PROPERTIES
Antidepressant, antiemetic, antifungal, anti-inflammatory, antimicrobial, antiseptic, antiviral, aphrodisiac, astringent, calmative, carminative, cicatrizant, deodorant, digestive, diuretic, febrifuge, fungicidal, insect repellent, insecticide, sedative

USES
Effective in treating hemorrhoids, yeast infections, and fungal infections, including athlete's foot; ideal for use in perfumes and skin-care products

BLENDS WELL WITH
Bergamot, clary sage, davana, geranium, lavender, mandarin, myrrh, palmarosa, rose geranium, Spanish sage, spikenard, sweet orange, tangerine, yuzu

PRECAUTIONS
Generally regarded as safe.

PEPPERMINT
Mentha piperita

CRISP, MINTY
COST: $

Peppermint has been cultivated throughout human history, with evidence of its use found in an Egyptian tomb that was dated to 1000 BCE. Greek mythology describes peppermint's origin as the result of an act of jealousy: Pluto's jealous wife, Persephone, trod a nymph called Mentha into the ground in a fit of rage. Pluto transformed Mentha into an herb for people to enjoy for eternity.

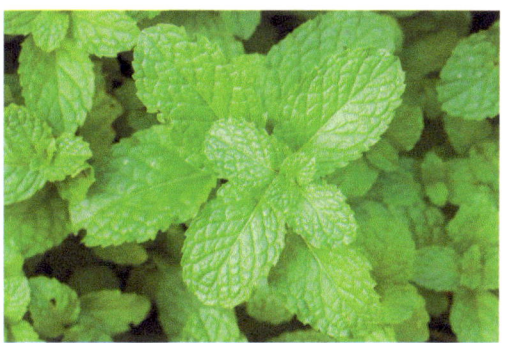

MEDICINAL PROPERTIES
Analgesic, anti-inflammatory, antiseptic, antispasmodic, astringent, carminative, cholagogue, cordial, decongestant, emmenagogue, expectorant, febrifuge, nervine, stimulant, stomachic, sudorific, vasoconstrictor, vermifuge

USES
Effective in treating headaches and indigestion; ideal for making salves to treat sunburn, itching, and skin inflammation

BLENDS WELL WITH
Benzoin, eucalyptus (any species), fir needle, German chamomile, juniper berry, lavender, lemon, mandarin, marjoram, melissa, niaouli, pine, ravintsara, rosemary, tangerine

PRECAUTIONS
Do not use during pregnancy. Not recommended for use on children less than six years old. Peppermint can cause skin irritation and irritate mucous membranes.

PETITGRAIN
Citrus aurantium

FRESH, SLIGHTLY BITTER FLORAL SCENT
COST: $

Petitgrain essential oil is an outstanding antidepressant that is ideal for easing mild, long-term disorders, including seasonal affective disorder (SAD). It stimulates clear thinking, relieves stress, and eliminates brain fog. If you blend petitgrain and neroli, you'll be enjoying two unique essential oils from the same tree.

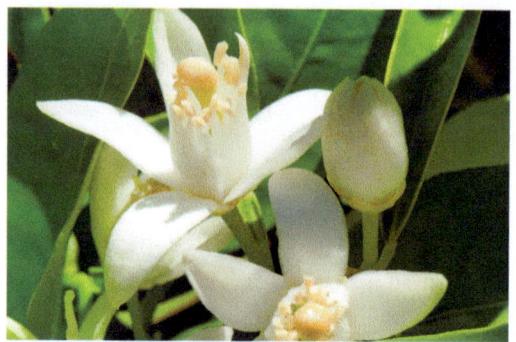

MEDICINAL PROPERTIES
Antidepressant, antiseptic, antispasmodic, deodorant, digestive, nervine, sedative, stomachic

USES
Effective in treating respiratory infections, asthma, and congestion; ideal for making uplifting bath and body products that promote balanced skin

BLENDS WELL WITH
Atlas cedarwood, balsam of Peru, bergamot, black pepper, cedarwood, clove bud, coriander, cypress, elemi, frankincense, mandarin, may chang, neroli, patchouli, rose, rosewood, sweet orange, tangerine, vetiver, yuzu

PRECAUTIONS
Generally regarded as safe.

PINE
Pinus sylvestris

FRESH, GREEN-FOREST SCENT
COST: $

While many think of pine trees simply as a source of wood, they have been used for many things throughout history. Native Americans and others used their rich, delicious seeds as an important source of protein and fat, and employed the needles as a source of vitamin C to prevent scurvy. Among the many medicinal uses of its essential oil are relief from arthritis, muscle, and joint pain, and the treatment of respiratory illnesses.

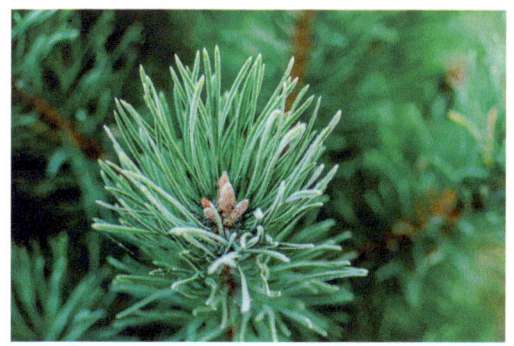

MEDICINAL PROPERTIES
Analgesic, antibacterial, antiseptic, antiviral, cholagogue, deodorant, diuretic, expectorant, insecticide, rubefacient, stimulant, sudorific, vermifuge

USES
Effective in treating colds, coughs, sinusitis, and bronchitis; ideal for making soothing salves to ease muscle and joint pain

BLENDS WELL WITH
Atlas cedarwood, bay laurel, cedarwood, clary sage, eucalyptus (all species), fir needle, juniper, lavender, lemon, niaouli, ravensara leaf, rosemary, Spanish sage, spikenard

PRECAUTIONS
Not recommended for use during pregnancy due to the increased risk of skin sensitization. Pine can cause skin irritation.

RAVENSARA LEAF
Ravensara aromatica,
Agathophyllum aromatica

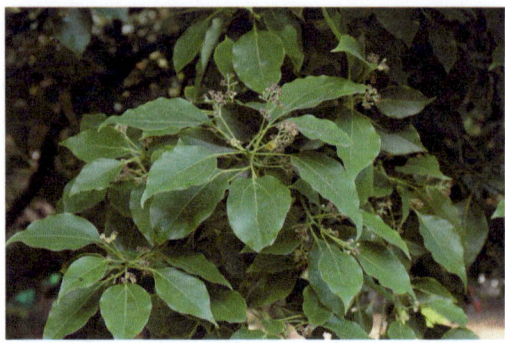

FRUITY, SLIGHTLY MEDICINAL SCENT
COST: $

Ravensara leaf essential oil comes from Madagascar, where it is believed to be a cure-all in much the same way that tea tree oil is esteemed in Australia. It is a good choice for pain relief, including headaches, muscle and joint soreness, toothaches, and earaches. Some sources confuse ravensara leaf with ravintsara. Although the two varieties have similar-sounding species names, they are of different genera and offer different properties.

MEDICINAL PROPERTIES
Analgesic, anti-allergenic, antibacterial, antidepressant, antifungal, antiseptic, antispasmodic, antiviral, aphrodisiac, disinfectant, diuretic, expectorant, relaxant

USES
Effective in treating minor wounds, water retention, and eczema; ideal for diffusing to ease stress, nervousness, and insomnia

BLENDS WELL WITH
Atlas cedarwood, bay laurel, bergamot, black pepper, cardamom, cedarwood, clary sage, cypress, eucalyptus (any species), frankincense, geranium, ginger, grapefruit, lavender, lemon, mandarin, marjoram, palmarosa, pine, rosemary, rosewood, sandalwood, tea tree, thyme

PRECAUTIONS
Do not use during pregnancy. Ravensara leaf can cause skin irritation.

RAVINTSARA
Cinnamomum camphora

EARTHY, FRESH SCENT
COST: $$

Often referred to as Ho wood, ravintsara essential oil comes from the roots, stumps, wood, and branches of a tree traditionally used to craft handles for Japanese knives and swords. Today, the wood is often used to build cabinets and provide architectural trim pieces. In China, statues of Buddha are often carved from Ho wood.

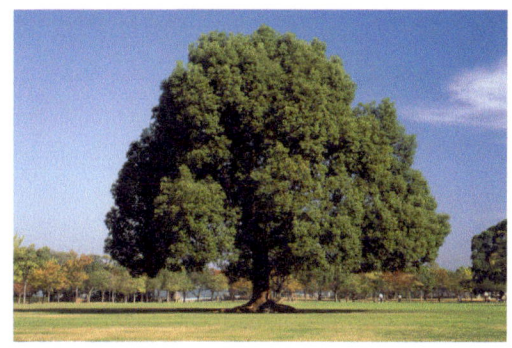

MEDICINAL PROPERTIES
Antibacterial, antifungal, anti-inflammatory, antiseptic, antispasmodic, antiviral, carminative, diuretic, expectorant, stimulant

USES
Effective in treating cold sores, chicken pox, and viral infections; ideal for diffusing and vaporizing to treat respiratory illnesses

BLENDS WELL WITH
Basil, cajuput, German chamomile, helichrysum, lavender, lemon, peppermint, Roman chamomile, rosewood, sandalwood, spearmint, ylang-ylang

PRECAUTIONS
Ravintsara can cause skin irritation.

ROMAN CHAMOMILE
Anthemis nobilis

SWEET, HERBAL SCENT
COST: $$$

Roman chamomile offers a pleasant scent that reminds many people of ripe apples. In aromatherapy, it is highly prized for its skin-healing properties and its ability to calm frayed nerves. If you suffer from PMS or are feeling irritable or impatient, this is an excellent oil to try.

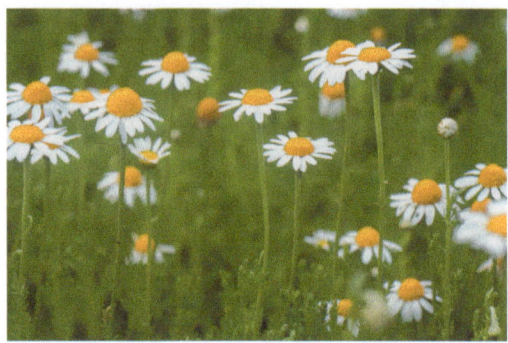

MEDICINAL PROPERTIES

Analgesic, antibiotic, antidepressant, anti-inflammatory, antiseptic, antispasmodic, bactericidal, carminative, cholagogue, cicatrizant, digestive, emmenagogue, febrifuge, nervine, sedative, stomachic, sudorific, tonic, vermifuge, vulnerary

USES

Effective in treating dry or chapped skin, infant teething, acne, eczema, and dermatitis; ideal in blends for alleviating indigestion

BLENDS WELL WITH

Bergamot, cajuput, carrot seed, clary sage, cucumber seed, elemi, eucalyptus (any species), frankincense, geranium, grapefruit, jasmine, lavender, lemon, neroli, palmarosa, rose, rose geranium, rosewood, tea tree

PRECAUTIONS

Do not use during pregnancy. Roman chamomile can cause skin irritation.

ROSE
Rosa damascena

SWEET, FLORAL SCENT
COST: $$$$

Inside each bottle of pure rose essential oil, which is also sometimes called rose otto, you'll find the power of more than one thousand roses, all picked at the peak of their potency. A little drop goes a long way, helping prevent scarring, rejuvenating aging or dry skin, and soothing the discomfort of eczema and other painful disorders. If you find the cost of pure rose or rose otto prohibitive, but want to experience the fragrance, you'll find that many top retailers offer delightful prediluted rose oils for a fraction of the cost.

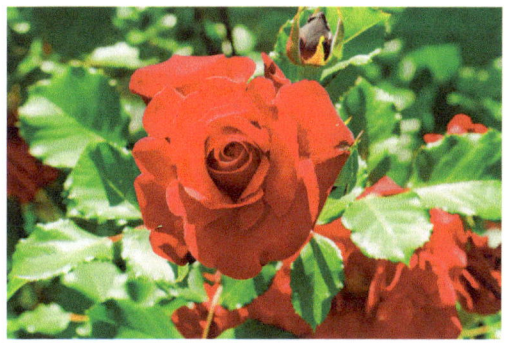

MEDICINAL PROPERTIES
Antidepressant, anti-inflammatory, antiseptic, antispasmodic, antiviral, aphrodisiac, astringent, bactericidal, cicatrizant, depurative, emmenagogue, hemostatic, laxative

USES
Effective in treating impotence, depression, anger, and stress; ideal for making soothing bath and body products

BLENDS WELL WITH
Balsam of Peru, bergamot, clove bud, davana, frankincense, galbanum, geranium, jasmine, melissa, myrrh, palmarosa, patchouli, rosewood, yuzu

PRECAUTIONS
Do not use during pregnancy.

ROSE GERANIUM
Pelargonium graveolens

GREEN, FLORAL SCENT
COST: $$

Sometimes referred to as bourbon geranium, rose geranium essential oil has a light, rosy scent with minty undertones. Rose geranium's ability to stimulate the adrenal cortex (the outer part of the adrenal gland) makes it useful in lifting depression and alleviating anxiety. It stimulates the lymph system to aid in detoxification, and it helps balance dry and oily skin.

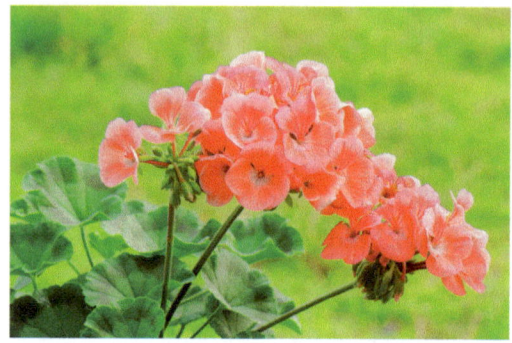

MEDICINAL PROPERTIES
Antidepressant, antiseptic, astringent, cicatrizant, cytophylactic, deodorant, diuretic, hemostatic, styptic, vermifuge, vulnerary

USES
Effective in treating sunburn, PMS, and painful periods; ideal for making nourishing bath and body products

BLENDS WELL WITH
Basil, bergamot, carrot seed, cedarwood, citronella, clary sage, cucumber seed, grapefruit, jasmine, lavender, lemon, lime, mandarin, neroli, patchouli, rosemary, sweet orange

PRECAUTIONS
Not recommend for use during pregnancy owing to rose geranium's hormone-balancing properties.

ROSEMARY
Rosmarinus officinalis

REFRESHING, HERBAL SCENT
COST: $

The rosemary plant has the intriguing ability to stimulate memory and facilitate clear thinking. In ancient Greece, scholars wore sprigs of rosemary while studying, as it helped them retain information. Diffusing rosemary essential oil can sharpen your focus and aid with productivity while promoting a sense of calm confidence.

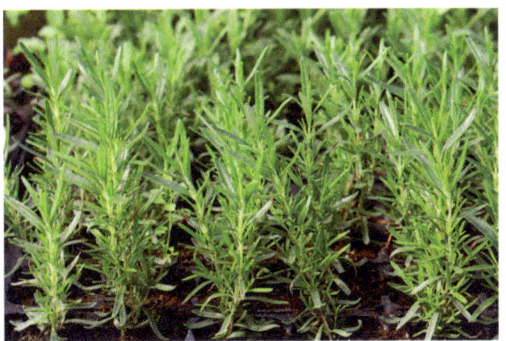

MEDICINAL PROPERTIES
Analgesic, antibacterial, antidepressant, antifungal, antimicrobial, antioxidant, antiseptic, antispasmodic, astringent, carminative, cicatrizant, digestive, diuretic, emmenagogue, hypertensive, stimulant, sudorific, vulnerary

USES
Effective in treating digestive complaints, muscle pain, and dandruff; ideal for making bath and body products to balance skin and nourish hair

BLENDS WELL WITH
Balsam of Peru, basil, bay laurel, bergamot, cajuput, clary sage, clove bud, elemi, fennel seed, juniper berry, lemon, niaouli, peppermint, petitgrain, Spanish sage, spearmint, tea tree

PRECAUTIONS
Do not use during pregnancy. Do not use if diagnosed with epilepsy. Rosemary is quite stimulating; using it within three or four hours of bedtime can cause wakefulness.

ROSEWOOD
Aniba rosaeodora

SPICY, WOODY SCENT
COST: $$

Also known as pau-rosa, Brazilian rosewood, or bois de rose, rosewood essential oil comes from the wood of the Brazilian rosewood tree, which is endangered in the wild. When shopping for this beautiful, nourishing oil, be sure to select a brand that is ethically harvested from a rosewood farm. These managed plantations provide rosewood for carving and furniture making, and they are careful to plant more trees than they harvest.

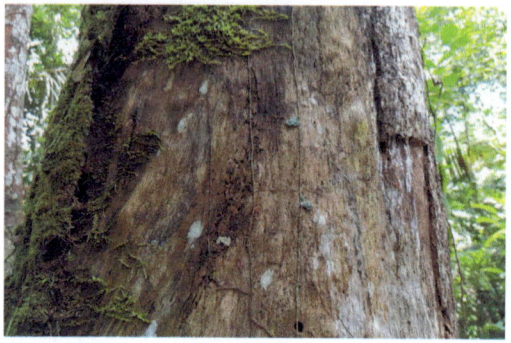

MEDICINAL PROPERTIES
Analgesic, antibacterial, antidepressant, antimicrobial, antiseptic, aphrodisiac, calmative, deodorant, emollient, euphoriant, stimulant

USES
Effective in treating dry, chapped skin; ideal for making nourishing bath and body products that lift the spirits

BLENDS WELL WITH
Benzoin, bergamot, clary sage, copaiba, davana, jasmine, lavender, lemon, mandarin, may chang, neroli, palmarosa, petitgrain, rose, sweet orange, tangerine, vetiver, ylang-ylang, yuzu

PRECAUTIONS
Generally regarded as safe.

SANDALWOOD
Santalum album

SWEET, WOODY SCENT
COST: $$$$

Sandalwood essential oil comes from the dead roots and wood of very old *Santalum album* trees. Prized as a perfume material since ancient times, it is also used in incense sticks and for making furniture. Like rosewood, sandalwood trees are subject to poaching and improper harvesting; however, most well-known essential oil companies take care to source their product ethically, from farmers who raise the trees.

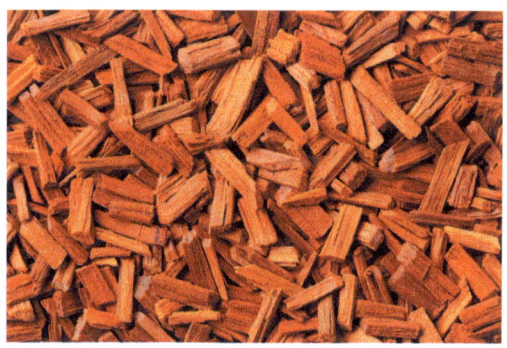

MEDICINAL PROPERTIES
Antidepressant, anti-inflammatory, antiseptic, antispasmodic, aphrodisiac, astringent, carminative, cicatrizant, digestive, diuretic, expectorant, insect repellent, nervine, sedative, stomachic, tonic, vermifuge, vulnerary

USES
Effective in treating psoriasis, eczema, and dry skin; ideal for diffusing to create an enticing, romantic atmosphere

BLENDS WELL WITH
Bergamot, black pepper, geranium, jasmine, lavender, myrrh, neroli, rose, vetiver, ylang-ylang, yuzu

PRECAUTIONS
Generally regarded as safe. Sandalwood essential oil gets stronger over time; a tiny drop goes a long way.

SPANISH SAGE
Salvia lavandulaefolia

STRONG, HERBACEOUS SCENT
COST: $$

Spanish sage is among a few different types of essential oils marketed as "sage" and is not to be confused with Dalmatian sage (*Salvia officinalis*). It is a very potent oil that calls for a light, judicious hand, but it proves effective as a mood lifter, memory aid, and remedy for dealing with PMS, painful periods, and menopause symptoms.

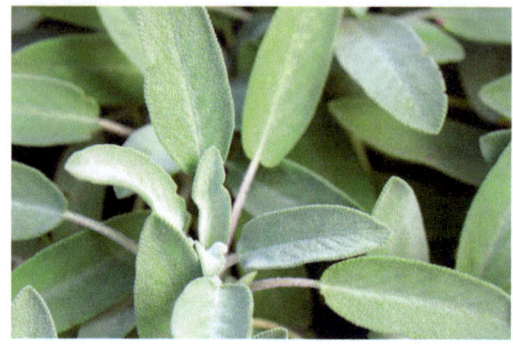

MEDICINAL PROPERTIES
Anti-inflammatory, antimicrobial, antioxidant, antiseptic, emmenagogue

USES
Effective in treating hot flashes, night sweats, insomnia; ideal for adding to salves for easing aches and pains

BLENDS WELL WITH
Bergamot, lavender, lemon, lime, sweet orange, rosewood, sandalwood

PRECAUTIONS
Do not use during pregnancy or breastfeeding. Do not use if diagnosed with epilepsy or high blood pressure.

SPEARMINT
Mentha spicata, M. viridis

SWEET, MINTY SCENT
COST: $

A gentler substitute for peppermint essential oil, spearmint oil calms itching, relieves coughs and colds, eases indigestion, and has a marvelously uplifting effect on the mind. A Mediterranean native that is now cultivated worldwide, spearmint was used by ancient Greeks, who enjoyed the scent in their bathwater. During medieval times, it was used to whiten teeth and soothe sore gums, much in the way fresh, minty toothpaste is used today.

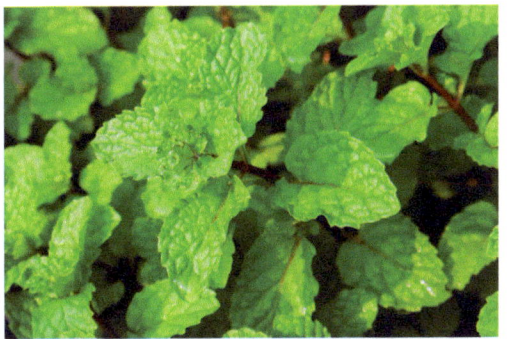

MEDICINAL PROPERTIES
Antidepressant, antiseptic, antispasmodic, astringent, carminative, decongestant, digestive, diuretic, expectorant, insecticide, stimulant, stomachic

USES
Effective in treating halitosis, hiccups, and headaches; ideal for making balms to treat acne and itching

BLENDS WELL WITH
Basil, bay laurel, benzoin, eucalyptus (any species), jasmine, lavender, lemon, lime, mandarin, niaouli, peppermint, rosemary, sweet orange, tangerine

PRECAUTIONS
Do not use spearmint if breastfeeding, as it can reduce lactation. Spearmint is unique in that it can sometimes weaken homeopathic remedies; if you take a homeopathic remedy, ensure that spearmint is compatible before using it.

SPIKENARD
Nardostachys jatamansi

MUSKY, WOODY SCENT
COST: $$$

A favorite of ancient Egyptians, spikenard was also mentioned in the Bible's Song of Solomon as well as in the book of John. It was often used to make tea for treating nervousness and heart palpitations, and in India, Ayurvedic practitioners use it to aid healthy liver function. Spikenard essential oil is sometimes called false valerian; like the real thing, it can promote deep, restful sleep.

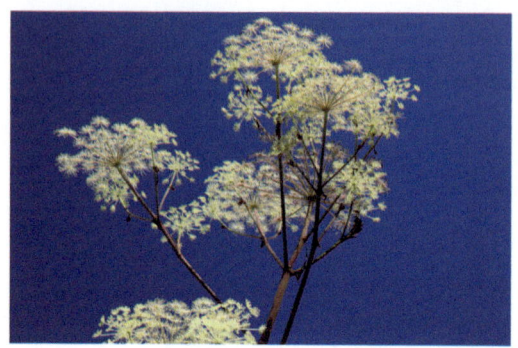

MEDICINAL PROPERTIES
Antibacterial, antifungal, anti-inflammatory, antioxidant, antiseptic, antispasmodic, deodorant, digestive, diuretic, febrifuge, laxative, sedative

USES
Effective in treating insomnia, stress, and nervousness; ideal for making bath and body products to soothe and nourish dry or aging skin

BLENDS WELL WITH
Cardamom, cinnamon leaf, clary sage, coriander, fennel seed, lavender, neroli, patchouli, pine, vetiver

PRECAUTIONS
Not recommended for use during pregnancy owing to spikenard's deeply relaxing effect. Do not use on children less than six years old.

SPRUCE
Picea mariana

FRESH, FOREST SCENT
COST: $

Also known as black spruce, *Picea mariana* is a slow-growing coniferous tree that is part of the pine family. The provincial tree of Labrador and Newfoundland, it is native to North America's boreal forests. There are a few other spruce oils on the market with similar properties, but black spruce offers the sweetest, lightest aroma among them.

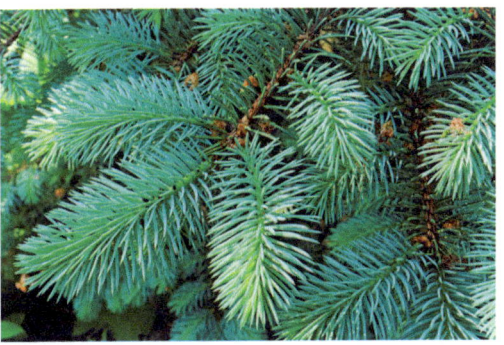

MEDICINAL PROPERTIES
Anti-inflammatory, antiseptic, antispasmodic, antitussive, astringent, diuretic, expectorant, nervine, vulnerary

USES
Effective in colds, coughs, flu, and respiratory ailments; ideal for making warming salves to treat joint and muscle pain

BLENDS WELL WITH
Atlas cedarwood, benzoin, cedarwood, clary sage, cypress, eucalyptus (any species), fir needle, frankincense, galbanum, lavender, lemon, palo santo, petitgrain, pine, rose, rosemary, rosewood, sandalwood

PRECAUTIONS
Spruce gets stronger with age; it can cause skin sensitization when oxidized. Use up within six months of opening for topical use, and reserve older oil for inhalation and household cleaning purposes.

SWEET ORANGE
Citrus sinensis

SWEET, CITRUS SCENT
COST: $

Oranges make a fantastic snack, but historically, they have also been put to medicinal and cosmetic uses. In ancient China, dried oranges were a popular remedy for a bloated stomach, and the peel was used to relieve coughing. Sweet orange's essential oil has an enticing aroma that is good for more than just air fresheners; it (and other citrus oils) have been successfully used to curb cigarette cravings.

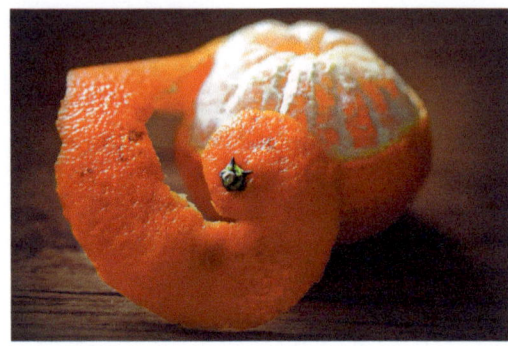

MEDICINAL PROPERTIES
Antibacterial, antidepressant, anti-inflammatory, antiseptic, antiviral, aperitive, astringent, carminative, cholagogue, digestive, diuretic, fungicidal, hypotensive, stomachic, tonic

USES
Effective in treating colds, flu, and digestive ailments; ideal for making air fresheners and cleaning products

BLENDS WELL WITH
Anise, allspice, black pepper, caraway seed, cardamom, cinnamon leaf, clove bud, copaiba, elemi, fennel seed, frankincense, galbanum, ginger, rosewood, sandalwood, tagetes, vetiver

PRECAUTIONS
Phototoxic: Do not apply to skin that will be exposed to direct sunlight. Use up within six months of opening for topical use, and reserve older oil for inhalation and household cleaning purposes.

TAGETES
Tagetes minuta

SHARP, GREEN HERBAL SCENT
COST: $

Sometimes referred to as marigold or Mexican marigold, tagetes is not to be confused with calendula. A very strong insect repellent and insecticide, tagetes is native to Africa, where branches of it can sometimes be seen hanging near homes to deter mosquitoes and flies. Also known as khaki bush, tagetes is now grown throughout France and North America, where its essential oil is popular with the perfume industry.

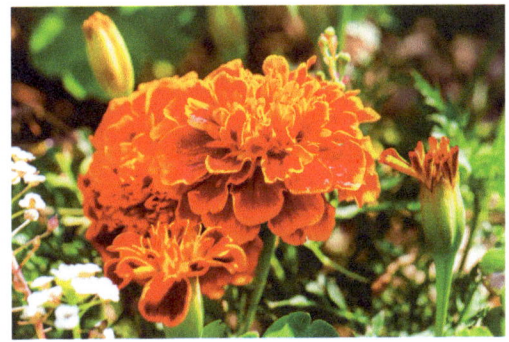

MEDICINAL PROPERTIES
Antibiotic, antimicrobial, antiseptic, antispasmodic, insect repellent, insecticide, sedative

USES
Effective in treating coughs, colds, and bronchitis; ideal for making insect repellents

BLENDS WELL WITH
Bergamot, clary sage, jasmine, lavender, lemon, lime, mandarin, neroli, sweet orange

PRECAUTIONS
Not recommended for use during pregnancy owing to the risk of skin sensitization. Tagetes can cause skin irritation, particularly in those with sensitive skin. Phototoxic: do not apply to skin that will be exposed to direct sunlight.

TANGERINE
Citrus reticulata blanco

SWEET, CITRUS SCENT
COST: $

Tangerine oil is closely related to mandarin essential oil, and the two are often used interchangeably despite subtle differences in fragrance. Tangerine's aroma is sweeter and a bit heavier than that of mandarin, which is light and almost candy-like. Both bring feelings of joy and relieve stress, and both are ideal for use around children. Like mandarin, tangerine is not typically phototoxic.

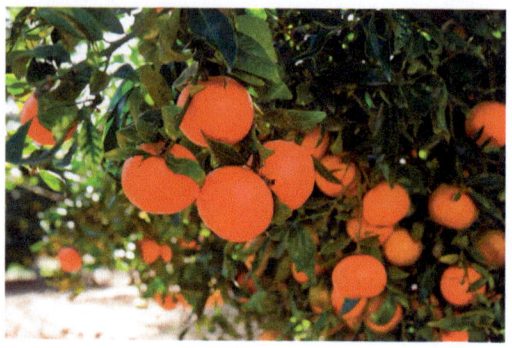

MEDICINAL PROPERTIES
Antiseptic, antispasmodic, cytophylactic, depurative, sedative, stomachic, tonic

USES
Effective in treating stress, nervousness, and depression; ideal for making air fresheners and scented bath and body products

BLENDS WELL WITH
Allspice, bergamot, caraway seed, cardamom, clary sage, clove bud, elemi, frankincense, ginger, myrrh, neroli, ylang-ylang

PRECAUTIONS
Generally regarded as safe.

TEA TREE
Melaleuca alternifolia

LIGHT, CAMPHOR SCENT
COST: $

One of the most potent immune-stimulating essential oils available, tea tree comes from New South Wales, in Australia, where Indigenous Peoples first enjoyed its many medicinal purposes. During World War II, tea tree was so important to the Allies that tea tree cutters and producers were exempt from military service. Soldiers and sailors used it the same way as it is employed today—to treat minor wounds, infections, and more.

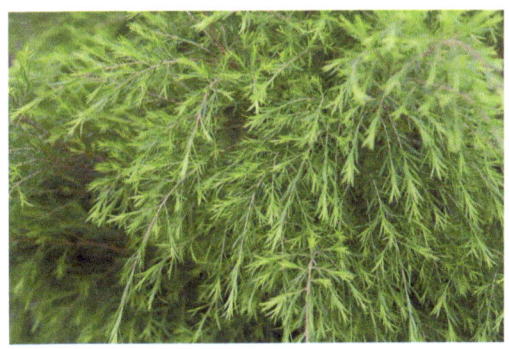

MEDICINAL PROPERTIES
Antimicrobial, antiseptic, antiviral, bactericide, cicatrizant, expectorant, fungicide, insect repellent, insecticide, stimulant, sudorific

USES
Effective in treating minor wounds, sinusitis, and respiratory ailments; ideal for making powerful antiseptic household cleaners

BLENDS WELL WITH
Cinnamon leaf, clary sage, clove bud, eucalyptus (any species), geranium, lavender, lemon, myrrh, oregano, rosemary, rosewood, thyme

PRECAUTIONS
Generally regarded as safe.

THYME
Thymus vulgaris

SPICY, HERBACEOUS SCENT
COST: $$

Thyme has a long history of culinary use, as well as an interesting medicinal background. Ancient Greeks used it to repel insects, and Romans believed bathing in thyme-scented water would impart courage and vigor. Thyme essential oil is spicy and must be used judiciously. In salves and compresses, it improves circulation, making it ideal for treating sprains, bruises, and muscle aches.

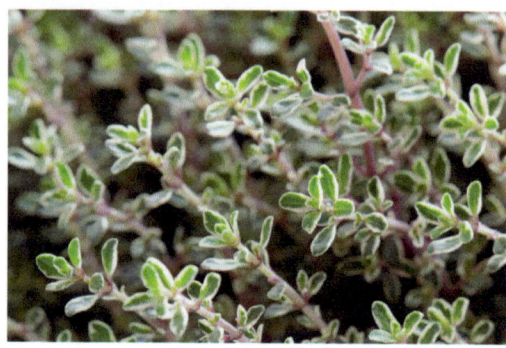

MEDICINAL PROPERTIES
Antibacterial, antifungal, antimicrobial, antioxidant, antiseptic, antispasmodic, antitoxic, antitussive, astringent, cicatrizant, disinfectant, expectorant, hypertensive, insect repellent, insecticide, stimulant, sudorific

USES
Effective in treating diarrhea, infectious colitis, and upper respiratory infections; ideal for making insect repellents

BLENDS WELL WITH
Balsam of Peru, bay laurel, bergamot, black pepper, clary sage, fir needle, grapefruit, juniper berry, lemon, lime, lavender, pine, rosemary, Spanish sage

PRECAUTIONS
Do not use on children less than six years old.

VALERIAN
Valerian officinalis

COMPLEX MUSKY SCENT
COST: $$

Valerian's power to calm the central nervous system comes from two sesquiterpenes: valerone and valerenic acid. A drop or two of this potent essential oil applied to the feet or temples promotes sound, refreshing sleep, as do herbal sleep aids containing valerian.

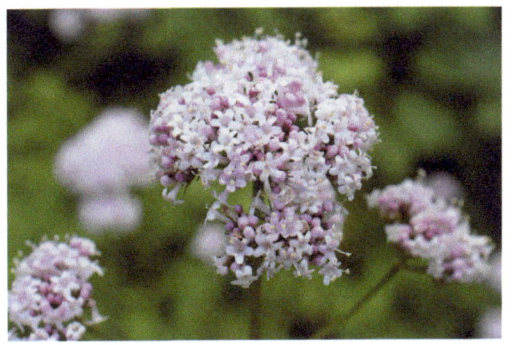

MEDICINAL PROPERTIES
Antispasmodic, bactericidal, carminative, diuretic, hypnotic, hypotensive, nervous system depressant, sedative

USES
Effective in treating insomnia, nervous tension, and exhaustion; ideal for making calming bath and body products

BLENDS WELL WITH
Atlas cedarwood, cedarwood, clary sage, lavender, mandarin, patchouli, petitgrain, pine, rose, rosemary, rosewood, sandalwood, tangerine

PRECAUTIONS
Do not use during pregnancy. Do not use with antidepressants, pharmaceutical sedatives, or alcohol.

VETIVER
Chrysopogon zizanioides

SWEET, WOODY SCENT
COST: $

Vetiver is a perennial tufted grass native to the tropics, where it is used to weave fragrant mats, baskets, and window coverings, and also for erosion control in wet areas. Besides its many practical uses, vetiver essential oil is widely employed by the fragrance industry. In aromatherapy, it is called the "oil of tranquillity" for its ability to ward off depression while calming nervousness and stress.

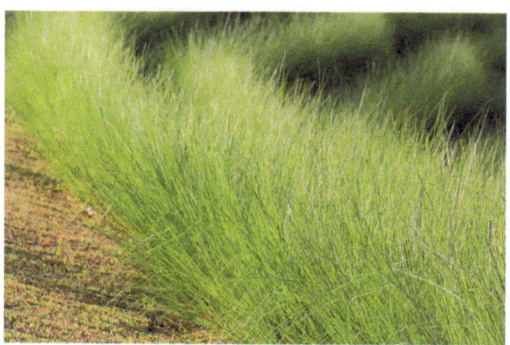

MEDICINAL PROPERTIES
Analgesic, anti-inflammatory, antiseptic, antispasmodic, aphrodisiac, astringent, calmative, cicatrizant, detoxifier, insect repellent, nervine, sedative, stomachic, tonic, vulnerary

USES
Effective in treating ADHD, stress, and postpartum depression; ideal for making soothing products to ease the pain of arthritis, rheumatism, muscle strains, and more

BLENDS WELL WITH
Benzoin, cardamom, clary sage, fennel seed, grapefruit, jasmine, mandarin, marjoram, maychang, neroli, patchouli, petitgrain, sweet orange, tangerine, ylang-ylang

PRECAUTIONS
Generally regarded as safe.

VITEX BERRY
Vitex agnus-castus

MINTY HERBAL SCENT WITH BERRY UNDERTONES
COST: $$$

Also known as chaste tree, chasteberry, or monk's pepper, vitex berry has a long traditional use as a hormone balancer, particularly for those who are suffering from PMS, painful periods, or menopause symptoms. It has a progesterone-like effect on the body and must be used in small increments.

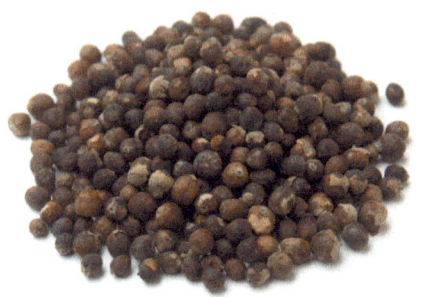

MEDICINAL PROPERTIES
Anaphrodisiac, diaphoretic, diuretic, emmenagogue, febrifuge, galactagogue, sedative, vulnerary

USES
Effective in treating cramps, breast tenderness, and depression associated with PMS; ideal for making treatments for period-related acne and for easing turbulent emotions

BLENDS WELL WITH
Clary sage, geranium, lavender, may chang, rose, rose geranium, valerian

PRECAUTIONS
Do not use during pregnancy. Do not use in conjunction with birth control pills or hormone-replacement therapies. Do not use on children.

YLANG-YLANG
Cananga odorata

SWEET FLORAL SCENT
COST: $$

Sometimes referred to as "poor man's jasmine," ylang-ylang has a beautifully haunting scent that makes it a favorite with perfumeries. Pronounced *ee-lang ee-lang*, ylang-ylang means "flower of flowers." Like jasmine, neroli, and other heady florals, a little bit of the essential oil goes a long way.

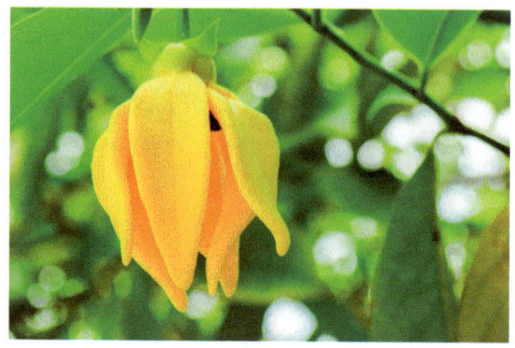

MEDICINAL PROPERTIES
Antidepressant, antiseborrheic, antiseptic, aphrodisiac, hypotensive, nervine, sedative

USES
Effective in treating stress, nervousness, and anxiety; ideal for making romantic, relaxing bath and body products

BLENDS WELL WITH
Bergamot, cypress, davana, grapefruit, lavender, lemon, mandarin, petitgrain, rosewood, sandalwood, tangerine, vetiver, yuzu

PRECAUTIONS
Generally regarded as safe; however, overuse can cause nausea and headaches.

YUZU
Citrus junos

FLORAL CITRUS SCENT
COST: $$$

Yuzu is a citrus fruit that is very popular in Japan, where it is made into marmalade, blended into ice cream, and enjoyed whole. The aromatic rinds are sometimes added to a hot bath, where they are used to refresh the mind and ward off colds and the flu. Yuzu is an excellent oil to diffuse when you're feeling stressed, burned out, or frustrated.

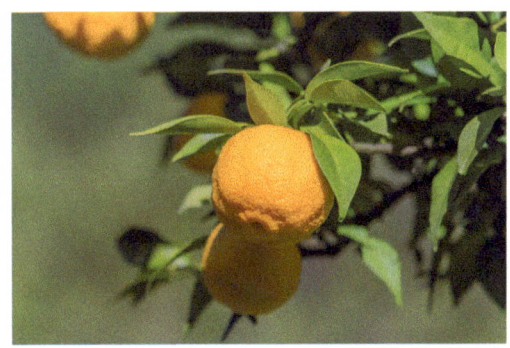

MEDICINAL PROPERTIES
Antidepressant, antiseptic, antispasmodic, calmative, cicatrizant, deodorant, digestive, febrifuge, vulnerary

USES
Effective in treating colds and flu; ideal for blending personal fragrances and making uplifting bath and body products

BLENDS WELL WITH
Basil, benzoin, clary sage, cypress, davana, frankincense, ginger, jasmine, neroli, patchouli, petitgrain, palmarosa, rose, rosewood, sandalwood, vetiver, ylang-ylang

PRECAUTIONS
Phototoxic: Do not apply to skin that will be exposed to direct sunlight.

PART THREE

Recipes, Remedies, and Applications for Health and Wellness

Aromatherapy has been used for centuries to improve health and fight illness. Today, it serves as a complementary therapy to Western medicine. For minor ailments, many people choose to turn to natural solutions like aromatherapy at home, instead of using over-the-counter pharmaceutical products.

Aromatherapy remedies may include salves, lotions, massage oils, baths, and a host of other applications. These aromatherapy remedies may help reduce the toxic load placed on your body from over-the-counter medications, and they tend to be less expensive. However, if you are pregnant or breastfeeding or have a serious illness, talk to your primary health care provider about the use of aromatherapy, as it may be contraindicated with certain medications or conditions.

Essential oils should be capped tightly and stored in a cool, dark place. Unless otherwise noted, any treatments you make with essential oils that are not used immediately should be treated the same way.

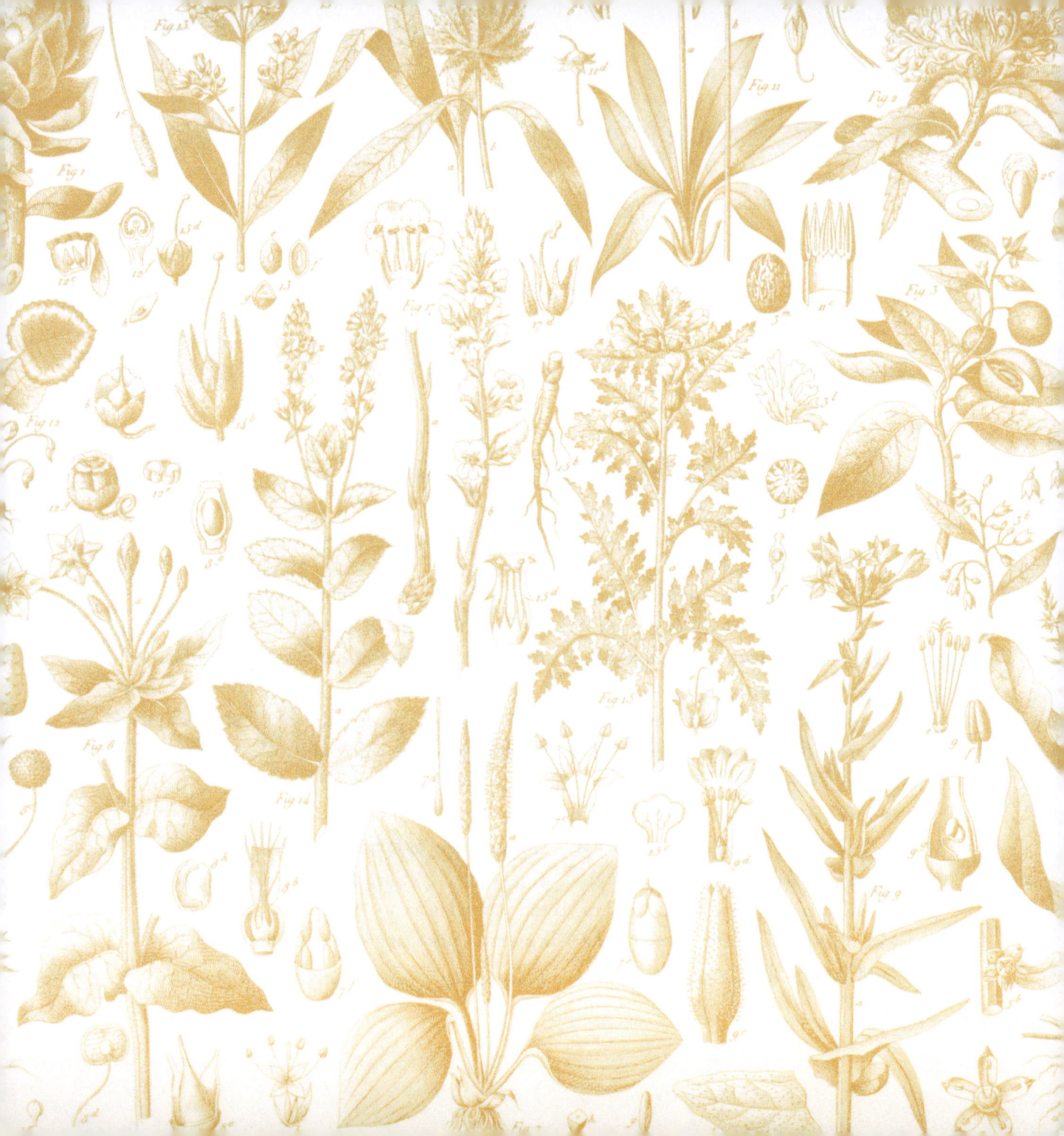

CHAPTER FOUR

CHRONIC CONDITIONS, DISEASES, AND ILLNESSES

Asthma   132

Bronchitis   134

Canker Sores   136

Colds   138

Congestion   140

Fever   142

Fibromyalgia   144

Halitosis   146

Laryngitis and Sore Throat   148

Pinkeye   150

Sinusitis   152

ASTHMA

With wheezing and shortness of breath that can lead to feelings of panic, asthma sufferers experience intense physical and emotional discomfort. Aromatherapy treatments help address both issues. Keep in mind that asthma is a serious illness, so be sure to let your doctor know that you're using aromatherapy alongside prescribed treatments.

Cajuput-Bergamot Diffusion
MAKES 1 TREATMENT

Cajuput essential oil is a strong decongestant that promotes easy breathing, and bergamot essential oil addresses fear and stress. Both offer antispasmodic properties to help keep the muscles around the airway relaxed.

2 drops bergamot essential oil
1 drop cajuput essential oil

1. Add the essential oils to your diffuser according to the manufacturer's instructions.
2. Run the diffuser nearby.
3. Repeat as needed.

Relaxing Clary Sage–Lavender Chest Rub

MAKES ABOUT 2 FLUID OUNCES (¼ CUP)

Clary sage and lavender essential oils offer anti-inflammatory, antispasmodic, and sedative properties that provide relief while offering a potent calming effect. Avoid driving or attempting tasks that require concentration after use.

¼ cup coconut oil, melted
30 drops lavender essential oil
15 drops clary sage essential oil

1. In a small bowl, combine the coconut oil and essential oils. Whisk to blend thoroughly, and then transfer the rub to a small jar with a lid.
2. Every 5 minutes or so, stir with a thin rod. Allow the mixture to cool completely before capping.
3. With your fingertips, apply ½ teaspoon of the salve to your chest, and massage the area.
4. Repeat up to three times daily, as needed.

Synergistic Asthma Inhaler

MAKES 1 REUSABLE INHALER

Refreshing pine, eucalyptus, tea tree, thyme, frankincense, and myrrh essential oils combine to help you expel mucus and breathe easier, while relaxing the muscles surrounding the airway.

6 drops eucalyptus essential oil (any species)
6 drops pine essential oil
6 drops tea tree essential oil
4 drops frankincense essential oil
4 drops myrrh essential oil
4 drops thyme essential oil

1. In a small bottle with a lid, combine the essential oils. Shake well to blend.
2. Apply the blend to the cotton wick of an aromatherapy inhaler.
3. Hold the inhaler beneath your nose, and inhale slowly through both nostrils to a count of five. Hold your breath for another count of five, and then exhale slowly.
4. Repeat as needed to prevent and soothe symptoms.

SUBSTITUTION TIP: If you don't have an inhaler, you can transfer the blend to a small, dark glass bottle and inhale directly from the bottle, or place 3 drops of the blend in your diffuser.

Keep in mind that asthma is a serious illness, so be sure to let your doctor know that you're using aromatherapy alongside prescribed treatments.

BRONCHITIS

With a painful cough, sore throat, and shortness of breath caused by swollen bronchial tubes, bronchitis can make you feel miserable. Antibiotics might be necessary, so see your doctor. Aromatherapy treatments can help by easing breathing and providing gentle comfort.

Allspice–Sweet Orange Diffusion

MAKES 1 TREATMENT

Allspice and sweet orange help ease breathing while killing bacteria. Because allspice is a spicy oil that can irritate mucous membranes, don't inhale directly from the diffuser.

1 drop allspice essential oil
3 drops sweet orange essential oil

1. Add the essential oils to your diffuser according to the manufacturer's instructions.
2. Run the diffuser nearby for 30 minutes three or four times daily until recovered.

SUBSTITUTION TIP: If you don't have sweet orange essential oil on hand, you can use bergamot oil instead.

Anise–Caraway Seed Vapor

MAKES 1 TREATMENT

Anise and caraway seed essential oils are potent antibacterial agents; they also provide a calming influence while helping expel phlegm.

1 cup near-boiling water
1 drop anise essential oil
2 drops caraway seed essential oil

1. Pour the hot water into a large mug, and then add the essential oils.
2. Hold the mug in front of you and occasionally breathe in the vapors as you relax.
3. Continue until the water cools.
4. Repeat two or three times daily, until recovered.

Soothing Spearmint-Hyssop Gargle

MAKES 8 FLUID OUNCES (1 CUP)

Hyssop and spearmint essential oils offer antiseptic and expectorant properties, which help bring comfort and promote healing.

1 cup less 2 tablespoons distilled water
2 tablespoons unflavored vodka
3 drops hyssop essential oil
2 drops spearmint essential oil

1. In a medium bottle or jar with a lid, combine the water, vodka, and essential oils.
2. Shake well to blend, and then shake again before each use.
3. Gargle with 1 tablespoon of the blend for 30 seconds, being careful not to swallow.
4. Spit out when finished.
5. Repeat two or three times daily, until recovered.

CANKER SORES

Also known as aphthous ulcers, canker sores develop along the base of the gums and throughout the soft tissues of the mouth, appearing as small, red bumps that burst, leaving shallow yellowish or white lesions behind.

Dill Seed Balm

MAKES 1 FLUID OUNCE (2 TABLESPOONS)

Dill seed essential oil helps canker sores by easing pain and speeding healing. Although some sources state that this oil is edible, it is best to avoid swallowing it.

2 tablespoons fractionated coconut oil
10 drops dill seed essential oil

1. In a small bottle or jar with a lid, combine the coconut oil and essential oil. Shake well to blend.
2. With a cotton swab, apply 1 drop of the blend to the canker sore. Use a new swab for each sore.
3. Repeat the treatment once or twice daily, until recovered.

Oregano Salve and Compress

MAKES ½ FLUID OUNCE (1 TABLESPOON)

Oregano essential oil relieves discomfort and helps prevent infection by killing bacteria. Because this oil can irritate mucous membranes, it must be heavily diluted before using on canker sores.

1 tablespoon fractionated coconut oil
1 drop oregano essential oil

1. In a small bottle or jar with a lid, combine the coconut oil and essential oil. Shake well to blend.
2. Apply 1 drop of the blend to a cotton ball or a piece of gauze and then position it over the canker sore.
3. Hold the compress in place for 3 or 4 minutes.
4. Repeat the treatment two or three times daily, until recovered.

Tea Tree Rinse

MAKES ABOUT 4 FLUID OUNCES (½ CUP)

Tea tree essential oil brings quick pain relief and helps prevent canker sores from becoming infected.

7 tablespoons distilled water
1 tablespoon fractionated coconut oil
8 drops tea tree essential oil

1. In a small bottle or jar with a lid, combine the water, coconut oil, and essential oil. Shake well to blend, and then shake again before each use.
2. Rinse your mouth with 1 teaspoon of the blend for 30 seconds to 1 minute, focusing on the area where canker sores are present, being very careful not to swallow the mixture. Spit out when finished. (Flush the drain with hot water.)
3. Repeat two or three times daily, until recovered.

COLDS

Chest congestion, coughing, and stuffy or runny noses are all symptoms of the common cold—for which there is no known cure. Aromatherapy brings relief without the unpleasant side effects that often accompany drugstore remedies.

Bay Laurel–Lavender Diffusion

MAKES 1 TREATMENT

Bay laurel is a powerful antiseptic and antispasmodic essential oil that can help purify the air in your home while providing relief from coughing and congestion. Too much can irritate mucous membranes, however, so don't breathe directly from the diffuser.

2 drops bay laurel essential oil
1 drop lavender essential oil

1. Add the essential oils to your diffuser according to the manufacturer's instructions.
2. Run the diffuser nearby.
3. Repeat two or three times daily.

Caraway–Clove Bud Chest Rub

MAKES ABOUT 8 FLUID OUNCES (1 CUP)

Caraway and clove bud essential oils bring relief from relentless coughing and congestion via their antispasmodic and expectorant properties. As a bonus, this blend smells a bit nicer than classic eucalyptus-based rubs.

¼ cup coconut oil, melted
¼ cup shea butter
2 tablespoons sweet almond oil
2 tablespoons beeswax, melted
25 drops clove bud essential oil
25 drops caraway essential oil

1. In a medium bowl, combine the coconut oil, shea butter, almond oil, beeswax, and essential oils. Whisk to blend thoroughly.
2. Pour the mixture into a medium jar with a lid and allow to cool completely before capping.
3. When ready to use, use your fingertips to apply a dime-sized amount of the blend to the chest and massage the area, using light strokes.
4. Repeat two or three times daily, as needed.

May Chang–Lemon Lotion

MAKES ABOUT 8 FLUID OUNCES (1 CUP)

May chang and lemon essential oils offer some protection from viruses and bacteria, and this blend promotes a clear airway.

8 fluid ounces (1 cup) unscented body lotion or hand cream
20 drops lemon essential oil
10 drops may chang essential oil

1. In a medium bowl, combine the lotion and essential oils. Whisk to blend thoroughly, and then transfer the lotion to a medium jar with a lid or back into the empty lotion container.
2. Apply 1 teaspoon of the blend to your hands, arms, and shoulders. Use a little more, or less, as needed, and feel free to apply the lotion to other body parts.
3. Use as often as you like throughout the day, especially after washing your hands.

NOTE: Keep this lotion in a convenient location if you plan to use it all within 2 weeks; otherwise, store it in a glass jar in a cool, dark place.

CONGESTION

Often caused by allergies or experienced alongside common cold symptoms, congestion prevents you from breathing comfortably. Aromatherapy treatments help by thinning out mucus and promoting an open airway.

Caraway Seed–May Chang Shower Steam

MAKES 1 TREATMENT

Potent caraway seed and may chang essential oils combine with your shower's steam to deliver quick relief from congestion.

6 drops may chang essential oil
3 drops caraway seed essential oil

1. Apply the essential oils to a folded washcloth and position it on the shower floor, opposite the area where you stand.
2. Enjoy a hot, steamy shower and breathe deeply while your sinuses open.
3. Repeat the treatment once or twice daily while dealing with congestion.

SUBSTITUTION TIP: If you don't have these essential oils on hand, use 9 drops of eucalyptus (any species) or peppermint essential oil instead.

Copaiba–Spanish Sage Vapor

MAKES 1 TREATMENT

Copaiba and Spanish sage essential oils work together to open your airway. This is a pungent-smelling treatment, but it provides quick relief.

2 cups near-boiling water
1 drop copaiba essential oil
1 drop Spanish sage essential oil

1. Pour the hot water into a large bowl, and then add the essential oils.
2. Place a box of tissues nearby.
3. Sit comfortably in front of the bowl and drape a towel over your head and the bowl, creating a tent that concentrates the steam and vapors.
4. Emerge to blow your nose or breathe cool air as needed.
5. Try to spend 10 minutes with the treatment, then repeat it once or twice daily while you are recovering.

Soothing Spruce-Yuzu Massage

MAKES 1 FLUID OUNCE (2 TABLESPOONS)

Spruce and yuzu essential oils target bacteria while offering a clean, bracing fragrance that improves your mood while helping you breathe better.

2 tablespoons sweet almond oil
3 drops spruce essential oil
6 drops yuzu essential oil

1. In a small bottle or jar with a lid, combine the almond oil and essential oils. Shake well to blend.
2. With your fingertips or a cotton ball, apply ½ teaspoon of the blend to your chest and throat.
3. Repeat two or three times daily, until recovered.

SUBSTITUTION TIP: If you plan to spend time in the sun, replace the yuzu essential oil with 2 drops of peppermint or 4 drops of spearmint essential oil.

PREFERENCE TIP: Add an additional drop of spruce for a more woodsy scent or an additional 2 drops of yuzu for a more citrusy scent.

FEVER

While a fever is an expression of your body's natural defense against infection, it can make you feel quite uncomfortable. Aromatherapy treatments bring relief, but use good judgment by consulting your doctor to determine when medical intervention might be necessary.

Aromatic Eucalyptus Sponge Bath

MAKES 1 TREATMENT

Cool eucalyptus essential oil brings rapid relief from a fever's heat. Adults can use lemon eucalyptus or *Eucalyptus globulus*; seniors and children tolerate *Eucalyptus radiata* better.

2 cups ice-cold water

2 drops eucalyptus essential oil

1. In a large bowl, combine the cold water and essential oil. Soak a washcloth or body sponge in the mixture and wring it out so that it doesn't drip.

2. Run the washcloth or sponge across the forehead, the back of the neck, the armpits, and the chest. Wet the washcloth again when it becomes warm and reapply.

3. Repeat every 3 or 4 hours.

Cool Spearmint Compress

MAKES 1 TREATMENT

Bracing spearmint essential oil combines with cold water to bring comfort and help cool your fever.

½ cup distilled water

2 ice cubes

2 drops spearmint essential oil

1. In a small bowl, pour the water over the ice cubes, and then add the essential oil.
2. Soak a folded washcloth in the solution, and then place it on your forehead. Top the washcloth with a folded hand towel to catch any drips.
3. Leave the compress in place for 15 minutes.
4. Repeat as needed.

Cooling Peppermint Body Wrap

MAKES 1 TREATMENT

Refreshing peppermint essential oil combines with water and a clean twin sheet to create a cooling body wrap that helps bring body temperature down.

2 cups ice-cold water

2 drops peppermint essential oil

1. In a large bowl or basin, combine the cold water and essential oil.
2. Place a folded sheet in the bowl and allow it to absorb the water. Flip the sheet over to ensure that both sides are coated.
3. Wring out any excess water, and then unfold the sheet. Wrap it around your entire body, ensuring that the sheet makes contact with the skin.
4. Relax while sitting or lying on a few towels. Leave the wrap in place for at least 15 minutes, then repeat two or three times over the course of a day.

FIBROMYALGIA

Fibromyalgia brings several distressing symptoms with it, including muscle pain, fatigue, and headaches. Aromatherapy helps by soothing the discomfort while addressing stress and improving your emotional state.

Eucalyptus, Juniper, and Geranium Lotion

MAKES ABOUT 8 FLUID OUNCES (1 CUP)

Penetrating eucalyptus, woody juniper, and fragrant geranium essential oils combine to ease discomfort and bolster your immune system while promoting a positive mood.

8 fluid ounces (1 cup) unscented body lotion
16 drops geranium essential oil
8 drops eucalyptus essential oil (any species)
8 drops juniper essential oil

1. In a medium bowl, combine the lotion and the essential oils. Whisk to blend thoroughly, and then transfer the lotion to a medium jar with a lid or back into the empty lotion container.

2. Apply 1 teaspoon of the blend to your hands, arms, shoulders, and other body parts as desired, using a little more or less as needed.

3. Repeat as often as you like throughout each day, especially after washing your hands.

NOTE: Keep this lotion in a convenient location if you plan to use it all within 2 weeks; otherwise, store it in a glass bottle or jar in a cool, dark place.

Minty Lemon-Lavender Temple Rub

MAKES 150 ROLL-ON TREATMENTS

Brisk peppermint and bright lemon essential oils come together with a touch of lavender essential oil to ease pain and stress while offering an uplifting scent.

12 drops peppermint essential oil
20 drops lemon essential oil
20 drops lavender essential oil

1. In a small bottle, preferably with a roll-on applicator, combine the essential oils. Shake well to blend.
2. With your fingertips or the roller, apply 1 drop of the blend to each of your temples. This treatment can also be applied to sore spots.
3. Repeat as needed.

NOTE: Keep the bottle in a convenient location if you plan to use it up within a few weeks; otherwise, store it in a cool, dark place for up to a year.

Spicy Frankincense-Helichrysum Balm

MAKES ABOUT 4 FLUID OUNCES (½ CUP)

Clove bud, frankincense, and helichrysum essential oils offer analgesic properties that target pain and help relax tight muscle fibers.

¼ cup shea butter
2 tablespoons coconut oil, melted
1 tablespoon beeswax, melted
1 tablespoon sweet almond oil
20 drops clove bud essential oil
12 drops frankincense essential oil
12 drops helichrysum essential oil

1. In a small bowl, combine the shea butter, coconut oil, beeswax, almond oil, and essential oils. Whisk to blend thoroughly.
2. Pour the blend into a small jar with a lid and allow it to cool completely before capping.
3. Apply a pea-sized amount of the balm to each painful point, and massage the area, using light strokes.
4. Repeat once or twice daily, using a little more or less as needed to bring relief.

HALITOSIS

Spicy food, sinus infections, and dry mouth are a few of the many things that can lead to halitosis. Aromatherapy treatments work wonders for bad breath and cost far less than their commercial counterparts.

Citrus–Clove Bud Breath Drops

MAKES 150 TREATMENTS

Sweet orange, grapefruit, and clove bud essential oils combine to target bacteria and leave you with fresh-smelling breath.

1 tablespoon fractionated coconut oil
2 drops grapefruit essential oil
2 drops sweet orange essential oil
1 drop clove bud essential oil

1. In a small bottle with an orifice reducer, combine the coconut oil and essential oils. Shake well to blend.
2. Apply 1 drop of the blend to the underside of your tongue directly from the bottle, being careful not to touch the bottle to your mouth.
3. Repeat as needed to keep bad breath at bay.

NOTE: Keep in a convenient location if you plan to use it up within a few weeks; otherwise, store it in a cool, dark place for up to a year.

SUBSTITUTION TIP: If you prefer a minty scent, replace the citrus and clove bud essential oils with 5 drops of spearmint oil.

Lavender Mouthwash

MAKES 4 FLUID OUNCES (½ CUP)

Lavender essential oil makes short work of bacteria, leaving your breath with a pleasant fragrance. If the flavor of lavender doesn't appeal to you, this mouthwash can also be made with lemon or spearmint oil.

7 tablespoons distilled water
1 tablespoon brandy
4 drops lavender essential oil

1. In a small bottle or jar with a lid, combine the water, brandy, and essential oil. Shake well to blend, and then shake again before each use.
2. Swish your mouth with ½ tablespoon of the mouthwash for 30 seconds to 1 minute, being careful not to swallow. Spit out when finished.
3. Repeat two or three times daily.

Lavender-Spearmint Breath Spray

MAKES 4 FLUID OUNCES (½ CUP)

Lavender and spearmint essential oils kill bacteria while leaving you with fresh, fragrant breath. You can replace the vodka in this recipe with additional distilled water, if you'd prefer an alcohol-free breath spray.

7 tablespoons distilled water
1 tablespoon unflavored vodka
1 drop lavender essential oil
3 drops spearmint essential oil
3 drops liquid stevia

1. In a small bottle with a fine-mist spray top, combine the water, vodka, essential oils, and stevia. Shake well to blend, and then shake again before each use.
2. Apply 1 spritz to the inside of your mouth.
3. Repeat as often as needed to keep breath smelling fresh.

LARYNGITIS AND SORE THROAT

A bacterial infection can leave you with a sore throat, and an evening spent cheering loudly for your favorite team can cause inflammation in your voice box, resulting in laryngitis. Whatever the case, aromatherapy helps by soothing the pain and inflammation and by targeting any bacterial infection.

Lavender-Marjoram Sore Throat Spray

MAKES ABOUT 4 FLUID OUNCES (½ CUP)

Soothing lavender and marjoram combine with sea salt to ease pain, minimize inflammation, and kill bacteria.

½ cup warm water
½ teaspoon sea salt
4 drops marjoram essential oil
2 drops lavender essential oil

1. In a small bottle with a fine-mist spray top, combine the water, salt, and essential oils. Shake well to blend, and then shake again before each use.
2. Apply 2 to 3 spritzes to the back of your throat.
3. Repeat hourly, or as often as needed.

Lavender-Lemon Gargle

MAKES 8 FLUID OUNCES (1 CUP)

Refreshing lemon and soothing lavender essential oils offer antiseptic and analgesic properties; they help bring comfort while killing bacteria and promoting healing.

1 cup less 2 tablespoons distilled water
2 tablespoons unflavored vodka
3 drops lemon essential oil
2 drops lavender essential oil

1. In a medium bottle or jar with a lid, combine the water, vodka, and essential oils. Shake well to blend, and then shake again before each use.
2. Pour 1 tablespoon of the blend into a glass, and then gargle for 30 seconds, being careful not to swallow. Spit out when finished.
3. Repeat two or three times daily, until recovered.

Soothing Bergamot-Lavender Neck Wrap

MAKES 1 TREATMENT

Fragrant bergamot and lavender essential oils combine with potent tea tree essential oil to provide comfort while delivering a powerful antibacterial punch.

2 cups hot tap water
3 drops lavender essential oil
2 drops bergamot essential oil
1 drop tea tree essential oil

1. In a large bowl, combine the water and essential oils. Soak a soft cloth in the water and wring it out.
2. Wrap the cloth securely around your neck and cover it with a second towel to hold the heat in. Remove the wrap before it cools completely.
3. Repeat as often as you like.

PINKEYE

Also known as conjunctivitis, pinkeye is normally caused by the same viruses that send colds, sore throats, and other illnesses around schools and communities. Aromatherapy treatments help ease the itch while also helping stop the virus, without actually touching the eye.

Cool Chamomile Compress
MAKES 1 TREATMENT

Chamomile offers antiseptic and anti-inflammatory action, but it is milder than other pinkeye treatments. If you feel a telltale itch in your eye but don't yet have full-blown conjunctivitis, this is a good remedy to try.

¼ cup distilled water

3 drops Roman or German chamomile essential oil

1. In a shallow bowl, combine the water and essential oil. Fold a washcloth lengthwise and use it to absorb the mixture from the bowl.
2. Wring out any excess moisture, and then lie down with your eyes closed. Lay the compress over both eyes and leave it in place for 15 minutes.
3. Repeat two or three times daily, until the itch is gone.

Lavender–Tea Tree Compress

MAKES 1 TREATMENT

Lavender, tea tree, and *Eucalyptus globulus* essential oils offer a potent antibacterial effect when combined. Be very careful not to get any essential oil into the eye itself.

2 drops *Eucalyptus globulus* essential oil
1 drop lavender essential oil
1 drop tea tree essential oil

1. Fold a paper towel into quarters, and then apply the essential oils, one drop on top of each other.
2. Close the affected eye and place a cotton ball on the eyelid. Position the paper towel on top of the cotton ball.
3. Relax while holding the compress in place. Leave the treatment on the eye for 15 minutes, and then discard.
4. Repeat two or three times daily, until pinkeye is gone.

PREFERENCE TIP: If you would rather not use the compress, blend the essential oils with 4 drops of carrier oil and apply the blend to the cheekbone and side of the nose.

Synergistic Pinkeye Blend

MAKES ½ FLUID OUNCE (1 TABLESPOON)

Tea tree, lemon, frankincense, and cypress essential oils combine with other antiviral, antibacterial, and anti-inflammatory essential oils to stop pinkeye quickly. Do not attempt to apply the essential oils directly to eye tissue.

1 tablespoon fractionated coconut oil
9 drops lemon essential oil
9 drops tea tree essential oil
4 drops frankincense essential oil
4 drops helichrysum essential oil
4 drops lavender essential oil
2 drops cypress essential oil
2 drops *Eucalyptus globulus* essential oil
2 drops lemongrass essential oil

1. In a small bottle or jar with a lid, combine the coconut oil and the essential oils. Shake well to blend.
2. Carefully apply 1 drop of the blend to the top of the cheekbone, directly beneath the affected eye. Apply 1 more drop to the side of the nose, on the same side as the affected eye.
3. Repeat two or three times daily, until pinkeye is gone.

SINUSITIS

When sinuses become inflamed and irritated, chronic congestion and discomfort result. Aromatherapy addresses pain, congestion, inflammation, and infection, often eliminating the need for potentially toxic medicines. If pain worsens or symptoms persist despite your best efforts, see your doctor for something stronger.

Eucalyptus-Spearmint Vapor
MAKES 1 TREATMENT

Eucalyptus and spearmint essential oils work together to clear sinuses and kill bacteria, while the warm steam moisturizes your sinuses.

2 cups near-boiling water
1 drop eucalyptus essential oil (any species)
1 drop spearmint essential oil

1. Pour the hot water into a large bowl, and then add the essential oils. Place a box of tissues nearby.
2. Sit comfortably in front of the bowl and drape a towel over your head and the bowl, creating a tent that concentrates the steamy vapors. Emerge to blow your nose or breathe cool air as needed.
3. Try to spend 10 minutes with the treatment, then repeat it once or twice daily while you are recovering.

Synergistic Sinusitis Inhaler

MAKES 1 REUSABLE INHALER

With this handy inhaler, eucalyptus, cedarwood, oregano, and niaouli essential oils combine to clear your sinuses and ease your breathing whenever you take a sniff.

10 drops eucalyptus essential oil
5 drops cedarwood essential oil
5 drops oregano essential oil
3 drops niaouli essential oil

1. In a small bottle or jar with a lid, combine the essential oils. Shake well to blend.
2. Apply the blend to the cotton wick of the aromatherapy inhaler.
3. Hold the inhaler beneath your nose, and inhale slowly through both nostrils to a count of five. Hold your breath for another count of five, and then exhale slowly.
4. Repeat as needed to prevent and soothe symptoms.

SUBSTITUTION TIP: If you don't have an inhaler, you can transfer the blend to a small, dark glass bottle and inhale directly from the bottle, or place 3 drops of the blend in your diffuser.

Synergistic Sinusitis Shower Melts

MAKES 10 MELTS

Eucalyptus, ginger, thyme, and tea tree essential oils combine with the steam from your hot shower to deliver quick relief from symptoms while addressing inflammation and targeting infection.

2½ cups baking soda
½ cup tap water
20 drops ginger essential oil
20 drops eucalyptus essential oil (all species)
20 drops thyme essential oil
20 drops tea tree essential oil

1. Preheat the oven to 350°F and line a standard muffin tin with ten cupcake liners.
2. In a small bowl, combine the baking soda and water. Stir until it forms a thick paste.
3. Evenly divide the paste among the muffin cups. Bake for 20 minutes or until the melts are dried through.
4. Allow the melts to cool completely, and then peel off the paper liners. To each melt add 2 drops of each essential oil. Transfer the melts immediately to several widemouth jars or a large storage container and cover with lids.
5. Place 1 melt in the shower stall just before stepping in. Breathe deeply while you enjoy the fragrant steam.
6. Repeat once or twice daily while sinusitis persists.

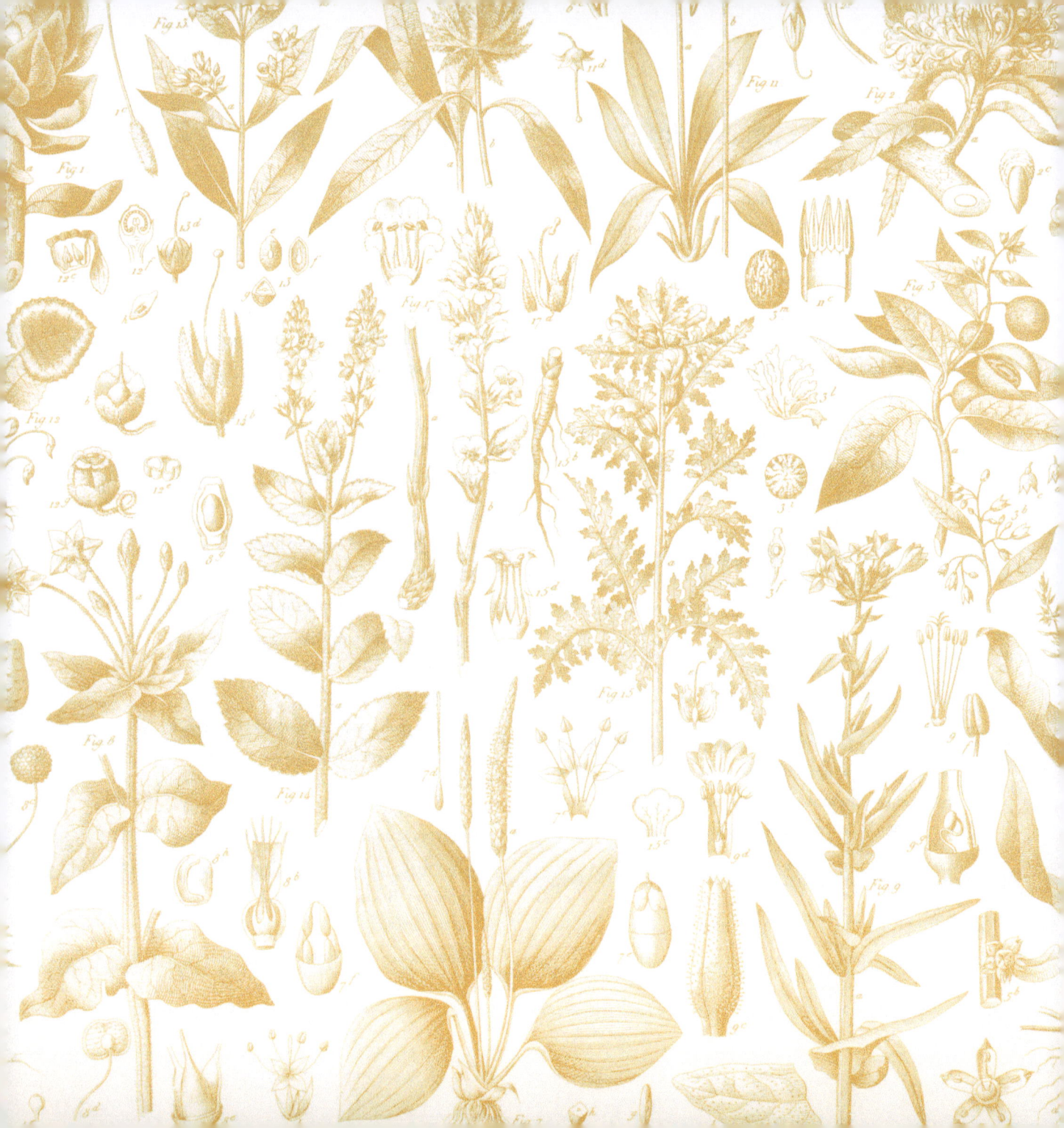

CHAPTER FIVE

ACHES AND PAINS

Backache 156

Cuts and Scrapes 158

Hangover 160

Headache 162

Joint Pain 164

Motion Sickness 166

Muscle Cramps 168

Muscle Soreness 170

Neck Pain 172

Nosebleed 174

Sprain 176

Toothache 178

BACKACHE

Strain, pregnancy, and long hours spent in a seated position are some of the things that can cause a backache. Aromatherapy provides prompt relief.

Cedarwood Massage Oil

MAKES ABOUT 1 FLUID OUNCE (2 TABLESPOONS)

Cedarwood essential oil offers an antispasmodic property that helps muscle fibers relax. It is also a mild sedative that makes for a pleasant massage.

2 tablespoons sweet almond oil
20 drops cedarwood essential oil

1. In a small bottle or jar with a lid, combine the almond oil and essential oil. Shake well to blend.
2. With your fingertips, apply ½ teaspoon of the blend to the achy portion of your back, and massage the area, using light pressure.
3. Repeat as needed.

Cinnamon Leaf–Ginger Salve

MAKES ABOUT 4 FLUID OUNCES (½ CUP)

Spicy cinnamon leaf and ginger essential oils offer analgesic and antispasmodic properties that ease discomfort while providing penetrating warmth. The benzoin essential oil increases pain relief while lending a note of vanilla fragrance to the blend.

¼ cup grapeseed oil
¼ cup sweet almond oil
2 tablespoons beeswax, melted
½ tablespoon vitamin E oil
10 drops ginger essential oil
5 drops cinnamon leaf essential oil
4 drops benzoin essential oil

1. In a small bowl, combine the grapeseed oil, almond oil, beeswax, vitamin E oil, and essential oils. Stir well to blend, and then transfer the mixture to a widemouth glass jar with a lid and allow the mixture to cool completely before capping.

2. Apply ½ teaspoon of the blend to the achy portion of your back and massage the area. Use a little more or less as needed.

3. Repeat two or three times daily, while discomfort persists.

Lavender-Benzoin Bath Salts

MAKES 8 TREATMENTS

Benzoin and lavender essential oils combine with Epsom salts to offer quick pain relief. This blend is strongly sedative, so it's best for times when you don't need to drive or focus on important tasks.

1 tablespoon fractionated coconut oil
16 drops benzoin essential oil
16 drops lavender essential oil
4 cups Epsom salts

1. In a large bowl, combine the coconut oil and essential oils. Add the Epsom salts and stir well to blend. Transfer the bath salts to a large jar with a lid.

2. Draw a hot bath and dissolve ½ cup of the bath salts in the water. Soak in the bath for at least 15 minutes.

3. Repeat as needed.

CUTS AND SCRAPES

Kitchens, backyards, and playgrounds are hot spots for cuts and scrapes. Simple aromatherapy treatments help prevent infection while easing pain and promoting healing.

Lavender Neat Treatment
MAKES 1 TREATMENT

Lavender essential oil soothes minor cuts and scrapes quickly while also serving as a natural antiseptic and helping skin heal faster. Be sure to conduct a patch test before using this undiluted treatment.

1 drop lavender essential oil, or as needed

1. Wash the wound and pat it dry.
2. Apply the lavender essential oil by dripping it directly onto the wound from the bottle, being careful not to touch the bottle to the wound. Use another drop or two if you have a large cut and need additional coverage.

Patchouli-Myrrh Antiseptic Gel

MAKES ABOUT 4 FLUID OUNCES (½ CUP)

Patchouli and myrrh essential oils smell marvelous, but that's not all; they also help minor wounds heal faster while preventing infection.

½ cup aloe vera gel
8 drops myrrh essential oil
6 drops patchouli essential oil

1. In a small bowl, combine the aloe vera and essential oils. Whisk to blend thoroughly, and then transfer the gel to a small jar and cover with the lid.
2. Wash the affected area and gently pat it dry. With your fingertips or a cotton swab, apply a pea-sized amount of the gel to the wound and allow it to melt in.
3. Repeat two or three times daily, as needed.

Tagetes-Rosewood Balm

MAKES ABOUT 2 FLUID OUNCES (¼ CUP)

Tagetes and rosewood essential oils provide analgesic and antiseptic properties that combine to bring relief from pain while helping prevent infection.

2 tablespoons coconut oil, melted
1 tablespoon beeswax, melted
1 tablespoon sweet almond oil
10 drops rosewood essential oil
10 drops tagetes essential oil

1. In a small bowl, combine the coconut oil, beeswax, almond oil, and essential oils. Whisk to blend thoroughly.
2. Pour the blend into a small jar with a lid and allow it to cool completely before capping.
3. Wash the affected area and gently pat it dry. With your fingertips or a cotton swab, apply a pea-sized amount of the balm to the wound and allow it to melt in.
4. Repeat two or three times daily, as needed.

HANGOVER

When you've indulged in a few too many drinks, your pounding head and churning stomach can make it difficult to face the day ahead. Aromatherapy can help by promoting detoxification, restoring your sense of balance, and helping your head feel clearer.

Citrus-Mint Diffusion

MAKES 1 TREATMENT

Cheerful citrus and fresh peppermint essential oils help you clear the cobwebs from your head, plus they provide some relief from nausea.

1 drop lemon essential oil
1 drop peppermint essential oil
1 drop sweet orange essential oil

1. Add the essential oils to your diffuser according to the manufacturer's instructions.
2. Run the diffuser nearby.
3. Repeat as needed throughout the day.

SUBSTITUTION TIP: If you like, try other citrus scents, such as bergamot, lime, grapefruit, or mandarin essential oil in this blend.

Detoxifying Massage Oil

MAKES ABOUT 4 FLUID OUNCES (½ CUP)

Soothing lavender, crisp citrus, and cooling peppermint essential oils combine to cheer you up and support the detoxification process.

½ cup fractionated coconut oil
20 drops lavender essential oil
20 drops lemon essential oil
20 drops mandarin essential oil
20 drops peppermint essential oil

1. In a small bottle or jar with a lid, combine the coconut oil and essential oils. Shake well to blend.
2. Apply 1 teaspoon of the blend to your chest, arms, and shoulders, and lightly massage the areas of application while breathing deeply. Then massage 1 drop of the oil into each of your temples.

Restorative Shower Melts

MAKES 10 MELTS

Bracing basil, soothing patchouli, and comforting lavender, lemon, and peppermint essential oils bring you back to your senses, especially when combined with a hot, steamy shower.

2½ cups baking soda
½ cup tap water
10 drops basil essential oil
20 drops lavender essential oil
20 drops peppermint essential oil
20 drops patchouli essential oil
30 drops lemon essential oil

1. Preheat the oven to 350°F and line a standard muffin tin with ten cupcake liners.
2. In a large bowl, combine the baking soda and water. Stir until it forms a thick paste.
3. Evenly divide the paste among the muffin cups and bake for 20 minutes or until thoroughly dried.
4. Allow the melts to cool completely, and then peel off the paper liners. To each melt add 1 drop of the basil, 2 drops of the lavender, 2 drops of the peppermint, 2 drops of the patchouli, and 3 drops of the lemon essential oils. Transfer the melts to widemouth glass jars or a large storage container and close with lids.
5. Place 1 melt in the shower stall just before stepping in. Breathe deeply while you enjoy the fragrant steam.

HEADACHE

Stress, tension, and dehydration are among the top causes of headaches. Aromatherapy treatments help ease the pain while you determine the root cause of the headache and address it.

Lavender, Marjoram, and Basil Balm for Tension Headaches

MAKES 100 TREATMENTS

Warming basil, marjoram, and lavender essential oils help tight head and neck muscles relax, easing the pain and allowing you to relax.

1 tablespoon fractionated coconut oil
18 drops lavender essential oil
12 drops marjoram essential oil
6 drops basil essential oil

1. In a small bottle, preferably with a roll-on applicator, combine the coconut oil and essential oils. Shake well to blend.
2. With your fingertips or the roller, apply 1 drop to each of your temples, and gently massage the areas while breathing deeply.
3. Apply 2 to 3 drops of the blend to the base of your neck and massage the area. If you can pinpoint any sore spots on your head, apply 1 drop to each of them, as well.

NOTE: Keep in a convenient location if you plan to use it up within a few weeks; otherwise, store it in a cool, dark place for up to a year.

Rosemary, Basil, and Mint Shower Melts for General Headaches
MAKES 10 MELTS

Bracing rosemary, basil, and peppermint essential oils relieve headaches quickly, especially when combined with the steam from your hot shower.

2½ cups baking soda
½ cup tap water
10 drops rosemary essential oil
10 drops basil essential oil
20 drops peppermint essential oil

1. Preheat the oven to 350°F and line a standard muffin tin with ten cupcake liners.
2. In a medium bowl, combine the baking soda and water. Stir into a thick paste.
3. Evenly divide the paste among the muffin cups and bake for 20 minutes or until thoroughly dried.
4. Allow the melts to cool completely, and then peel off the paper liners. To each melt add 1 drop of the rosemary, 1 drop of the basil, and 2 drops of the peppermint essential oils. Transfer the melts immediately to widemouth glass jars or a large storage container and cover with lids.
5. Place 1 melt in the shower stall just before stepping in. Breathe deeply while you enjoy the fragrant steam.
6. Repeat once or twice daily while dealing with headaches.

Rosemary-Eucalyptus Vapor for Sinus Headaches
MAKES 1 TREATMENT

Rosemary and eucalyptus essential oils work together to open your airways, take the pressure off your sinuses, and stop your pain. This is a relaxing treatment, but you'll feel wide awake afterward.

2 cups near-boiling water
1 drop rosemary essential oil
1 drop eucalyptus essential oil (any species)

1. Pour the hot water into a large bowl and then add the essential oils. Place a box of tissues nearby.
2. Sit comfortably in front of the bowl and drape a towel over your head and the bowl, creating a tent that concentrates the steam and vapors. Emerge to blow your nose or breathe cool air as needed.
3. Try to spend 10 minutes with the treatment, and then repeat it once or twice daily while dealing with sinus headaches.

JOINT PAIN

Many conditions can cause joint pain. Once your doctor has determined the cause, you can use aromatherapy treatments alone or alongside medication, physical therapy, and other physician-recommended remedies.

Benzoin Balm

MAKES ABOUT 2 FLUID OUNCES (¼ CUP)

Benzoin essential oil improves circulation and gently warms tissue, helping ease pain and promote healing.

2 tablespoons shea butter
1 tablespoon coconut oil, melted
1 tablespoon hemp oil
40 drops benzoin essential oil

1. In a small bowl, combine the shea butter, coconut oil, hemp oil, and essential oil. Whisk to blend thoroughly, and then transfer the balm to a small jar and cover with a lid.
2. Apply ½ teaspoon of balm to the affected joint, and massage the area, using light pressure and circular motions. Use a little more or less of the balm as needed to cover the painful area.
3. Repeat as often as needed to keep pain to a minimum.

Peppermint-Pine Liniment

MAKES ABOUT 4 FLUID OUNCES (½ CUP)

Brisk peppermint and pine essential oils combine with soothing chamomile essential oil to penetrate deep into tissue, targeting inflammation while encouraging tight, stiff joints to relax.

¼ cup aloe vera gel
2 tablespoons fractionated coconut oil
2 tablespoons rubbing alcohol
40 drops peppermint essential oil
20 drops German or Roman chamomile essential oil
20 drops pine essential oil

1. In a small bowl, combine the aloe vera, coconut oil, rubbing alcohol, and essential oils. Whisk to blend thoroughly, and then transfer the liniment to a small jar and cover with a lid.
2. Apply 1 teaspoon of the liniment to the affected area, using a little more or less as needed.
3. Repeat two or three times daily while joint pain persists.

Spruce Compress

MAKES 1 TREATMENT

Fragrant spruce essential oil is a potent anti-inflammatory agent with cortisone-like effects. When combined with soothing heat, it eases pain quickly.

6 drops fractionated coconut oil
6 drops spruce essential oil

1. In the palm of your hand, combine the coconut oil and essential oil.
2. Apply the blend to the affected joint, and massage the area, using small circular motions.
3. Sit or lie down and cover the affected joint with a warm heating pad, following the manufacturer's instructions for safe use. Leave the heating pad in place for at least 15 minutes.
4. Repeat two or three times daily while pain persists.

MOTION SICKNESS

Queasiness and vomiting make motion sickness unbearable for the sufferer and unpleasant for fellow travelers, as well. Because it can be difficult to stop the symptoms of motion sickness once they begin, it's best to start using these treatments before movement takes place, and to continue using them throughout your journey.

Ginger Inhaler

MAKES 1 REUSABLE INHALER

Ginger is such a reliable remedy for motion sickness that it is often called the *traveler's friend*. This inhaler makes it quick and easy to prevent symptoms on the road and in the air.

12 drops ginger essential oil

1. Apply the essential oil to the wick of an aromatherapy inhaler.
2. Hold the inhaler beneath your nose and inhale slowly through both nostrils to a count of five. Hold your breath for another count of five, and then exhale slowly. Do this six to seven times every 30 minutes or so, beginning an hour before you set off on your journey.
3. Repeat as needed to prevent and soothe symptoms.

SUBSTITUTION TIP: If you don't have an inhaler, you can put the ginger in a small, dark glass bottle and inhale directly from the bottle, or place 3 drops of the ginger essential oil in your diffuser.

Peppermint-Basil Travel Gel

MAKES ABOUT 4 FLUID OUNCES (½ CUP)

If you tend to sweat and feel nauseated while traveling, peppermint, basil, and lavender can help by calming the muscle tissues and cooling the heat.

7 tablespoons aloe vera gel
1 tablespoon fractionated coconut oil
20 drops lavender essential oil
20 drops peppermint essential oil
12 drops basil essential oil

1. In a small bowl, combine the aloe vera, coconut oil, and essential oils. Whisk to blend thoroughly, and then transfer the gel to a small jar with a lid.
2. Apply ½ teaspoon of the gel to the back of your neck about 30 minutes before setting out on your travels.
3. Reapply every hour or so during travel.

Synergistic Traveler's Body Lotion

MAKES ABOUT 8 FLUID OUNCES (1 CUP)

Roman chamomile, ginger, peppermint, and lemon essential oils combine to quell nausea and keep you in a positive mood as you travel.

8 fluid ounces (1 cup) unscented body lotion or hand cream
30 drops ginger essential oil
20 drops lemon essential oil
10 drops peppermint essential oil
10 drops Roman chamomile essential oil

1. In a medium bowl, combine the lotion and essential oils. Whisk to blend thoroughly, and then transfer the lotion to a medium jar with a lid or back into the empty lotion container.
2. Apply 1 teaspoon of the lotion to your hands, arms, neck, and shoulders about 30 minutes before setting out. Use a little more or less as needed, and feel free to apply the lotion to other body parts.
3. Apply another ½ teaspoon or so hourly while traveling, targeting your hands and the back of your neck.

NOTE: Keep this lotion in a convenient location if you plan to use it all within 2 weeks; otherwise, store it in a glass bottle or jar in a cool, dark place.

MUSCLE CRAMPS

Cramps occur when muscles tighten involuntarily. Depleted mineral levels, dehydration, overexercise, and nerve irritation are some causes, so be sure to address these conditions while using aromatherapy treatments to bring relief.

Lavender-Marjoram Compress

MAKES 1 TREATMENT

Lavender and marjoram essential oils combine with soothing heat to promote relaxation while easing the pain that accompanies cramping.

½ teaspoon fractionated coconut oil
3 drops lavender essential oil
2 drops marjoram essential oil

1. In the palm of your hand, combine the coconut oil and the essential oils.
2. Apply the blend to the cramped muscle and massage it in, using deep, firm strokes.
3. Sit or lie down comfortably and cover the cramped muscle with a warm heating pad, following the manufacturer's instructions for safe use. Leave the heating pad in place for at least 15 minutes.
4. Repeat two or three times daily, or as needed.

Minty Lavender-Cypress Gel

MAKES ABOUT 4 FLUID OUNCES (½ CUP)

Peppermint, lavender, and cypress essential oils come together to ease inflammation and help relax tight, cramping muscles.

7 tablespoons aloe vera gel
1 tablespoon fractionated coconut oil
20 drops peppermint essential oil
16 drops cypress essential oil
12 drops lavender essential oil

1. In a small bowl, combine the aloe vera, coconut oil, and essential oils. Whisk to blend thoroughly, and then transfer the gel to a small jar and cover with the lid.
2. Apply 1 teaspoon of the gel to the affected area, using a little more or less as needed.
3. Repeat two or three times daily, or as needed.

NOTE: If you like, you can keep this gel in the refrigerator for an intense cooling sensation upon application; otherwise, store it in a cool, dark place.

Soothing Massage Oil

MAKES 1 FLUID OUNCE (2 TABLESPOONS)

Ginger, cinnamon leaf, and black pepper essential oils warm muscle fibers and encourage them to relax while simultaneously helping you feel less stressed.

2 tablespoons fractionated coconut oil
4 drops black pepper essential oil
4 drops cinnamon leaf essential oil
2 drops ginger essential oil

1. In a small bottle or jar with a lid, combine the coconut oil and essential oils. Shake well to blend.
2. Apply ½ teaspoon of the blend to the area where cramping is present, and massage it in, using deep, firm strokes.
3. Repeat two or three times daily, or as needed.

MUSCLE SORENESS

Repetitive or strenuous activity often leads to sore muscles. The discomfort may make you want to reach for an over-the-counter pain reliever, but give aromatherapy a try instead.

Benzoin–Black Pepper Muscle Balm

MAKES ABOUT 4 FLUID OUNCES (½ CUP)

Benzoin and black pepper essential oils improve circulation and provide a warming sensation, helping ease your discomfort so that you can rest or get on with your day.

2 tablespoons beeswax, melted
2 tablespoons coconut oil, melted
2 tablespoons shea butter
1 tablespoon avocado oil
1 tablespoon sweet almond oil
40 drops benzoin essential oil
20 drops black pepper essential oil

1. In a small bowl, combine the beeswax, coconut oil, shea butter, avocado oil, almond oil, and essential oils. Whisk to blend thoroughly, and then transfer the balm to a small jar and cover with the lid.

2. Apply 1 teaspoon of balm to the sore area, using a little more or less as needed.

3. Repeat every 2 or 3 hours to stay comfortable until recovered.

Fir Needle Gel

MAKES ABOUT 4 FLUID OUNCES (½ CUP)

Fir needle stops muscle pain quickly, and its bright, uplifting aroma helps you deal with any accompanying mental fatigue.

7 tablespoons aloe vera gel
40 drops fir needle essential oil

1. In a small bowl, combine the aloe vera and essential oil. Whisk to blend thoroughly, and then transfer the gel to a small jar and cover with a lid.
2. Apply 1 teaspoon of the gel to the affected area, using a little more or less as needed.
3. Repeat two or three times daily.

NOTE: If you like, you can keep this gel in the refrigerator for an intense cooling sensation upon application; otherwise, store it in a cool, dark place.

Synergistic Pain-Relief Compress

MAKES 1 TREATMENT

Warm ginger, cinnamon leaf, and cajuput essential oils combine with comforting German chamomile essential oil and soothing heat to provide deep, penetrating relief for sore muscles.

1 teaspoon avocado oil
4 drops cinnamon leaf essential oil
3 drops cajuput essential oil
3 drops German chamomile essential oil
2 drops ginger essential oil

1. In the palm of your hand, combine the avocado oil and essential oils.
2. Apply the blend to the sore area, and massage it in. (For a larger area, double or triple the ingredients, and combine in a jar.)
3. Relax and cover the sore area with a warm heating pad, following the manufacturer's instructions for safe use. Leave the heating pad in place for at least 15 minutes.
4. Repeat once or twice daily, until recovered.

NECK PAIN

Stress, poor ergonomics, and muscle strain are among the chief causes of neck pain. Aromatherapy treatments offer quick, nontoxic relief by reducing inflammation, promoting relaxation, and dissipating stress.

Juniper-Peppermint Gel

MAKES ABOUT 4 FLUID OUNCES (½ CUP)

Juniper berry and peppermint essential oils stop pain quickly while targeting inflammation and helping dispel unpleasant emotions such as stress and anxiety.

7 tablespoons aloe vera gel
1 tablespoon fractionated coconut oil
20 drops juniper berry essential oil
20 drops peppermint essential oil

1. In a small bowl, combine the aloe vera, coconut oil, and essential oils. Whisk to blend thoroughly, and then transfer the gel to a small jar and cover with a lid.
2. Apply ½ teaspoon of the blend to the back of your neck, and massage the area, using deep up-and-down strokes.
3. Repeat two or three times daily.

NOTE: If you like, you can keep this gel in the refrigerator for an intense cooling sensation upon application; otherwise, store it in a cool, dark place.

Marjoram–Fir Needle Compress

MAKES 1 TREATMENT

Relaxing marjoram and fir needle essential oils combine with heat to improve circulation, soothe spasms, and stop pain quickly. The uplifting fragrance helps with stress, too.

½ teaspoon fractionated coconut oil
1 drop fir needle essential oil
1 drop marjoram essential oil

1. In the palm of your hand, combine the coconut oil and essential oils.
2. Apply the blend to the back of your neck, and gently massage the area.
3. Sit or lie down and cover your neck area with a warm heating pad, following the manufacturer's instructions for safe use. Leave the heating pad in place for at least 15 minutes.
4. Repeat two or three times daily, or as needed.

Synergistic Pain-Relief Blend

MAKES ABOUT 12 TREATMENTS

Warming basil, cool peppermint, lavender, cypress, and marjoram essential oils combine to increase blood flow and stop pain while targeting stress, muscle tension, spasms, and cramping.

2 tablespoons sweet almond oil
12 drops cypress essential oil
12 drops lavender essential oil
6 drops basil essential oil
6 drops marjoram essential oil
6 drops peppermint essential oil

1. In a small bottle or jar with a lid, combine the almond oil and essential oils. Shake well to blend.
2. With your fingers, apply ½ teaspoon of the blend to the base of your skull and the back and sides of your neck. Massage the area, using deep, kneading motions.
3. Repeat every 2 or 3 hours, or as often as needed.

NOSEBLEED

Dry air and trauma are two main contributors to nosebleeds. As long as your nose hasn't been broken, aromatherapy can likely help. If you have chronic nosebleeds, consult with your doctor to rule out an underlying cause.

Cypress Nasal Compress
MAKES 1 TREATMENT

Cypress essential oil is a vasoconstrictor, meaning that it narrows the blood vessels. This narrowing effect helps stop a nosebleed.

1 drop cypress essential oil

1. Apply the cypress essential oil to a facial tissue.
2. Lie down or tilt your head back, tuck the tissue into the affected nostril, and pinch your nostrils slightly together while breathing through your mouth. Leave the compress in place for 15 minutes, even if it seems like the bleeding has stopped.

Lavender Nasal Salve

MAKES ½ FLUID OUNCE (1 TABLESPOON)

If your nosebleeds are occurring because of overexposure to dry air, this salve can help. The lavender essential oil heals the nasal lining, while the coconut oil provides deep moisture where it's needed most.

1 tablespoon fractionated coconut oil
10 drops lavender essential oil

1. In a small bottle, combine the coconut oil and essential oil. Shake to blend.
2. With a cotton swab, apply 1 drop of the salve to the inner lining of the nose, focusing on the central portion that divides the nostrils.
3. Repeat once or twice daily, as long as dry air conditions are present.

Lemon-Lavender Nasal Compress

MAKES 1 TREATMENT

Lemon essential oil is a hemostatic, meaning it encourages blood to clot faster. Lavender essential oil and an ice pack applied to the back of the neck soothe pain and encourage faster healing.

2 drops tap water
1 drop lemon essential oil
4 drops lavender essential oil

1. Moisten a cotton ball with the water and add the lemon essential oil. Insert the cotton ball into the affected nostril.
2. Apply the lavender essential oil directly to the back of your neck.
3. Wrap an ice pack in a towel and lie down with the ice pack under your neck. Rest for at least 15 minutes, and then remove the cotton ball.
4. Repeat as needed.

SPRAIN

Painful, swollen ligament injuries occur when trauma causes a joint to move in a direction other than the one that it's meant to move. When combined with traditional first-aid measures, including rest, ice, compression, and elevation, aromatherapy eases pain and helps you heal faster. Seek medical attention if you suspect you've broken a bone, or if swelling and pain fail to decrease after a day or two.

Minty Helichrysum-Chamomile Compress

MAKES 1 TREATMENT

A soothing combination of peppermint, helichrysum, and chamomile essential oils brings quick pain relief and promotes healing, while a cold compress helps minimize swelling.

4 drops helichrysum essential oil
2 drops carrier oil of choice
2 drops German or Roman chamomile
2 drops peppermint essential oil

1. In the palm of your hand, combine the essential oils.
2. Apply the blend to the sprain site, and gently massage the area. (Use another drop or two of each oil if you need to cover a large area.)
3. Wrap an ice pack in a hand towel, and then elevate the injury before laying the compress over the sprained area.
4. Leave the compress in place for 30 minutes, removing it periodically if your skin starts to feel uncomfortably numb.
5. Repeat every hour or so during the first day to help the swelling come down.

Synergistic First-Aid Gel and Sprain Compress

MAKES ABOUT 4 FLUID OUNCES (½ CUP)

Ginger, helichrysum, and lavender essential oils work together to stop pain and promote healing. On the first day of treatment, use this blend with an ice pack. Do not apply heat on the first day of sprain treatment. On the second and third days, you can alternate between using a heating pad and applying an ice pack.

7 tablespoons aloe vera gel
1 tablespoon fractionated coconut oil
36 drops lavender essential oil
24 drops helichrysum essential oil
12 drops ginger essential oil

1. In a small bowl, combine the aloe vera, coconut oil, and essential oils. Whisk to blend thoroughly, and then transfer the gel to a small jar and cover with the lid.

2. Apply 1 teaspoon of the gel to the affected area, using a little more or less as needed. Cover the area either with an ice pack or a warm heating pad, following the manufacturer's instructions for safe use. Leave the ice pack or heating pad in place for 15 to 20 minutes.

3. Reapply the gel each time you apply a heating pad or ice pack, ensuring that you keep the injury elevated as much as possible.

NOTE: You can keep this gel in the refrigerator; otherwise, store it in a cool, dark place.

Synergistic Healing Balm

MAKES ABOUT 4 FLUID OUNCES (½ CUP)

Lavender, marjoram, and peppermint essential oils help improve circulation while providing pain relief. This balm is ideal for application under compression bandages, as long as no broken skin is present.

¼ cup shea butter
2 tablespoons coconut oil, melted
2 tablespoons sweet almond oil
36 drops lavender essential oil
24 drops marjoram essential oil
12 drops peppermint essential oil

1. In a small bowl, combine the shea butter, coconut oil, almond oil, and essential oils. Whisk to blend thoroughly, and then transfer the balm to a small jar and cover with the lid.

2. Apply 1 teaspoon of the balm to the sprain, using a little more or less as needed to cover as needed. Massage the balm in using light, gentle strokes, and then cover with a compression bandage.

3. Repeat each time you rebandage the sprain.

TOOTHACHE

The best practice is to get to the dentist as soon as possible when suffering from a toothache, but it can take time to obtain an appointment. While you're waiting, aromatherapy treatments can provide you with much-needed relief.

Chamomile-Peppermint Compress

MAKES 1 TREATMENT

Soothing chamomile and peppermint essential oils combine to ease dental pain quickly. A cotton ball holds the treatment in place. There's no need to rinse after this treatment; the small amount of oil in your mouth gets absorbed by the oral tissues.

6 drops distilled water
1 drop peppermint essential oil
1 drop Roman chamomile essential oil

1. In a small dish, combine the water and essential oils. Saturate a cotton ball in the blend.
2. Apply the cotton ball to the affected tooth and keep it in place for 10 to 15 minutes.
3. Repeat as needed to keep pain to a minimum.

Clove Bud Neat Treatment

MAKES 1 TREATMENT

Clove bud essential oil is such an effective numbing agent that it has a time-honored place in the history of dentistry. Just a drop delivers immediate relief. There's no need to worry about putting this in your mouth; your oral tissues will absorb it.

1 drop clove bud essential oil

1. With a pipette or glass dropper, apply the essential oil directly to the painful tooth.
2. Breathe through your mouth to prevent saliva from washing the treatment away while it is absorbed. You should be able to return to normal nose breathing within a minute or two.
3. Repeat two or three times daily, as needed.

Synergistic Toothache Blend

MAKES ABOUT 1 FLUID OUNCE (2 TABLESPOONS)

If tooth pain occurs because a wisdom tooth is erupting, or you want to try something other than pain medication following an uncomfortable dental procedure, a topical application of clove bud, chamomile, and lemon essential oils can often bring comfort.

2 tablespoons sweet almond oil
90 drops German chamomile essential oil
30 drops clove bud essential oil
30 drops lemon essential oil

1. In a small bottle or jar with a lid, combine the almond oil and essential oils. Shake well to blend.
2. With your fingertips, apply ½ teaspoon of the blend to the outside portion of your cheek and/or jawline where pain is greatest. Massage well until the blend is absorbed.

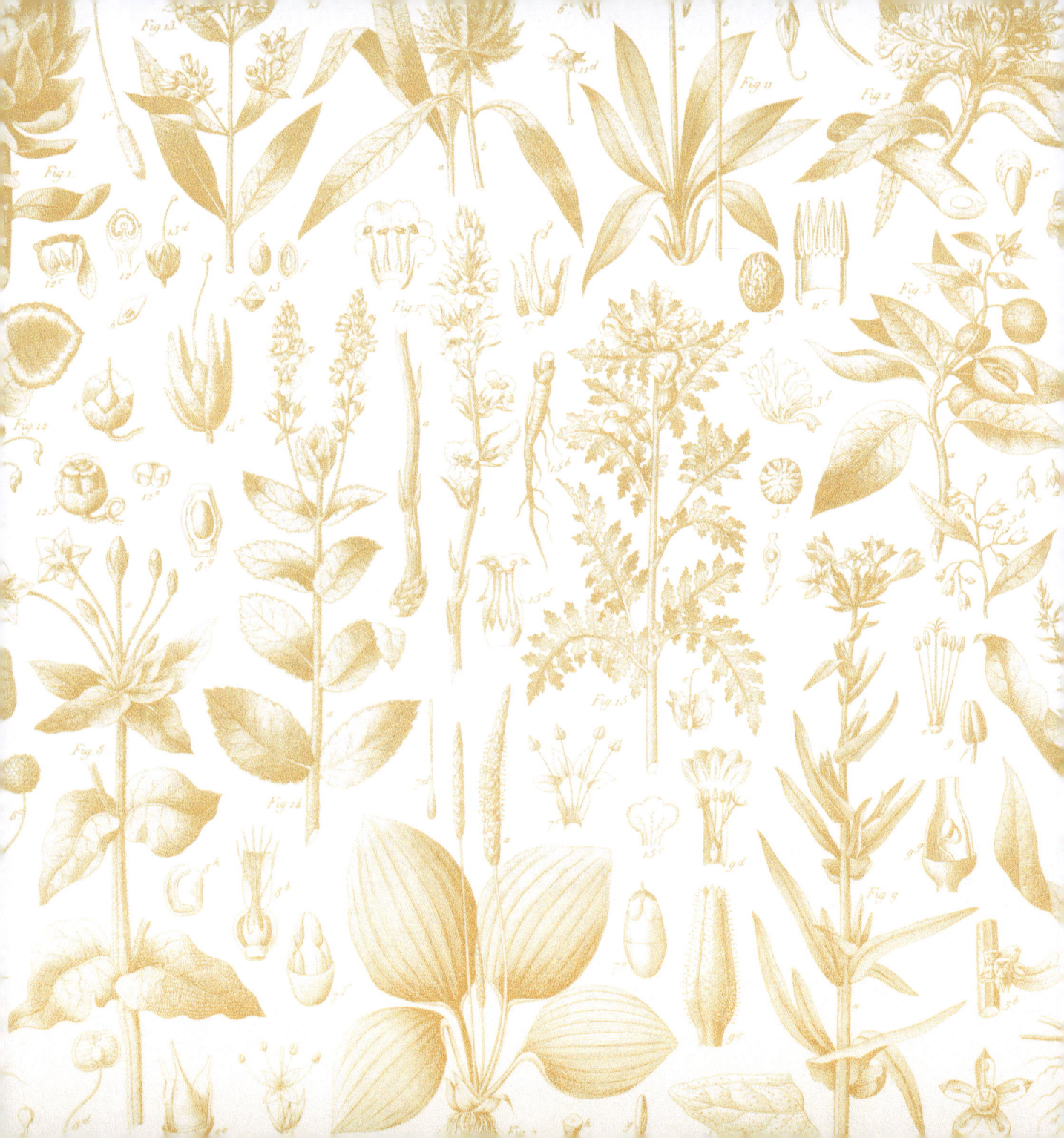

CHAPTER SIX

SKIN CONDITIONS AND CONCERNS

Blisters   182

Boils   184

Burns   186

Chapped Lips   188

Cold Sores   190

Diaper Rash (for Infants)   192

Eczema   194

Hives   196

Psoriasis   198

Stretch Marks   200

Warts   202

BLISTERS

Aromatherapy treatments are ideal for blisters caused by friction, but if you've been burned or have a large, painful blister, you should see your doctor before using essential oils.

Lavender Neat Treatment
MAKES 1 TREATMENT

Lavender is one of a few essential oils that can be applied neat. Its analgesic and antiseptic properties combine to bring healing and quick relief from pain. Be sure to conduct a patch test before using this neat treatment.

1 drop lavender essential oil

1. Wash the affected area, and then pat it dry.
2. Apply the lavender essential oil by dripping it directly onto the blister from the bottle, being careful not to touch the bottle to the blister.
3. Repeat the treatment every 3 or 4 hours, or as needed.

Myrrh-Helichrysum Compress

MAKES 1 TREATMENT

Myrrh and helichrysum essential oils combine with cold water to bring rapid pain relief while providing protection from infection.

½ cup distilled water
2 ice cubes
1 drop helichrysum essential oil
1 drop myrrh essential oil

1. In a small bowl, pour the water over the ice cubes, and then add the essential oils.
2. Soak a folded washcloth in the solution, and then place it on the blister. Top the washcloth with a folded hand towel to catch any drips.
3. Leave the compress in place for 15 minutes. Allow your skin to air-dry after removal.
4. Repeat as needed.

PREFERENCE TIP: If you want to treat your blistered foot to a healing footbath instead, make this treatment in a shallow basin large enough to accommodate your foot. Double or triple the ingredients as needed. Soak your foot for 15 minutes, and then allow it to air-dry.

Roman Chamomile–Tea Tree Balm

MAKES ½ FLUID OUNCE (1 TABLESPOON)

Roman chamomile and tea tree essential oils combine to offer quick pain relief and protection from infection. If your blister has popped, this is a good remedy to apply.

1 tablespoon fractionated coconut oil
10 drops Roman chamomile essential oil
10 drops tea tree essential oil

1. In a small bottle with a lid, combine the coconut oil and essential oils. Shake well to blend.
2. Apply the blend by dripping 1 or 2 drops directly onto the blister, being careful not to touch the bottle to the blister.
3. Repeat the treatment every 3 or 4 hours, or as needed.

BOILS

Red, painful, and inflamed, boils often develop along the hairline, on the buttocks, in the groin area, or under the arms. If a boil worsens, enlarges, or begins to develop red streaks, seek medical attention, and save aromatherapy treatment for another time.

Chamomile-Helichrysum Gel
MAKES 1 FLUID OUNCE (2 TABLESPOONS)

Comforting chamomile and helichrysum essential oils combine with aloe vera gel to soothe and heal painful boils. You can use this blend on boils that have drained, as well as on those that are still developing.

2 tablespoons aloe vera gel
6 drops German or Roman chamomile essential oil
4 drops helichrysum essential oil

1. In a small bowl, combine the aloe vera and essential oils. Whisk to blend thoroughly, and then transfer the blend to a small jar with a lid.
2. With a cotton swab, apply 1 drop of the blend to the boil.
3. Repeat as often as needed, especially after bathing or showering.

NOTE: If you like, you can keep this gel in the refrigerator for an intense cooling sensation upon application; otherwise, store it in a cool, dark place.

Synergistic Hot Compress

MAKES 1 TREATMENT

Antibacterial juniper berry, chamomile, tea tree, and lavender essential oils combine to create a strong disinfectant that kills germs while putting a stop to pain and swelling. Hot water opens the pores to speed delivery.

½ cup hot tap water
2 drops lavender essential oil
2 drops tea tree essential oil
1 drop juniper berry essential oil
1 drop Roman or German chamomile essential oil

1. In a small bowl, combine the hot water and essential oils.
2. Soak a folded washcloth in the blend and apply it to the boil. Top the washcloth with a folded hand towel to catch any drips.
3. Leave the compress in place for 15 minutes.
4. Repeat two or three times daily, until the boil is gone.

Tea Tree Steam Treatment

MAKES 1 TREATMENT

Tea tree essential oil and steam from a hot towel work together to kill bacteria and speed healing. Be sure that the water you use is steaming, but not so hot that it scalds your skin.

1 drop tea tree essential oil
1 cup near-boiling water

1. With a cotton swab, apply the tea tree essential oil to the boil.
2. Dip a folded washcloth into the hot water and wring it out. Gently place the cloth over the boil, and, without applying pressure, keep it in place until the heat dissipates.
3. Repeat two or three times daily, until the boil is gone.

BURNS

Aromatherapy treatments are appropriate for first-degree burns. If you have a large second-degree burn with blisters, or if a third-degree burn has damaged skin and underlying tissue, seek emergency medical treatment.

Chamomile–Tea Tree Balm
MAKES ABOUT 1 FLUID OUNCE (2 TABLESPOONS)

Chamomile and tea tree essential oils can help older burns heal faster while preventing infection.

2 tablespoons fractionated coconut oil
12 drops Roman or German chamomile essential oil
6 drops tea tree essential oil

1. In a small bottle or jar with a lid, combine the coconut oil and essential oils. Shake well to blend.
2. With a cotton swab, apply 1 drop of the blend to the burn.
3. Repeat two or three times daily, until recovered.

Lavender-Geranium Compress

MAKES 1 TREATMENT

Lavender and geranium essential oils come together with healing aloe and a cold compress to relieve pain and improve healing.

½ **teaspoon aloe vera gel**
2 drops lavender essential oil
1 drop geranium essential oil

1. In a small bowl, combine the aloe vera and essential oils. Stir well to blend.
2. Apply the entire blend to the burn. Wrap the ice pack in a soft cloth and lay it over the burn. Leave the pack in place for 5 to 10 minutes, or longer if needed.
3. Repeat the treatment every 2 or 3 hours, up to three times daily.

Lavender Neat Treatment

MAKES 1 TREATMENT

When applied immediately after you've gotten a minor burn, lavender essential oil helps stop pain and speed healing. Be sure to conduct a patch test before using this neat treatment.

1 drop lavender essential oil

1. Gently wash the burn with cold water, and then pat it dry.
2. Drop the essential oil onto the burn.
3. Repeat every 2 or 3 hours, until pain stops.

CHAPPED LIPS

Because your lips don't contain oil glands, they chap more easily than the rest of your skin. Luxurious aromatherapy treatments help heal and moisturize your lips, and they don't contain any harmful petroleum products, as many commercial lip balms do.

Basic Lip Balm

MAKES 1 FLUID OUNCE (2 TABLESPOONS)

Lips can chap and crack easily, especially during extreme weather. This lip balm uses moisturizing coconut oil to protect and soothe your lips.

1 tablespoon grated beeswax
1 tablespoon coconut oil
5 drops of your favorite essential oil

1. Fill a small saucepan with a few inches of water and set it on the stove over low heat. Fit a small metal or glass bowl into the pan so that it sits just above the water. Put the beeswax in the bowl and wait until it melts. Then stir in the coconut oil.

2. Remove the bowl from the heat and stir in the essential oil, using a metal spoon or glass stirring rod.

3. Transfer the mixture to a small jar with a lid and allow the lip balm to harden before capping.

4. Smooth over your lips with a finger two or three times per day.

NOTE: Store the container in a cool, dark location for up to a year. Or carry it with you so it's handy. It will last for about 6 months.

PREFERENCE TIP: If you prefer a harder texture for your lip balm, double the amount of beeswax in the recipe.

Lavender-Peppermint Lip Salve

MAKES 100 TREATMENTS

Refreshing peppermint and healing lavender essential oils combine with fractionated coconut oil to soothe irritation while offering a deep, moisturizing effect.

1 tablespoon fractionated coconut oil
8 drops lavender essential oil
1 drop peppermint essential oil

1. In a small bottle, preferably with a roll-on applicator, combine the coconut oil and essential oils. Shake well to blend.
2. With your fingertips or the roller, apply 2 to 3 dabs to lips. Reapply as needed throughout the day, and again at bedtime.

NOTE: Keep in a convenient location if you plan to use it up within a few weeks; otherwise, store it in a cool, dark place for up to a year.

Lemon-Lavender Lip Balm

MAKES 1 FLUID OUNCE (2 TABLESPOONS)

This recipe uses fragrant lemon and lavender essential oils to soothe and protect lips, but you can play with your own scents.

1 tablespoon grated beeswax
1 tablespoon coconut oil
5 drops lemon essential oil
5 drops lavender essential oil

1. Fill a small saucepan with a few inches of water and set it on the stove over low heat. Fit a small metal or glass bowl into the pan so that it sits just above the water.
2. Put the beeswax in the bowl and wait until it melts. Then stir in the coconut oil.
3. Remove the bowl from the heat and stir in the essential oils using a metal spoon or glass stirring rod.
4. Quickly pour the mixture into a small lip balm tube or tin before it hardens.
5. Smooth a dab of the lip balm on your lips as needed throughout the day.

NOTE: Store any unopened lip balm for up to a year in a cool, dark location. Opened containers will last for up to 6 months.

SUBSTITUTION TIP: For a nourishing and spicy-scented variation, substitute ginger and ylang-ylang essential oils for the lemon and lavender. Equal parts iris and geranium essential oils can also be substituted.

COLD SORES

Also known as fever blisters, cold sores are caused by the herpes simplex virus, and are extremely contagious. Aromatherapy treatments don't cure the virus, but they do provide relief and can sometimes shorten the duration of an outbreak.

Melissa Neat Treatment

MAKES 1 TREATMENT

Melissa is a potent antiviral essential oil that can help shorten the duration of a cold sore. Applying it at the first sign of a telltale tingle can keep an outbreak to a minimum. Be sure to conduct a patch test before using this neat treatment.

1 drop melissa essential oil

1. With a cotton swab, apply the melissa essential oil to the affected area.
2. Use a new swab for each affected area.
3. Repeat three or four times daily.

SUBSTITUTION TIP: If you don't have melissa essential oil, try 1 drop of lavender essential oil instead.

Soothing Niaouli-Hops Balm

MAKES ABOUT 1 FLUID OUNCE (2 TABLESPOONS)

Niaouli and hops essential oils, together with fractionated coconut oil, help bring quick comfort to cold sores while promoting faster healing.

2 tablespoons fractionated coconut oil
10 drops hops essential oil
10 drops niaouli essential oil

1. In a small bottle or jar with a lid, combine the coconut oil and essential oils. Shake well to combine.
2. With a cotton swab, apply 1 drop of the blend to each affected area, using a new cotton swab for each area.
3. Repeat two or three times daily.

Synergistic Cold Sore Ointment

MAKES 1 FLUID OUNCE (2 TABLESPOONS)

Tea tree, peppermint, lavender, and lemon essential oils work together to bolster your immune system and keep a cold sore from growing larger.

2 tablespoons coconut oil, melted
3 drops lavender essential oil
2 drops tea tree essential oil
2 drops lemon essential oil
1 drop peppermint essential oil

1. In a small bowl, combine the coconut oil and essential oils. Whisk to blend thoroughly, and then transfer the ointment to a small jar with a lid.
2. With a cotton swab, apply 1 drop of the blend to the cold sore, using a new swab for each affected area.
3. Repeat three or four times daily.

DIAPER RASH (FOR INFANTS)

A painful, angry-looking diaper rash can happen despite your best efforts to keep your infant dry. Aromatherapy treatments help soothe the sting and promote healing, and they're completely nontoxic.

Frankincense-Myrrh Barrier Cream

MAKES 4 FLUID OUNCES (½ CUP)

Soothing frankincense and myrrh essential oils blend with rich coconut oil to stop bacteria while providing a light layer of protection from moisture.

¼ cup coconut oil, melted
¼ cup shea butter
4 drops frankincense essential oil
4 drops myrrh essential oil

1. In a small bowl, combine the coconut oil, shea butter, and essential oils. Whisk to blend thoroughly, and then transfer the cream to a small jar with a lid. Allow it to cool completely before capping.
2. With your fingertips or a cotton ball, apply ½ teaspoon of the cream to the baby's diaper region. Use a little more or less, ensuring that you spread a thin layer over the entire affected area.
3. Repeat treatment at each diaper change.

PREFERENCE TIP: If you would prefer a much thicker barrier cream, replace the coconut oil and shea butter with ½ cup of softened lanolin.

Lavender-Neroli Baby Powder

MAKES 4 FLUID OUNCES (½ CUP)

Calming lavender and neroli essential oils combine with naturally absorbent arrowroot powder to prevent the accumulation of excess moisture and stop bacteria from spreading, without the dangers associated with the use of talcum powder.

½ cup arrowroot powder
4 drops lavender essential oil
2 drops neroli essential oil
1 teaspoon uncooked rice (optional; for humidity control)

1. In a small bowl, combine the arrowroot and essential oils. Whisk to blend thoroughly.
2. Sift the mixture into a second bowl to remove any lumps. Transfer the blend to a small jar or a metal sugar shaker. Add the rice, if using, and cover with the lid.
3. After each diaper change, apply ½ teaspoon of the powder to the baby's diaper area. Use a little more or less to ensure that you've left a thin coating of powder on all vulnerable surfaces.

SUBSTITUTION TIP: If you don't have neroli essential oil, use 2 drops of Roman chamomile or 6 drops of the lavender essential oil.

Lavender–Roman Chamomile Cleansing Wipes

MAKES 80 TO 100 DISPOSABLE WIPES

Healing lavender and Roman chamomile essential oils come together with aloe to soothe irritated skin while leaving your baby fresh and clean.

1 roll premium paper towels
2 cups distilled water
1 tablespoon natural baby shampoo
1 tablespoon aloe vera gel
1 tablespoon olive oil
10 drops lavender essential oil
10 drops Roman chamomile essential oil

1. With a sharp plain-edged knife, cut the paper towel roll in half horizontally.
2. In a large bowl, combine the water, shampoo, aloe vera, olive oil, and essential oils. Stir well.
3. Place one half-roll of the toweling into the bowl, allowing the paper to absorb some of the liquid. Flip the half-roll over to ensure even absorption. Repeat the process with the other half-roll of the toweling.
4. Pull the cardboard cores out of each half-roll to allow you to pull wipes up from the center. Place each half-roll of wipes in a 1-gallon zip-top bag.
5. Use as needed, as you would other cleansing wipes, during diaper changes.

ECZEMA

Itchy, inflamed skin calls for gentle treatment. Aromatherapy treatments can help resolve redness and discomfort inside the elbows, on the backs of the knees, and other places where eczema tends to appear.

Cooling Oregano–Cucumber Seed Spray

MAKES ABOUT 4 FLUID OUNCES (½ CUP)

Brisk oregano and cucumber seed essential oils combine with soothing aloe and refreshing witch hazel to ease the itching and inflammation that accompany eczema.

¼ cup distilled water
2 tablespoons alcohol-free witch hazel
2 tablespoons aloe vera gel
12 drops cucumber seed essential oil
3 drops oregano essential oil

1. In a small bottle with a fine-mist spray top, combine the water, witch hazel, aloe vera, and essential oils. Shake well to blend, and then shake again before each use.
2. Apply 1 spritz to each patch of eczema.
3. Repeat twice daily.

Geranium-Lavender Balm

MAKES ABOUT 4 FLUID OUNCES (½ CUP)

Geranium and lavender essential oils soothe irritation and promote healing. Coconut oil is particularly soothing because it has anti-inflammatory properties of its own.

½ cup coconut oil, melted
32 drops lavender essential oil
16 drops geranium essential oil

1. In a small bowl, combine the coconut oil and essential oils. Whisk to blend thoroughly, and then transfer the balm to a small jar with a lid.
2. With your fingertips, apply a pea-sized amount to each affected area, using a little more or less as needed to leave a thin layer of the balm on the skin. Repeat as needed.

CHILD-FRIENDLY TIP: If you are making this balm for a child less than 6 years old, omit the geranium essential oil.

Soothing Palmarosa-Lavender Bath Salts

MAKES 8 TREATMENTS

Lavender and palmarosa essential oils ease inflammation, especially when combined with warm water and Epsom salts.

1 tablespoon fractionated coconut oil
16 drops lavender essential oil
8 drops palmarosa essential oil
4 cups Epsom salts

1. In a large bowl, combine the coconut oil and essential oils. Add the Epsom salts and stir well to blend. Transfer the bath salts to a large jar with a lid.
2. Draw a warm (not hot) bath and dissolve ½ cup of the bath salts in the water. Soak in the bath for at least 15 minutes.
3. Repeat two or three times weekly while working to resolve eczema.

HIVES

Sometimes caused by allergies or intense periods of stress, hives can be as small as the tip of a pen to several inches across, and they sometimes connect to form even larger areas of red, angry itchiness. Aromatherapy treatments bring toxin-free comfort quickly; if a fever is present, call your doctor.

Calming Ravintsara Balm

MAKES ABOUT 1 FLUID OUNCE (2 TABLESPOONS)

Ravintsara essential oil calms pain and itching, and helps compromised skin heal. Its aroma brings quick relaxation, so if stress is to blame for your hives, this is a very good treatment to try.

2 tablespoons fractionated coconut oil
36 drops ravintsara essential oil

1. In a small bottle or jar with a lid, combine the coconut oil and essential oil. Shake well to blend.
2. With a cotton ball, apply 1 drop of the blend to each affected area. Use a little more or less as needed to cover all the hives.

CHILD-FRIENDLY TIP: If you're making this blend for a child less than 6 years old, replace the ravintsara with lavender essential oil.

Roman Chamomile–Lavender Spritz

MAKES ABOUT 8 FLUID OUNCES (1 CUP)

Soothing lavender and Roman chamomile essential oils combine with astringent witch hazel to bring fast relief from itching.

½ cup distilled water
½ cup alcohol-free witch hazel
20 drops lavender essential oil
20 drops Roman chamomile essential oil

1. In a medium bottle with a fine-mist spray top, combine the water, witch hazel, and essential oils. Shake well to blend, and then shake again before each use.
2. Apply 1 spritz to each affected area every 1 or 2 hours, as needed.

Soothing Myrrh Bath

MAKES 8 TREATMENTS

Myrrh essential oil combines with baking soda to ease pain and inflammation and to help stop the intense, burning itch that often accompanies hives.

2 tablespoons fractionated coconut oil
32 drops myrrh essential oil
4 cups baking soda

1. In a large bowl, combine the coconut oil and essential oil. Stir with a thin utensil to blend.
2. Add the baking soda and whisk to blend thoroughly. Transfer the mixture to a large jar with a lid.
3. Draw a lukewarm bath and add ½ cup of the bath blend. Soak in the bath for at least 15 minutes. Repeat once or twice daily, until hives are gone.

PSORIASIS

Psoriasis causes skin cells to grow about five times faster than normal, inducing thick, flaking, itchy patches called *plaques*. Aromatherapy treatments don't cure psoriasis, but they provide relief from discomfort.

Cajuput–Cucumber Seed Gel

MAKES ABOUT 4 FLUID OUNCES (½ CUP)

Refreshing cajuput and cucumber seed essential oils combine with cool aloe vera gel to soothe inflammation and stop itching.

7 tablespoons aloe vera gel
1 tablespoon fractionated coconut oil
24 drops cucumber seed essential oil
12 drops cajuput essential oil

1. In a small bowl, combine the aloe vera, coconut oil, and essential oils. Whisk to blend thoroughly, and then transfer the gel to a small jar with a lid.

2. Apply ½ teaspoon of the blend to the affected area, using a little more or less as needed.

3. Repeat two or three times daily during flare-ups.

NOTE: If you like, you can keep this gel in the refrigerator for an intense cooling sensation upon application; otherwise, store in a cool, dark place.

German Chamomile Bath Salts

MAKES 8 TREATMENTS

Chamomile, bergamot, and lavender essential oils combine with Dead Sea salt and moisturizing fractionated coconut oil to soothe inflammation and stop itching.

3 tablespoons fractionated coconut oil
24 drops lavender essential oil
12 drops German chamomile essential oil
6 drops bergamot essential oil
4 cups Dead Sea salt
1 cup oat flour

1. In a large bowl, combine the coconut oil and essential oils. Add the salt and stir well to blend. Add the flour and stir again, until completely incorporated. Transfer the bath salts to a large jar with a lid.

2. Draw a warm bath and add ½ cup of the bath salts. Soak in the bath for at least 15 minutes.

3. Repeat once or twice weekly while psoriasis is active.

Helichrysum Spray

MAKES ABOUT 8 FLUID OUNCES (1 CUP)

Helichrysum essential oil is a potent anti-inflammatory, plus it helps damaged tissue repair itself quickly. If stress plays a part in your psoriasis, you'll appreciate its ability to promote relaxation, too.

½ cup distilled water
½ cup alcohol-free witch hazel
24 drops helichrysum essential oil

1. In a medium bottle with a fine-mist spray top, combine the water, witch hazel, and essential oil. Shake well to blend, and then shake again before each use.

2. Apply 1 spritz to each affected area.

3. Repeat every 1 or 2 hours, as needed.

STRETCH MARKS

When skin distends or contracts rapidly owing to pregnancy, an adolescent growth spurt, or weight gain/loss, combined with hormonal changes that occur at the same time, off-color striations, commonly known as stretch marks, develop. Aromatherapy treatments can't make them disappear overnight, but they can help bring your skin closer to its former smooth appearance.

Galbanum Cream

MAKES ABOUT 8 FLUID OUNCES (1 CUP)

Cocoa butter and shea butter moisturize deeply, while the galbanum essential oil strengthens skin and improves its appearance.

½ cup cocoa butter

½ cup shea butter

32 drops galbanum essential oil

1. In a medium bowl, combine the cocoa and shea butters and the essential oil. Blend with an electric hand mixer, and then transfer the cream to a medium jar with a lid.
2. Apply 1 teaspoon of the cream to the affected areas, using a little more or less as needed.
3. Repeat once or twice daily, until stretch marks fade.

Geranium-Neroli Cream
MAKES ABOUT 8 FLUID OUNCES (1 CUP)

Neroli and geranium essential oils help damaged skin heal, and when applied to fresh, purple stretch marks, they can help minimize the appearance of the light-colored scars that appear later.

¾ cup shea butter
¼ cup jojoba oil
20 drops geranium or rose geranium essential oil
10 drops neroli essential oil

1. In a medium bowl, combine the shea butter, jojoba oil, and essential oils. Blend with an electric hand mixer, and then transfer the cream to a medium jar with a lid.
2. Apply 1 teaspoon of the cream to the affected areas, using a little more or less as needed.
3. Repeat once or twice daily, until stretch marks fade.

Post-Pregnancy Stretch Mark Slather
MAKES 4 FLUID OUNCES (½ CUP)

This body butter should not be used while pregnant: myrrh can induce premature labor or even miscarriage. Use only after you have delivered your baby.

2 tablespoons coconut oil
2 tablespoons cocoa butter
2 tablespoons shea butter
1 tablespoon sweet almond oil
3 drops vitamin E oil
8 drops neroli essential oil
6 drops myrrh essential oil
2 drops patchouli essential oil

1. Fill a small saucepan with a few inches of water and set it on the stove over low heat. Fit a small metal or glass bowl into the pan so that it sits just above the water.
2. Put the coconut oil, cocoa and shea butters, almond oil, and vitamin E in the bowl, whisking constantly as the butters melt.
3. Remove the bowl from the heat and stir in the essential oils, using a metal spoon or glass stirring rod.
4. Let the mixture cool, then spoon the body butter into a small jar with a lid.
5. Gently spread 1 or 2 tablespoons of the lotion onto stretch marks a few times per week.

NOTE: Store the tightly sealed container in a cool, dark place for up to a year.

WARTS

A wart is a small skin growth with either a smooth or a textured surface. Warts, which are caused by the human papillomavirus (HPV), are relatively common. The virus is highly contagious, so it's a good idea to treat a wart as soon as you notice one developing.

Lavender Neat Treatment for Post-Wart Removal
MAKES 1 TREATMENT

When warts fall off, they often leave a small hole behind. Lavender essential oil provides protection from infection and encourages the skin to heal faster. Be sure to conduct a patch test before using this neat treatment.

1 drop lavender essential oil

1. With a cotton swab, apply the lavender essential oil to the hole.
2. Repeat the treatment two or three times daily, until the site is healed.

Oregano Neat Treatment

MAKES 1 TREATMENT

Oregano essential oil kills the virus and irritates the wart tissue, causing it to shrink and fall off. Be very careful not to get any undiluted oregano oil onto the surrounding healthy skin. Be sure to conduct a patch test before using this neat treatment.

2 drops carrier oil of choice
1 drop oregano essential oil

1. Coat the skin surrounding the wart with the carrier oil.
2. With a cotton swab, apply the oregano essential oil to the wart. Cover the wart with a bandage.
3. Repeat the treatment once or twice daily until the wart falls off, usually within 5 to 10 days.

Tea Tree Neat Treatment

MAKES 1 TREATMENT

Tea tree essential oil dries out warts and kills the virus, encouraging the skin to heal. Additionally, it serves as an antiseptic, preventing the area from becoming infected. Be sure to conduct a patch test before using this neat treatment.

1 drop tea tree essential oil

1. With a cotton swab, apply the tea tree essential oil directly onto the wart.
2. Repeat two or three times daily until the wart disappears, usually within 1 or 2 weeks.

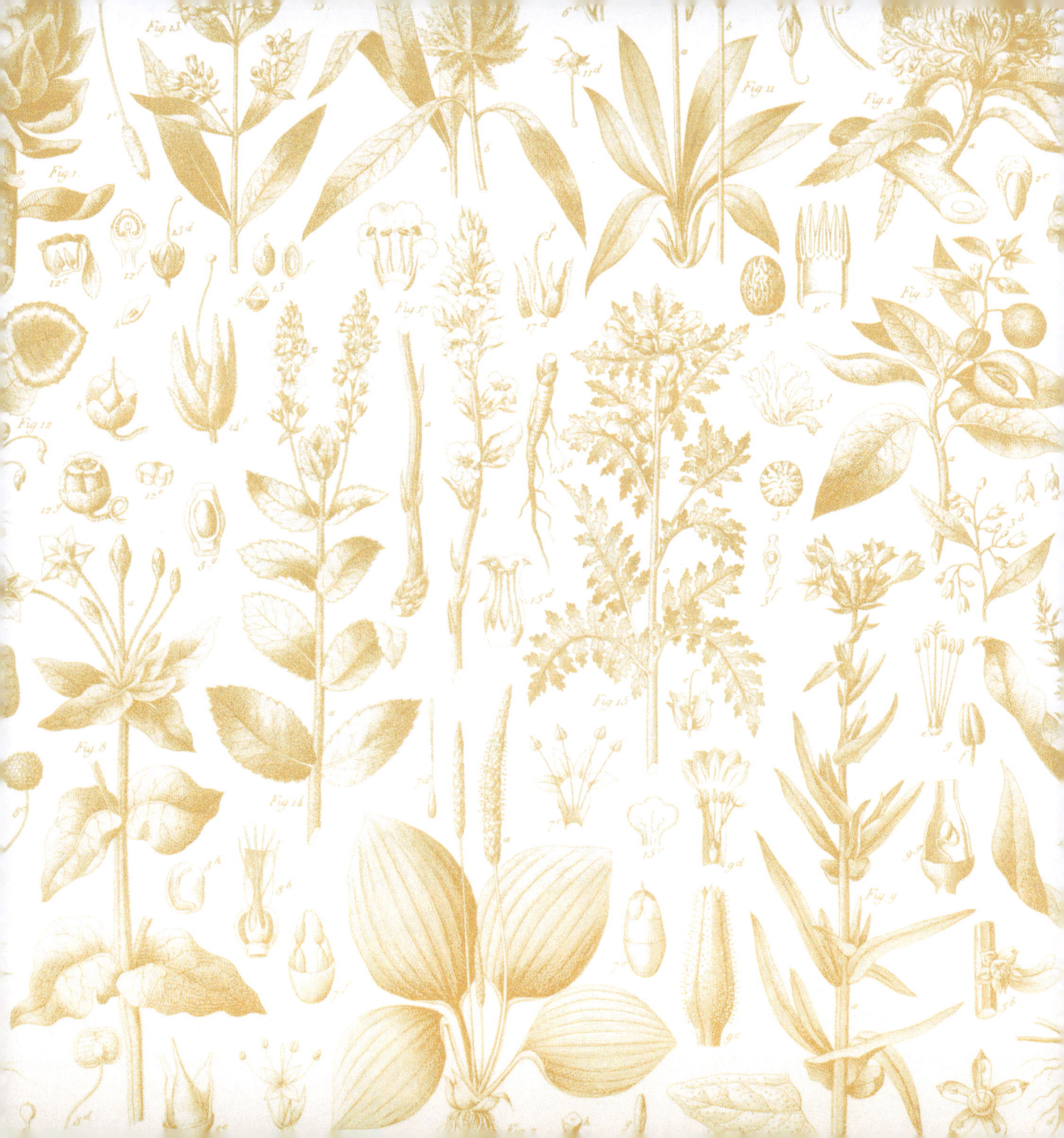

CHAPTER SEVEN

STRESS, WELL-BEING, AND SLEEP

Anxiety 206

Concentration 208

Exhaustion 210

Insomnia 212

Moodiness 214

Nervousness 216

Relaxation 218

Stress 220

ANXIETY

Whatever its cause, anxiety is a disruptive emotion that makes life seem difficult. Aromatherapy helps by promoting feelings of peace and tranquility.

Calming Temple Rub
MAKES 150 TREATMENTS

Soothing and uplifting essential oils combine to produce a sense of calm confidence. This blend is ideal for carrying along in a bag or briefcase.

1 tablespoon sweet almond oil
10 drops lavender essential oil
10 drops rose geranium essential oil
10 drops sandalwood essential oil
4 drops ylang-ylang essential oil

1. In a small bottle, preferably with a roll-on applicator, combine the almond oil and essential oils. Shake well to blend.
2. With your fingertips or the roller, apply 1 drop to each temple and gently massage the area.
3. Repeat as needed.

NOTE: Keep in a convenient location if you plan to use it up within a few weeks; otherwise, store it in a cool, dark place for up to a year.

Relaxing Lavender-Vetiver-Rose Bedtime Lotion

MAKES 16 TREATMENTS

When anxious thoughts cause restlessness, this trio creates a soothing fragrance that helps you put your worries to bed so you can rest.

8 fluid ounces (1 cup) unscented body lotion
40 drops lavender essential oil
40 drops vetiver essential oil
4 drops rose essential oil or rose absolute

1. In a medium bowl, combine the lotion and essential oils. Whisk to blend thoroughly, and then transfer the lotion to a medium jar with a lid or back into the empty lotion container.
2. Apply 1 tablespoon of lotion to your hands, arms, and shoulders as you are preparing for bed. Breathe deeply while relaxing.
3. Repeat nightly as necessary.

NOTE: Keep this lotion on your nightstand if you plan to use it all within 2 weeks; otherwise, store it it in a glass bottle or jar in a cool, dark place.

SUBSTITUTION TIP: You can use prediluted rose essential oil in this blend for a fraction of the cost. You'll need about 20 drops of the prediluted oil for each drop of the pure or the absolute.

Yuzu–Ylang-Ylang Diffusion

MAKES 10 TREATMENTS

This blend relies on yuzu and ylang-ylang essential oils to address two main components of anxiety by uplifting the spirit and relieving stress.

24 drops yuzu essential oil
6 drops ylang-ylang essential oil

1. In a small bottle with a lid, combine the essential oils. Shake well to blend. Add 3 drops of the blend to your diffuser according to the manufacturer's instructions.
2. Run the diffuser nearby and enjoy.
3. Repeat as needed each day.

PREFERENCE TIP: If you prefer florals, add another 1 or 2 drops of ylang-ylang essential oil; for a stronger citrus scent, add 4 to 6 more drops of yuzu essential oil.

CONCENTRATION

Work, study, and driving a car all call for a high level of focus. Aromatherapy helps by stimulating memory and promoting alertness.

Basil, Rosemary, and Cypress Diffusion

MAKES 1 TREATMENT

This fragrant blend makes your home or office smell fantastic, and it improves your ability to work or study.

3 drops cypress essential oil
2 drops basil essential oil
1 drop rosemary essential oil

1. Add the essential oils to your diffuser according to the manufacturer's instructions.
2. Run the diffuser nearby.
3. Repeat as needed.

Grapefruit-Spearmint Spritz

MAKES ABOUT 4 FLUID OUNCES (½ CUP)

This fantastic blend calls for grapefruit and spearmint essential oils, which stimulate concentration while promoting a positive outlook. This blend also makes a fragrant room spray.

½ cup distilled water
30 drops grapefruit essential oil
20 drops spearmint essential oil

1. In a small bottle with a fine-mist spray top, combine the water and essential oils. Shake well to blend, and then shake again before each use.
2. Apply 1 spritz of the blend to your hair or skin, or mist your clothing instead if you plan to be in the sun.
3. Repeat as often as you like.

Rosemary-Lemon Hand Cream

MAKES ABOUT 4 FLUID OUNCES (½ CUP)

A blend of rosemary and lemon essential oil makes for an irresistible fragrance that doubles as an aromatherapy treatment to promote concentration.

4 fluid ounces (½ cup) unscented hand cream or body butter
30 drops lemon essential oil
16 drops rosemary essential oil

1. In a small bowl, combine the lotion and essential oils. Whisk to blend thoroughly, and then transfer the cream to a bottle or jar and cover with the lid, or back into the empty hand cream container.
2. Apply ½ teaspoon to the palm of one hand, and then massage the blend into your skin while inhaling deeply.
3. Repeat as often as you like.

SUBSTITUTION TIP: If you plan to spend time in the sun, replace the lemon essential oil with 10 drops of peppermint essential oil.

EXHAUSTION

Exhaustion can take a serious toll on your mental and physical health, compounding other issues and making everything seem more difficult. Aromatherapy can help lessen the impact while you address the root cause.

Basil-Geranium Shower Steam

MAKES 1 TREATMENT

Uplifting basil and geranium essential oils combine with your shower's steam to deliver quick relief from exhaustion while elevating your mood.

6 drops geranium essential oil
2 drops basil essential oil

1. Apply the essential oils to a folded washcloth and position it on the shower floor, opposite the area where you stand.

2. Enjoy a hot, steamy shower and breathe deeply while you lather up with your favorite soap.

3. Repeat the treatment once daily while coping with exhaustion.

SUBSTITUTION TIP: If you don't have these essential oils on hand, use 2 drops of rosemary and 3 drops of peppermint essential oil instead.

Rosemary-Peppermint Temple Rub

MAKES 150 TREATMENTS

Soothing rosemary and invigorating peppermint essential oils come together with a touch of tangy lemon essential oil to create a wonderfully uplifting scent that sharpens your mind while improving your mood.

1 tablespoon sweet almond oil
20 drops lemon essential oil
10 drops peppermint essential oil
4 drops rosemary essential oil

1. In a small bottle, preferably with a roll-on applicator, combine the almond oil and essential oils. Shake well to blend.
2. With your fingertips or the roller, apply 1 drop of the blend to each of your temples, and gently massage the area.
3. Repeat two or three times daily.

NOTE: Keep in a convenient location if you plan to use it up within a few weeks; otherwise, store it in a cool, dark place for up to a year.

SUBSTITUTION TIP: If you plan to spend time in the sun, omit the lemon essential oil from this blend, or wear a hat that blocks the sun from hitting your temples.

Uplifting Citrus-Basil Diffusion

MAKES 1 TREATMENT

Crisp, cheerful citrus essential oils improve your mood, while basil essential oil acts as a strong mental stimulant. This blend smells delightful, making it enjoyable in your home or at the office.

1 drop basil essential oil
1 drop grapefruit essential oil
1 drop lemon essential oil
1 drop mandarin essential oil

1. Add the essential oils to your diffuser according to the manufacturer's instructions.
2. Run the diffuser nearby.
3. Repeat two or three times daily, as needed.

INSOMNIA

Instead of reaching for pharmaceuticals, give aromatherapy a try the next time sleeplessness takes over. These comforting remedies work best when you focus on relaxing. You can make natural sleep easier by turning off electronics an hour before bedtime.

Lavender-Chamomile Nighttime Shower Melts

MAKES 10 MELTS

Lavender and Roman chamomile essential oils help you fall asleep quickly, especially when combined with the steam from your hot shower. This treatment is ideal for travel, or for anyone who doesn't care much for baths.

2½ cups baking soda
½ cup tap water
40 drops lavender essential oil
40 drops Roman chamomile essential oil

1. Preheat the oven to 350°F and line a standard muffin tin with ten cupcake liners.

2. In a large bowl, combine the baking soda and water. Stir into a thick paste, evenly divide the paste among the ten muffin cups, and bake for 20 minutes or until dried through.

3. Allow the melts to cool completely, and then peel off the paper liners. To each melt add 4 drops of lavender and 4 drops of Roman chamomile essential oil. Transfer the melts immediately to widemouth glass jars or a large storage container. Cover with the lids.

4. Place 1 melt in the shower stall just before stepping in. Breathe deeply while you enjoy the fragrant steam.

5. Repeat nightly as needed.

Spikenard-Rose Bath Salts

MAKES 8 TREATMENTS

Spikenard and rose essential oils combine with soothing Epsom salts to promote deep relaxation. Spikenard is a highly effective sedative, so finish important tasks before enjoying this treatment.

2 tablespoons fractionated coconut oil
40 drops spikenard essential oil
4 drops rose essential oil or 20 drops prediluted rose oil
4 cups Epsom salts

1. In a large bowl, combine the coconut oil and essential oils. Add the Epsom salts and stir well to blend. Transfer the bath salts to a large jar with a lid.
2. Draw a hot bath and add ½ cup of the bath salts.
3. Soak in the bath for 15 to 20 minutes.
4. Repeat nightly as needed.

Valerian-Cedarwood Bedtime Balm

MAKES ABOUT 4 FLUID OUNCES (½ CUP)

Valerian essential oil promotes deep, peaceful sleep. Cedarwood essential oil tempers its intensely woody, earthy aroma, which some people dislike. Don't drink alcohol or use sleep aids alongside this treatment.

¼ cup coconut oil, melted
2 tablespoons shea butter
1 tablespoon sweet almond oil
1 tablespoon beeswax, melted
40 drops valerian essential oil
20 drops cedarwood essential oil

1. In a small bowl, combine the coconut oil, shea butter, almond oil, and beeswax, then stir in the essential oils. Whisk to blend thoroughly.
2. Pour the blend into a small jar with a lid and allow it to cool completely before capping.
3. With your fingertips, apply a dime-sized amount to your shoulder and neck area.
4. Repeat once nightly as needed to assist with falling asleep.

PREFERENCE TIP: Check the blend's aroma before allowing it to cool. If you dislike the fragrance, add 10 drops of lavender or lavandin essential oil.

MOODINESS

Discomfort, disease, medication side effects, or plain old bad days are among the causes of moodiness. If you are frequently irritable, have your doctor check for underlying illness; in the meantime, try these uplifting aromatherapy treatments.

Lemon, Rosemary, and Chamomile Diffusion

MAKES 1 TREATMENT

When stress and overwork are part of the equation, lemon, rosemary, and chamomile essential oils can perk you up, help you focus, and provide you with a bit more balance.

3 drops lemon essential oil
1 drop Roman or German chamomile essential oil
1 drop rosemary essential oil

1. Add the essential oils to your diffuser according to the manufacturer's instructions.
2. Run the diffuser nearby.

SUBSTITUTION TIP: If you need to go to sleep within 4 hours of using this diffusion blend, swap out the rosemary (which promotes alertness that can last for hours) for 1 drop of lavender essential oil.

Sandalwood-Vetiver Spray

MAKES ABOUT 8 FLUID OUNCES (1 CUP)

Sandalwood and vetiver essential oils lift your spirits quickly while promoting a sense of peaceful awareness. This blend smells so delicious that you might adopt it as your personal fragrance.

1 cup less 2 tablespoons distilled water
2 tablespoons alcohol-free witch hazel
30 drops sandalwood essential oil
20 drops vetiver essential oil

1. In a medium bottle with a fine-mist spray top, combine the water, witch hazel, and essential oils. Shake well to blend, and then shake again before each use.
2. Apply 1 spritz to each of the pulse points behind your ears, your inner elbows, and your wrists. You can also spritz clothing, your hair, or the air around you.
3. Repeat as needed.

Tangerine-Lavender Lotion

MAKES ABOUT 8 FLUID OUNCES (1 CUP)

Cheery tangerine and relaxing lavender essential oils combine to alter your mental state so that you feel a bit less cranky.

8 fluid ounces (1 cup) unscented body lotion or hand cream
30 drops tangerine essential oil
20 drops lavender essential oil

1. In a medium bowl, combine the lotion and essential oils. Whisk to blend thoroughly, and then transfer the lotion to a medium jar with a lid or back into the empty lotion container.
2. Apply 1 teaspoon of the blend to your hands, arms, and shoulders. Use a little more or less as needed, and feel free to apply the lotion to other body parts.
3. Use as often as you like throughout each day, especially after washing your hands.

NOTE: Keep this lotion in a convenient location if you plan to use it all within 2 weeks; otherwise, store it in a glass bottle or jar in a cool, dark place.

NERVOUSNESS

Nervousness is a state of hyper-awareness that may keep you physically and emotionally on edge. Whether you're chronically nervous or simply suffer from edginess before important events, aromatherapy can help ease the jitters and help you see things in a more positive light.

Calming Chamomile-Neroli Steam

MAKES 1 TREATMENT

Fragrant neroli and soothing Roman chamomile essential oils combine with the steam from your shower to deliver a heavenly fragrance and help bring you peace of mind.

6 drops Roman chamomile essential oil
3 drops neroli essential oil

1. Apply the essential oils to a folded washcloth and position it on the shower floor, opposite the area where you stand.
2. Enjoy a hot, steamy shower and breathe deeply while relaxing and dwelling on positive thoughts.
3. Repeat once or twice daily while dealing with nervousness.

Clary Sage–Citrus Diffusion

MAKES 1 TREATMENT

Clary sage and cheerful citrus essential oils combine with a touch of jasmine essential oil to calm your nerves and ground your emotions.

2 drops clary sage essential oil
2 drops prediluted jasmine essential oil
1 drop lemon essential oil
1 drop mandarin essential oil

1. Add the essential oils to your diffuser according to the manufacturer's instructions.
2. Run the diffuser nearby.
3. Repeat every 2 or 3 hours, or as needed.

Patchouli-Petitgrain Spritz

MAKES ABOUT 8 FLUID OUNCES (1 CUP)

Petitgrain and patchouli essential oils promote a sense of calm self-awareness while giving your mood a wonderful boost. You can use this spray on your skin, hair, and clothing, and even as an air freshener.

1 cup less 2 tablespoons distilled water
2 tablespoons alcohol-free witch hazel
14 drops patchouli essential oil
10 drops petitgrain essential oil

1. In a medium bottle with a fine-mist spray top, combine the water, witch hazel, and essential oils. Shake well to blend, and then shake again before each use.
2. Apply 1 spritz to your pulse points, targeting the areas behind your ears, on your inner wrists, and in the bend of each elbow.
3. Repeat as needed to take the edge off.

RELAXATION

Stress is linked to an enormous number of health problems, and taking time out to relax should be an important part of every day. Aromatherapy is an excellent tool for relaxation, and one that you'll eagerly look forward to using.

Everyday Citrus-Sandalwood Spritzer

MAKES ABOUT 8 FLUID OUNCES (1 CUP)

Snappy citrus essential oils combine with sweet sandalwood essential oil to keep you, your car, and your home smelling fantastic while promoting a sense of calm relaxation. While most relaxation treatments help you unwind, this one promotes clarity. It's just right for spraying in your car before a stressful commute.

1 cup less 2 tablespoons distilled water
2 tablespoons alcohol-free witch hazel
10 drops sandalwood essential oil
10 drops sweet orange essential oil
5 drops grapefruit essential oil
5 drops lemon essential oil
5 drops lime essential oil

1. In a medium bottle with a fine-mist spray top, combine the water, witch hazel, and essential oils. Shake well to blend, and then shake again before each use.

2. Apply three or four spritzes to your body, your clothing, your car's upholstery, or the air in your home or office.

3. Repeat as often as you like.

Lavender-Basil Bath Salts for Restless Legs Syndrome

MAKES 8 TREATMENTS

A warm Epsom salts bath spiked with soothing lavender and basil essential oils helps stop spasms, so you can relax and get that good night's rest you've been wanting.

2 tablespoons fractionated coconut oil
24 drops lavender essential oil
8 drops basil essential oil
4 cups Epsom salts

1. In a large bowl, combine the coconut oil and essential oils. Add the Epsom salts and stir well to blend. Transfer the bath salts to a large jar with a lid.
2. Draw a hot bath and add ½ cup of the bath salts. Soak in the bath for at least 15 minutes.
3. Repeat once daily while suffering from restless legs syndrome.

Synergistic Relaxation Diffusion

MAKES 40 TO 50 TREATMENTS

Rosewood, lavender, chamomile, and geranium essential oils combine with ylang-ylang, clary sage, and marjoram essential oils to deliver an intoxicating aroma that promotes relaxation.

36 drops lavender essential oil
30 drops rosewood essential oil
24 drops geranium or rose geranium essential oil
24 drops Roman chamomile essential oil
20 drops clary sage essential oil
20 drops ylang-ylang essential oil
16 drops marjoram essential oil

1. In a small bottle with a lid, combine the essential oils. Shake well to blend. With the cap secured, allow the different scents to marry for 24 to 48 hours before use.
2. Add 3 or 4 drops of the blend to your diffuser according to the manufacturer's instructions. Run the diffuser nearby.
3. Repeat as often as you'd like to create a relaxing atmosphere in your home or office.

STRESS

Often referred to as "the silent killer," stress is an uncomfortable state of emotional or mental strain that arises as the result of demanding or adverse circumstances. Aromatherapy treatments help ease the tension while you find healthy ways to decrease the amount of pressure in your life.

Benzoin-Bergamot Lotion
MAKES ABOUT 8 FLUID OUNCES (1 CUP)

Benzoin and bergamot essential oils help your mind relax without making you feel sleepy, plus the blend is a fantastic one for keeping skin in good shape.

8 fluid ounces (1 cup) unscented body lotion or hand cream
20 drops bergamot essential oil
10 drops benzoin essential oil

1. In a medium bowl, combine the lotion and essential oils. Whisk to blend thoroughly, and then transfer the lotion to a medium jar with a lid or back into the empty lotion container.

2. Apply 1 teaspoon of the lotion to your hands, arms, and shoulders. Use a little more or less as needed, and feel free to apply the lotion to other body parts.

3. Use as often as you like throughout the day, especially after washing your hands.

NOTE: Keep this lotion in a convenient location if you plan to use it all within 2 weeks; otherwise, store it in a glass bottle or jar in a cool, dark place.

Cardamom-Mandarin Temple Rub

MAKES 100 TREATMENTS

Warm, spicy cardamom essential oil blends with cheerful mandarin essential oil, uplifting your mood while alleviating stress. If you're feeling worried, depressed, or fatigued, this blend can help.

1 tablespoon sweet almond oil
20 drops mandarin essential oil
10 drops cardamom essential oil

1. In a small bottle, preferably with a roll-on applicator, combine the almond oil and essential oils. Shake well to blend.
2. With your fingertips or the roller, apply 1 drop to each of your temples, and then massage the areas gently while inhaling deeply.

NOTE: Keep in a convenient location if you plan to use it up within a few weeks; otherwise, store it in a cool, dark place for up to a year.

PREFERENCE TIP: If you like this fragrance and want to diffuse it, use a ratio of 1 drop cardamom essential oil to 2 drops mandarin essential oil to create a lovely blend for your home or office.

Grapefruit–Ylang-Ylang Diffusion

MAKES 36 TREATMENTS

Fresh, tangy grapefruit essential oil combines with grounding chamomile and sweet ylang-ylang essential oils to delight your senses and decrease your stress level. This blend is an excellent one for wearing in an aromatherapy pendant.

48 drops grapefruit essential oil
32 drops Roman chamomile essential oil
28 drops ylang-ylang essential oil

1. In a small bottle with a lid, combine the essential oils. Shake well to blend, then close with the lid. Allow the different scents to marry for at least 24 hours before use.
2. Add 3 drops of the blend to your diffuser according to the manufacturer's instructions.
3. Run the diffuser nearby.
4. Repeat as needed.

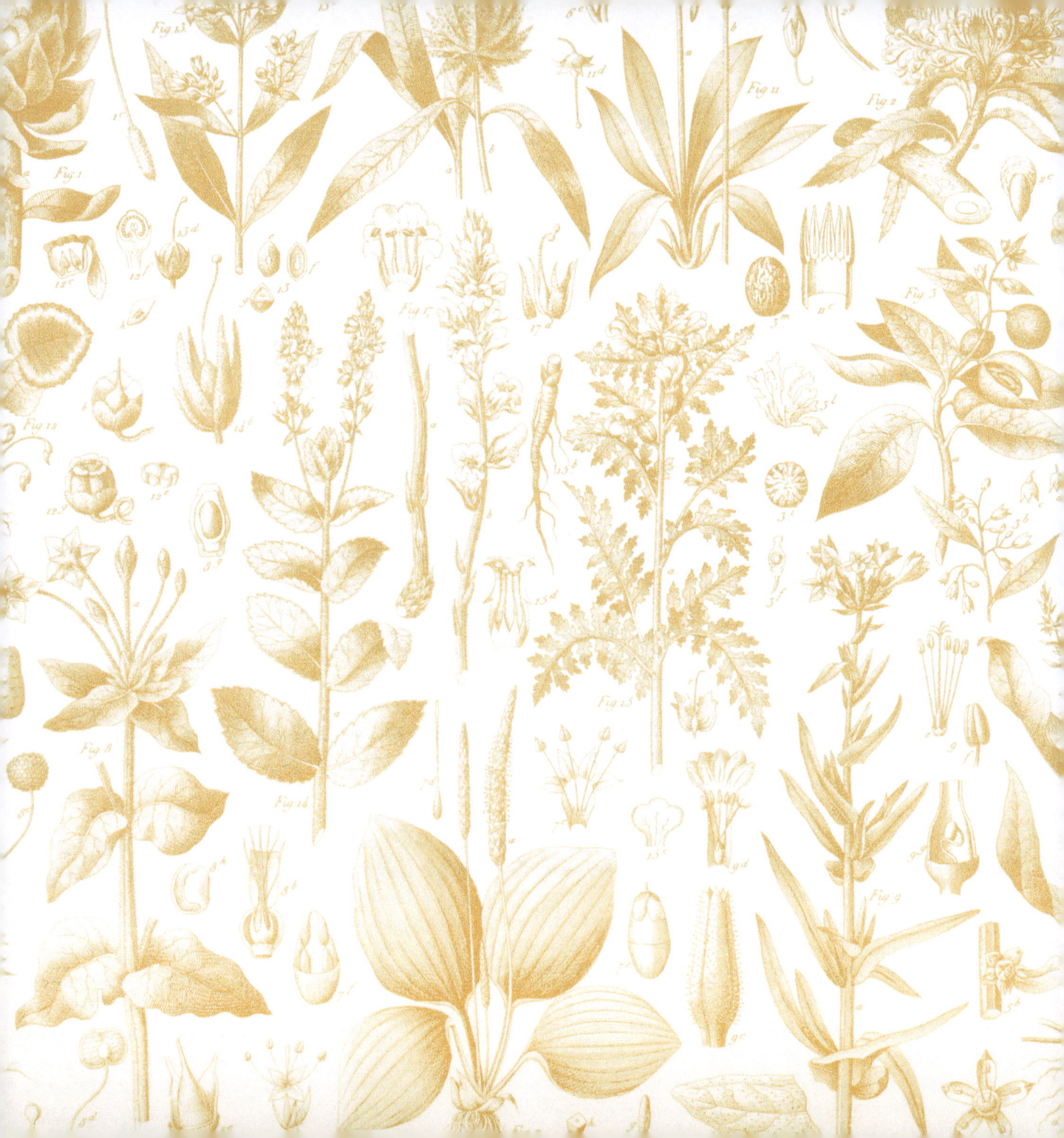

CHAPTER EIGHT

GUT HEALTH

Bloating   224

Constipation   226

Diarrhea   228

Heartburn   230

Hemorrhoids   232

Indigestion   234

Nausea and Vomiting   236

BLOATING

Overeating, drinking carbonated beverages, and eating too quickly are just a few of the habits that can lead to uncomfortable bloating. These gentle treatments help you feel like yourself again, with no unpleasant side effects.

Cinnamon Leaf–Fennel Seed Balm

MAKES ABOUT 2 FLUID OUNCES (¼ CUP)

Fennel seed and cinnamon leaf essential oils improve circulation and enhance digestion, helping get your bloated belly back down to size.

1 tablespoon coconut oil, melted
1 tablespoon hemp oil
1 tablespoon sweet almond oil
1 tablespoon shea butter
16 drops fennel seed essential oil
12 drops cinnamon leaf essential oil

1. In a small bowl, combine the coconut, hemp, and almond oils, the shea butter, and the essential oils. Whisk to blend thoroughly, and then transfer the balm to a small jar with a lid.

2. Apply 1 teaspoon of the balm to your abdomen, and massage the area, using firm clockwise strokes.

3. Repeat as often as needed.

Ginger–Black Pepper Digestive Massage

MAKES 1 TREATMENT

If overindulging in rich food is the cause of your bloating, try this quick treatment. Ginger and black pepper essential oils help move things along by improving circulation and speeding digestion.

1 tablespoon carrier oil of choice
3 drops black pepper essential oil
1 drop ginger essential oil

1. In a small bowl, combine the carrier oil and essential oils. Stir well to blend.
2. Apply the entire blend to your abdomen and massage the area, using clockwise motions.
3. Spend 15 minutes lying on your left side, if possible, to help the gas pass from your system more quickly.

Minty Orange-Chamomile Lotion

MAKES ABOUT 4 FLUID OUNCES (½ CUP)

Peppermint, sweet orange, and chamomile essential oils combine with unscented body lotion to enhance digestion and help prevent uncomfortable bloating.

4 fluid ounces (½ cup) unscented body lotion
15 drops Roman or German chamomile essential oil
15 drops sweet orange essential oil
10 drops peppermint essential oil

1. In a small bowl, combine the lotion and essential oils. Whisk to blend thoroughly, and then transfer the lotion to a bottle or jar with a lid, or back into the empty lotion container.
2. Apply 1 teaspoon of the lotion to your abdomen before eating a meal that's likely to trigger indigestion.
3. Repeat as needed.

NOTE: Keep this lotion in a convenient location if you plan to use it all within 2 weeks; otherwise, store it in a glass bottle or jar in a cool, dark place.

CONSTIPATION

Changes in routine, lack of dietary fiber, and not enough exercise are just a few causes of constipation. Aromatherapy helps by improving circulation and gently encouraging smooth muscle tissue in the digestive tract to function properly.

Peppermint–Fennel Seed Lotion

MAKES 1 TREATMENT

Peppermint and fennel seed essential oils stimulate the digestive tract and improve circulation, bringing relief from discomfort.

1 teaspoon unscented body lotion
4 drops peppermint essential oil
6 drops fennel seed essential oil

1. In the palm of your hand, combine the lotion and essential oils.
2. Apply the blend to your lower abdomen and massage the area, using clockwise strokes. Rest for at least 15 minutes, if possible.
3. Repeat once or twice daily while suffering from constipation.

Rosemary–Sweet Orange Compress

MAKES 1 TREATMENT

Rosemary and sweet orange essential oils promote relaxation and improve circulation, while heat promotes further relaxation.

½ teaspoon carrier oil of choice
8 drops sweet orange essential oil
4 drops rosemary essential oil

1. In a small bowl, combine the carrier oil and essential oils. Stir well to combine.
2. With your fingertips or a cotton ball, apply the entire treatment to your lower abdomen, focusing on the area located 2 inches below your navel.
3. Lie on your back and cover your abdomen with a warm heating pad, following the manufacturer's instructions for safe use. Relax for at least 15 minutes.
4. Repeat once or twice daily while suffering from constipation.

Synergistic Bath Blend

MAKES 8 TREATMENTS

Lemon, basil, and black pepper essential oils improve circulation, while hot water and Epsom salts encourage your muscles to relax.

4 cups Epsom salts
1 tablespoon sweet almond oil
16 drops lemon essential oil
8 drops basil essential oil
8 drops black pepper essential oil

1. In a large bowl, combine the Epsom salts, almond oil, and essential oils. Stir well to combine. Transfer the bath salts to a large jar and cover with a lid.
2. Draw a hot bath and add ½ cup of the blend. Spend at least 15 minutes soaking.
3. Repeat daily while suffering from constipation.

DIARRHEA

With its cramping and frequent, watery stools, diarrhea can make you feel miserable. Aromatherapy brings some relief by calming the inflammation and cramping, but it's important to stay hydrated and avoid trigger foods.

Copaiba-Coriander Compress

MAKES 1 TREATMENT

Copaiba and coriander essential oils combine with soothing heat to reduce spasms and bring comfort to an overworked digestive system.

½ teaspoon fractionated coconut oil
1 drop copaiba essential oil
1 drop coriander essential oil

1. In the palm of your hand, combine the coconut oil and essential oils.
2. Apply the blend to your lower abdomen and gently massage the area in a clockwise direction.
3. Lie down and cover your lower abdomen with a warm heating pad, following the manufacturer's instructions for safe use. Leave the heating pad in place for at least 15 minutes.
4. Repeat two or three times daily while suffering from diarrhea.

Synergistic Abdominal Massage Blend

MAKES 2 FLUID OUNCES (¼ CUP)

Ravensara leaf, *Eucalyptus radiata*, lavender, and marjoram essential oils combine to attack bacteria while improving circulation and relieving discomfort.

¼ cup fractionated coconut oil
4 drops lavender essential oil
4 drops marjoram essential oil
2 drops *Eucalyptus radiata* essential oil
2 drops ravensara leaf essential oil

1. In a small bottle or jar with a lid, combine the coconut oil and essential oils. Shake well to blend.
2. Apply ½ teaspoon of the blend to your abdomen. With the navel as the center starting point, gently massage the area, using clockwise strokes. Use a little more or less oil as needed, ensuring that you cover the entire abdomen.
3. Repeat once or twice daily while suffering from diarrhea.

PREFERENCE TIP: If you have time, cover your abdomen with a warm heating pad, following the manufacturer's instructions for safe use. Leave the heating pad in place for 15 minutes.

Triple-Spice Massage Blend

MAKES 1 FLUID OUNCE (2 TABLESPOONS)

Ginger, cinnamon leaf, and clove bud essential oils soothe your digestive system and improve circulation, helping you recover faster from a bout of diarrhea.

2 tablespoons fractionated coconut oil
4 drops ginger essential oil
2 drops cinnamon leaf essential oil
2 drops clove bud essential oil

1. In a small bottle or jar with a lid, combine the coconut oil and essential oils. Shake well to blend.
2. Apply ½ teaspoon of the blend to your lower abdomen, focusing on the area located about 2 inches below the navel, and massage the area, using light clockwise strokes.
3. Relax and breathe deeply, while sipping ginger or chamomile tea (if you have some available).
4. Repeat two or three times daily while suffering from diarrhea.

HEARTBURN

Heartburn occurs when stomach acid travels back up into the esophagus, usually after you've eaten a rich or spicy meal. Aromatherapy can cool the burn and make you more comfortable, but it's best to avoid trigger foods and overeating altogether; long-term exposure to stomach acid will damage your esophagus.

Minty Fennel Seed–Eucalyptus Lotion

MAKES ABOUT 4 FLUID OUNCES (½ CUP)

Fennel seed, ginger, and eucalyptus essential oils improve circulation and enhance digestion, while spearmint essential oil helps ease discomfort. Try using this blend before meals as a preventive measure.

4 fluid ounces (½ cup) unscented body lotion
16 drops fennel seed essential oil
16 drops ginger essential oil
12 drops spearmint essential oil
12 drops eucalyptus essential oil (any species)

1. In a small bowl, combine the lotion and essential oils. Whisk to blend thoroughly, and then transfer the lotion to a small jar with a lid, or back into the empty lotion container.
2. Apply 1 teaspoon of lotion to the upper abdominal area, and massage upward toward the chest.
3. Repeat two or three times daily, or as needed.

NOTE: Keep this lotion in a convenient location if you plan to use it all within 2 weeks; otherwise, store it in a glass bottle or jar in a cool, dark place.

Spearmint Compress

MAKES 1 TREATMENT

Cool spearmint essential oil combines with soothing heat to ease discomfort and stop any feelings of nausea that accompany heartburn.

½ teaspoon fractionated coconut oil
4 drops spearmint essential oil

1. In the palm of your hand, combine the coconut oil and essential oil.
2. Apply the blend to your upper abdomen and gently massage the area in a clockwise direction.
3. Lie down and cover your upper abdomen with a warm heating pad, following the manufacturer's instructions for safe use. Leave the heating pad in place for at least 15 minutes.
4. Repeat two or three times daily while suffering from heartburn.

Synergistic Heartburn Blend

MAKES ABOUT 4 FLUID OUNCES (½ CUP)

Anise, caraway, coriander, ginger, fennel seed, and peppermint essential oils combine to ease indigestion and stop the burn fast.

½ cup fractionated coconut oil
20 drops ginger essential oil
20 drops peppermint essential oil
14 drops caraway essential oil
14 drops coriander essential oil
10 drops anise essential oil
8 drops fennel seed essential oil

1. In a small bottle or jar with a lid, combine the coconut oil and essential oils. Shake well to blend.
2. With your fingertips, apply 1 teaspoon of the blend to your upper abdomen, chest, and throat, and gently massage the areas.
3. Lie on your left side and relax for 15 minutes.
4. Repeat once or twice daily while coping with heartburn.

SUBSTITUTION TIP: Peppermint can make heartburn worse in some individuals. If that's the case for you, make this recipe with spearmint essential oil in place of the peppermint.

HEMORRHOIDS

Pain, swelling, itching, and irritation are symptoms of swollen blood vessels in and around the rectum. Hemorrhoids can develop when you strain too much during bowel movements, as well as when you are pregnant or have been diagnosed with liver disease. Aromatherapy treatments bring relief and can help stop the swelling, but in severe cases, medical intervention may be the only answer.

Lemon-Cypress Compress
MAKES 1 TREATMENT

Lemon and cypress essential oils help soothe inflammation and shrink swelling. When combined with cold water, they bring rapid relief from discomfort.

½ cup distilled water
2 ice cubes
4 drops lemon essential oil
4 drops cypress essential oil

1. In a small bowl, pour the water over the ice cubes and then add the essential oils.
2. Roll a washcloth into a cylinder and soak it in the solution.
3. Lie flat on your stomach with a towel underneath your pelvic area to catch any drips. Position the rolled-up washcloth between the gluteus maximus muscles so that it is in contact with the inflamed tissue.
4. Leave the compress in place for 15 minutes. Allow your skin to air-dry after removal.
5. Repeat as needed until hemorrhoids resolve.

Neroli-Myrrh Wipes

MAKES 80 TO 100 DISPOSABLE WIPES

Neroli and myrrh essential oils come together with aloe and witch hazel to ease itching and soothe irritated skin while leaving you feeling fresh.

1 roll premium paper towels
1 cup distilled water
1 cup alcohol-free witch hazel
2 tablespoons aloe vera gel
1 tablespoon avocado oil
1 tablespoon fragrance-free liquid soap
20 drops myrrh essential oil
10 drops neroli essential oil

1. With a sharp plain-edged knife, cut the paper towel roll in half horizontally.

2. In a large bowl, combine the water, witch hazel, aloe vera, avocado oil, liquid soap, and essential oils. Stir well.

3. Place one half of the paper towel roll into the bowl, allowing the half-roll to absorb some liquid. Flip the half-roll over to ensure even absorption. Repeat the process with the other half of the paper towel roll.

4. Pull the cardboard cores out of the center of each half-roll to allow you to pull wipes up from the center. Place each half-roll of wipes in a 1-gallon zip-top bag.

5. Use wipes as needed, especially after bowel movements.

Roman Chamomile Salve for Bleeding Hemorrhoids

MAKES 1 FLUID OUNCE (2 TABLESPOONS)

Antiseptic tea tree and Roman chamomile essential oils help prevent infection, ease pain, and soothe irritated skin, while the avocado oil calms inflammation.

2 tablespoons avocado oil
8 drops Roman chamomile essential oil
2 drops tea tree essential oil

1. In a small bottle or jar with a lid, combine the avocado oil and essential oils. Shake well to blend.

2. Thoroughly cleanse the affected area. With a cotton cosmetic pad, apply ¼ teaspoon of the blend.

3. Repeat after bathing, showering, and bowel movements.

INDIGESTION

Uncomfortable belching, nausea, and a general sense of digestive distress are some of the hallmarks of indigestion. Aromatherapy brings quick comfort; however, if your symptoms are persistent, check with your doctor to rule out an underlying illness.

Cardamom Balm

MAKES ABOUT 4 FLUID OUNCES (½ CUP)

Cardamom essential oil improves circulation and stimulates healthy digestion. If you have overindulged, give this simple treatment a try.

½ cup coconut oil, melted

32 drops cardamom essential oil

1. In a small bowl, combine the coconut oil and essential oil. Whisk to blend thoroughly, and then transfer the balm to a small jar with a lid.
2. Apply 1 teaspoon of the mixture to the upper abdomen and lightly massage the area, using clockwise motions.
3. Repeat once or twice daily while suffering from indigestion.

Comforting Clove Bud Compress

MAKES 1 TREATMENT

Clove bud essential oil relaxes the smooth muscles of the digestive tract and prevents nausea, gas, and uncomfortable spasms. A warm compress brings additional relief.

1 teaspoon fractionated coconut oil
3 drops clove bud essential oil

1. In the palm of your hand, combine the coconut oil and essential oil.
2. Apply the blend to your abdomen and gently massage outward in a clockwise direction, beginning at the navel.
3. Lie down and cover your abdomen with a warm heating pad, following the manufacturer's instructions for safe use. Leave the heating pad in place for at least 15 minutes.
4. Repeat once or twice daily while suffering from indigestion.

Peppermint Massage

MAKES 1 TREATMENT

Peppermint relaxes the digestive muscles and improves circulation to help you get over indigestion quickly. If you're feeling a bit nauseous, this is a good treatment to try.

2 drops peppermint essential oil
2 drops carrier oil of choice

1. Apply the peppermint essential oil directly to the area located just beneath the sternum.
2. Apply the carrier oil over the peppermint oil and lightly massage the area.
3. Repeat once or twice daily while suffering from indigestion.

NAUSEA AND VOMITING

Certain medications, overconsumption of alcohol, and cancer treatments are just a few things that can cause nausea and/or vomiting. If you suffer from frequent nausea and haven't identified the cause, see your doctor to rule out a serious underlying illness. Aromatherapy can help reduce or eliminate symptoms in the meantime.

Copaiba-Chamomile Compress
MAKES 1 TREATMENT

Copaiba and German chamomile essential oils combine with soothing heat to stop stomach spasms and help you relax during your malady.

½ teaspoon fractionated coconut oil
2 drops copaiba essential oil
2 drops German chamomile essential oil

1. In the palm of your hand, combine the coconut oil and essential oils.
2. Apply the blend to your upper abdomen and gently massage the area in a clockwise direction.
3. Lie down and cover your upper abdomen with a warm heating pad, following the manufacturer's instructions for safe use. Leave the heating pad in place for at least 15 minutes.
4. Repeat two or three times daily while suffering from nausea.

Melissa-Spearmint Bath Salts

MAKES 8 TREATMENTS

Melissa and spearmint essential oils offer antispasmodic action and calm nerves, helping with both the physical and the emotional distress that accompanies nausea.

2 tablespoons sweet almond oil
24 drops melissa essential oil
4 drops spearmint essential oil
4 cups Epsom salts

1. In a large bowl, combine the almond oil and essential oils. Add the Epsom salts and stir well to blend. Transfer the bath salts to a large jar with a lid.
2. Draw a warm bath and add ½ cup of the bath salts. Soak in the bath for at least 15 minutes.
3. Repeat once daily, or as needed.

Soothing Sandalwood Lotion

MAKES ABOUT 8 FLUID OUNCES (1 CUP)

Sandalwood essential oil smells fantastic and is great for skin, plus it helps put a stop to nausea while relieving stress. Sandalwood oil also helps the body detoxify itself, so if dietary indiscretion is behind your discomfort, this is a good remedy to try.

8 fluid ounces (1 cup) unscented body lotion or hand cream
20 drops sandalwood essential oil

1. In a medium bowl, combine the lotion and essential oil. Whisk to blend thoroughly, and then transfer the lotion to a medium jar with a lid or back into the empty lotion container.
2. Apply 1 teaspoon of the blend to your hands, arms, and shoulders. Use a little more or less as needed, and feel free to apply the lotion to other body parts.
3. Use as often as you like.

NOTE: Keep this lotion in a convenient location if you plan to use it all within 2 weeks; otherwise, store it in a glass bottle or jar in a cool, dark place.

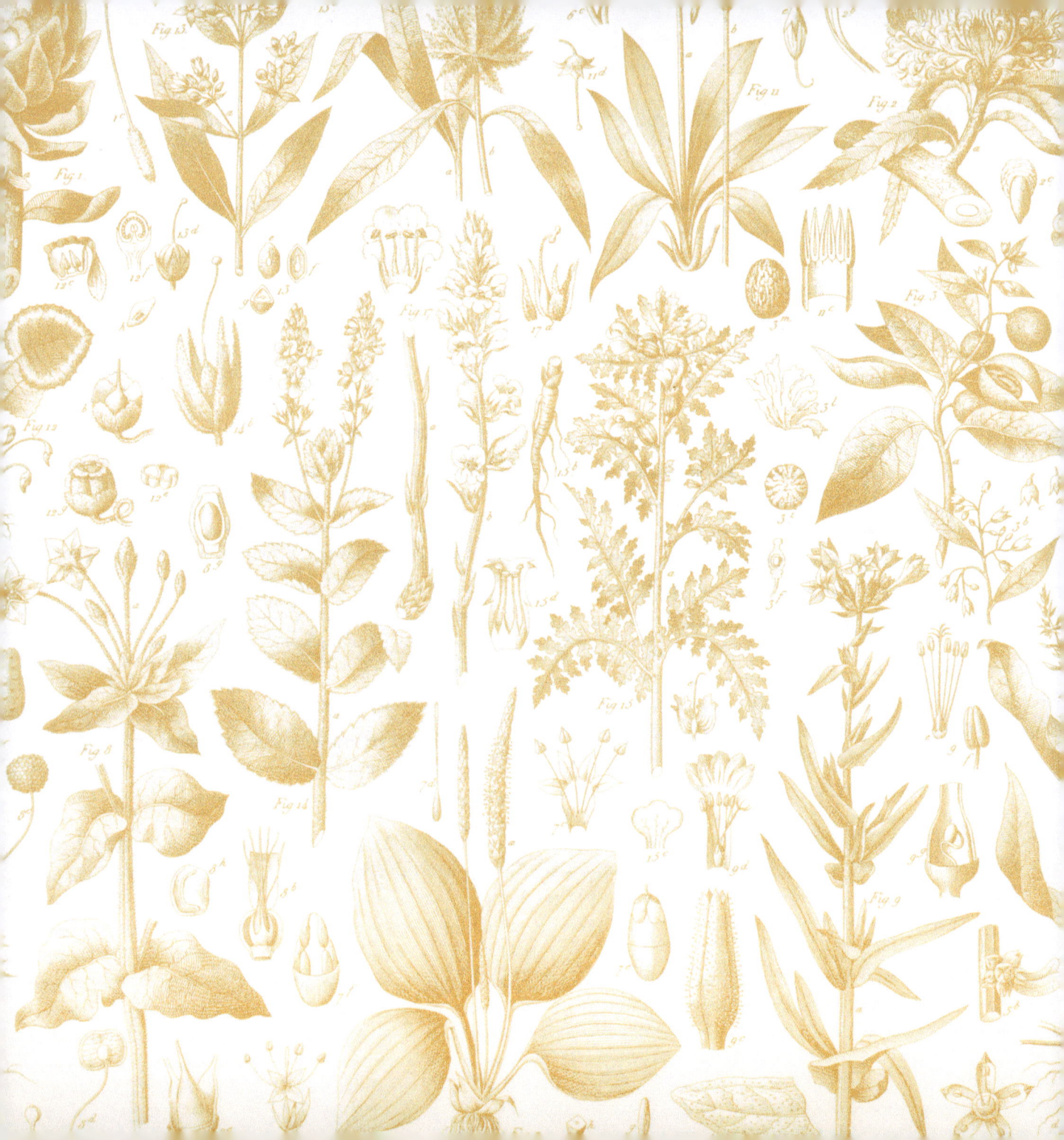

CHAPTER NINE

SEXUAL HEALTH

Arousal   240

Menopause   242

Menstrual Symptoms   244

Urinary Tract Infection (UTI)   246

Vaginal Yeast Infection   248

AROUSAL

Set the scene for romance with aromatherapy blends that enhance arousal by appealing to the senses and stimulating passion. These wonderful scents also address stress, making it much easier to focus on your partner.

Jasmine Linen Spray
MAKES 8 FLUID OUNCES (1 CUP)

Jasmine absolute offers a soothing, sensual scent that promotes feelings of love, peace, and emotional warmth. Use this spray to give your bedroom's curtains, carpet, and linens a lingering scent. It's nice as a hair and body spritz, too.

1 cup distilled water
4 drops jasmine absolute

1. In a medium bottle with a fine-mist spray top, combine the water and jasmine absolute. Shake well to blend, and then shake again before each use.
2. Spray liberally on linens, carpets, and curtains.

SUBSTITUTION TIP: Jasmine absolute is costly, so many companies offer this oil prediluted. If you use prediluted jasmine in this recipe, use 10 to 20 drops for each drop of jasmine absolute.

Rose-Davana Perfume

MAKES 150 TREATMENTS

Exotic davana and rose essential oils come together with a touch of tangerine essential oil to create a flirty scent. Davana is a unique oil, in that it smells different on everyone. Wear this on your pulse points for a unique, alluring fragrance.

1 tablespoon sweet almond oil
8 drops rose essential oil or rose absolute
8 drops mandarin essential oil
2 drops davana essential oil

1. In a small bottle, preferably with a roll-on applicator, combine the almond oil and essential oils. Shake well to blend.

2. With your fingertips or the roller, apply 1 drop to the pulse point behind each ear, and gently massage the area. If a stronger personal fragrance is desired, apply 1 drop to each wrist, your throat, or your inner elbows.

NOTE: Keep in a convenient location if you plan to use it up within a few weeks; otherwise, store it in a cool, dark place for up to a year.

Sensual Massage Oil

MAKES ABOUT 4 FLUID OUNCES (½ CUP)

This intoxicating blend includes ginger and ylang-ylang essential oils to promote feelings of intense happiness and heighten attraction. Sandalwood and patchouli essential oils promote euphoria, and the mandarin provides a yummy citrus note.

½ cup sweet almond oil
16 drops sandalwood essential oil
6 drops mandarin essential oil
4 drops patchouli essential oil
2 drops ginger essential oil
2 drops ylang-ylang essential oil

1. In a small bottle or jar with a lid, combine the almond oil and essential oils. Shake well to blend.

2. After bathing or showering, pat yourself dry and apply 1 teaspoon of the blend to your shoulders, neck, and upper arms, and massage it in. Add a little more to your legs and other areas, if you like.

MENOPAUSE

Although it can be uncomfortable, menopause is a normal part of the aging process. Aromatherapy can help with hot flashes, irritability, disrupted sleep, and other symptoms by stimulating the endocrine system and balancing the hormones, plus it can soothe specific symptoms.

Balancing Vitex Berry Lotion
MAKES ABOUT 8 FLUID OUNCES (1 CUP)

Vitex berry essential oil reduces the levels of estrogen in the body and increases the levels of progesterone, while rose and may chang essential oils lift the spirits and offer an irresistible fragrance. The vitex berry oil takes at least two months to have a real impact, so be sure to use this lotion daily.

8 fluid ounces (1 cup) unscented body lotion or hand cream
64 drops vitex berry essential oil
40 drops may chang essential oil
40 drops prediluted rose oil or 4 drops rose essential oil

1. In a medium bowl, combine the lotion and essential oils. Whisk to blend thoroughly, and then transfer the lotion to a medium jar with a lid or back into the empty lotion container.
2. Apply 1 teaspoon of the blend to your wrists and inner arms. Use a little more or less as needed, and feel free to apply the lotion to other body parts.
3. Use twice daily.

NOTE: Keep this lotion in a convenient location if you plan to use it all within 2 weeks; otherwise, store it in a glass bottle or jar in a cool, dark place.

Clary Sage Shower Melts

MAKES 24 MELTS

Comforting clary sage, geranium, and Roman chamomile essential oils combine with lavender essential oil and the steam from your shower to provide deep relaxation and relieve menopause symptoms.

5 cups baking soda
1 cup tap water
48 drops clary sage essential oil
24 drops geranium essential oil
24 drops lavender essential oil
24 drops Roman chamomile essential oil

1. Preheat the oven to 350°F and line 2 standard muffin tins with 24 cupcake liners (or make in 2 batches).
2. In a large bowl, combine the baking soda and water. Stir into a thick paste.
3. Evenly divide the paste among the muffin cups and bake for 20 minutes, or until dried through.
4. Allow the melts to cool completely, and then peel off the paper liners. To each melt add 2 drops of the clary sage, 1 drop of the geranium, 1 drop of the lavender, and 1 drop of the Roman chamomile essential oil. Transfer the melts immediately to several widemouth jars or a large storage container. Cover with lids.
5. Place 1 melt in the shower stall just before stepping in. Breathe deeply while you enjoy the fragrant steam.

Peppermint–Rose Geranium Gel for Hot Flashes

MAKES ABOUT 4 FLUID OUNCES (½ CUP)

Crisp peppermint essential oil combines with fragrant rose geranium essential oil to provide relief from hot flashes. Aloe vera gel provides an additional cooling sensation as it is absorbed by the skin.

7 tablespoons aloe vera gel
1 tablespoon fractionated coconut oil
40 drops rose geranium essential oil
20 drops peppermint essential oil

1. In a small bowl, combine the aloe vera, coconut oil, and essential oils. Whisk to blend thoroughly, and then transfer the gel to a small jar with a lid.
2. Apply a dime-sized amount of the blend to the back of your neck when you feel a hot flash coming. Use a little more or less as needed.
3. Repeat as needed throughout the day.

NOTE: If you like, you can keep this gel in the refrigerator for an intense cooling sensation upon application; otherwise, store it in a convenient location.

MENSTRUAL SYMPTOMS

Menstruation comes with its own set of complications. Cramping, bloating, and irregularity are a few of the most common. Remember to check in with your doctor at least once a year to ensure that your menstrual symptoms are not a sign of an underlying medical problem.

Cypress–German Chamomile Compress for Menstrual Cramps
MAKES 1 TREATMENT

Uplifting cypress and soothing German chamomile essential oils combine with heat to relax uterine muscle tissue and provide you with an emotional boost.

½ teaspoon fractionated coconut oil
5 drops cypress essential oil
5 drops geranium essential oil

1. In the palm of your hand, combine the coconut oil and essential oils.
2. Apply the blend to your lower abdomen, targeting the uterine area, and gently massage the blend in.
3. Lie down and cover your lower abdomen with a hot heating pad, following the manufacturer's instructions for safe use. Leave the heating pad in place for at least 15 minutes.
4. Repeat two or three times daily while suffering from cramps.

PREFERENCE TIP: If you'd like to use this compress at bedtime, add 2 to 4 drops of lavender essential oil to the blend for extra relaxation.

Fennel Seed–Grapefruit Massage for Bloating

MAKES ABOUT 4 FLUID OUNCES (½ CUP)

Soothing fennel seed and grapefruit essential oils improve circulation and encourage the body to release excess water, helping ease uncomfortable bloating.

2 tablespoons coconut oil, melted
2 tablespoons hemp oil
2 tablespoons sweet almond oil
2 tablespoons shea butter
64 drops grapefruit essential oil
32 drops fennel seed essential oil

1. In a small bowl, combine the coconut, hemp, and almond oils, the shea butter, and the essential oils. Whisk to blend thoroughly, and then transfer the message oil to a small jar with a lid.
2. Apply 1 teaspoon of the blend to the abdomen and massage the area, using light, gentle strokes. Apply 1 more teaspoon of the blend to your lower back, just above the buttocks, and massage in.
3. Repeat two or three times daily, until menstrual bloating subsides.

Synergistic Blend for Irregular Cycles

MAKES ABOUT 4 FLUID OUNCES (½ CUP)

A combination of Roman chamomile, geranium, fennel seed, vitex berry, and clary sage essential oils helps balance hormones and promotes regular menstruation. This blend often takes up to two months to start working, so be sure to use it daily.

½ cup sweet almond oil
60 drops clary sage essential oil
60 drops Roman chamomile essential oil
60 drops vitex berry essential oil
44 drops geranium essential oil
22 drops fennel seed essential oil

1. In a small bottle or jar with a lid, combine the almond oil and essential oils. Shake to blend.
2. Apply 1 drop of the blend to the inside of each elbow.
3. Repeat twice daily.

URINARY TRACT INFECTION (UTI)

Painful stinging upon urination and a constant feeling that you need to urinate even when your bladder is empty are two symptoms of a UTI. Aromatherapy treatments can help if you start to use them at the first sign of infection. If you have a fever or if the pain is getting worse, see your doctor.

Lavender Rinse

MAKES ABOUT 4 FLUID OUNCES (½ CUP)

Lavender essential oil stops pain and kills bacteria, especially when applied in a strong concentration like this one. If you notice any irritation, stop using this treatment.

½ cup distilled water

40 drops lavender essential oil

1. In a small bottle or jar with a lid, combine the water and essential oil. Shake well to blend, and then shake again before each use.
2. After urinating, draw at least 2 teaspoons of the blend into an oil-dispensing syringe, and then gently rinse the urethral opening. Be careful not to let the syringe come into contact with your body.
3. Repeat each time you urinate.

SUBSTITUTION TIP: If you don't have a syringe, you can use a cotton ball or cosmetic pad to apply the remedy. Be sure to completely saturate the urethral opening.

Synergistic Antibacterial Massage Blend

MAKES ABOUT 1 FLUID OUNCE (2 TABLESPOONS)

Fennel seed, tea tree, bergamot, cypress, and juniper berry essential oils offer strong antibacterial properties. Massaging your lower back and abdomen delivers the blend to the bladder.

2 tablespoons fractionated coconut oil
12 drops juniper berry essential oil
9 drops bergamot essential oil
9 drops tea tree essential oil
8 drops cypress essential oil
3 drops fennel seed essential oil

1. In a small bottle or jar with a lid, combine the coconut oil and essential oils. Shake well to blend.
2. At the first sign of discomfort, apply 1 teaspoon of the blend to your lower abdomen and lower back, and massage the blend in well.
3. If you have time, cover your lower abdomen with a hot heating pad, following the manufacturer's instructions for safe use. Leave the heating pad in place for 15 minutes.
4. Repeat twice daily.

Synergistic Antiseptic Bath Salts

MAKES 4 TREATMENTS

Bergamot, clove bud, juniper berry, eucalyptus, and cajuput essential oils are strong antiseptics that can help you fight off a UTI. The Epsom salts help by encouraging your body to release toxins.

2 tablespoons fractionated coconut oil
16 drops bergamot essential oil
16 drops clove bud essential oil
16 drops juniper berry essential oil
12 drops cajuput essential oil
12 drops *Eucalyptus globulus* essential oil
4 cups Epsom salts

1. In a large bowl, combine the coconut oil and essential oils. Add the Epsom salts and stir well to blend. Transfer the bath salts to a large jar with a lid.
2. Fill your bathtub with 4 inches of hot water and dissolve 1 cup of the bath salts in it. Soak in the bath for at least 20 minutes.
3. Repeat once daily.

VAGINAL YEAST INFECTION

Unbearable itching, irritation, and yeasty-smelling discharge are among the signs of a yeast infection caused by *Candida albicans*. This fungus naturally inhabits the body, only causing problems when its population grows out of control.

Lavender–Tea Tree Tampon

MAKES 1 TREATMENT

Lavender and tea tree essential oils offer potent antifungal action, quickly ridding the vagina of excess yeast.

1 tablespoon distilled water, warmed
2 drops lavender essential oil
2 drops tea tree essential oil
Tampons

1. In a small bowl, combine the water and essential oils. Soak an applicator-free tampon in the solution.
2. Insert the tampon into the vagina. Leave the tampon in place for 1 hour.
3. Repeat twice daily until the yeast infection is gone.

Lemon Salve

MAKES ABOUT 1 FLUID OUNCE (2 TABLESPOONS)

Lemon essential oil is an effective antifungal agent that makes short work of a yeast infection. Blended with fractionated coconut oil, it also soothes the burning and itching.

2 tablespoons fractionated coconut oil
16 drops lemon essential oil
Tampons

1. In a small bottle or jar with a lid, combine the coconut oil and essential oil. Shake well to blend.
2. Apply ½ teaspoon of the salve to an applicator-free tampon and insert it into the vagina. Leave the tampon in place for 2 hours.
3. Repeat three times daily, until the yeast infection is gone.

Synergistic Antifungal Douche

MAKES 1 TREATMENT

Rosemary, lavender, tea tree, and geranium essential oils combine with warm water and refreshing vinegar to kill excess yeast and soothe irritated tissue.

3 cups distilled water, heated to lukewarm
2 tablespoons distilled white vinegar
3 drops lavender essential oil
2 drops tea tree essential oil
2 drops rosemary essential oil
1 drop geranium essential oil

1. In a douche bag, combine the water, vinegar, and essential oils. Shake to blend.
2. In the shower, use the douche, following the manufacturer's instructions.
3. Repeat once daily until the yeast infection clears.

PART FOUR

Recipes, Remedies, and Applications for Beauty and Cosmetic Care

Beauty may be only skin deep, but when your cosmetics are enriched with essential oils, the benefits penetrate the skin, bringing you benefits at a deeper level. From frustrating pimples to painful cracked heels, common beauty problems are simple to solve with fragrant essential oils. If you're looking for a way to deal with dandruff, heal chapped lips, banish split ends, or strengthen brittle nails, this is the place to find it. Plus, making your own beauty products is not only fun—like playing with the best chemistry set ever—but it also allows you to detox your beauty routine and save money. As part of the planning process, remember to check each essential oil's profile to ensure it is suitable for you.

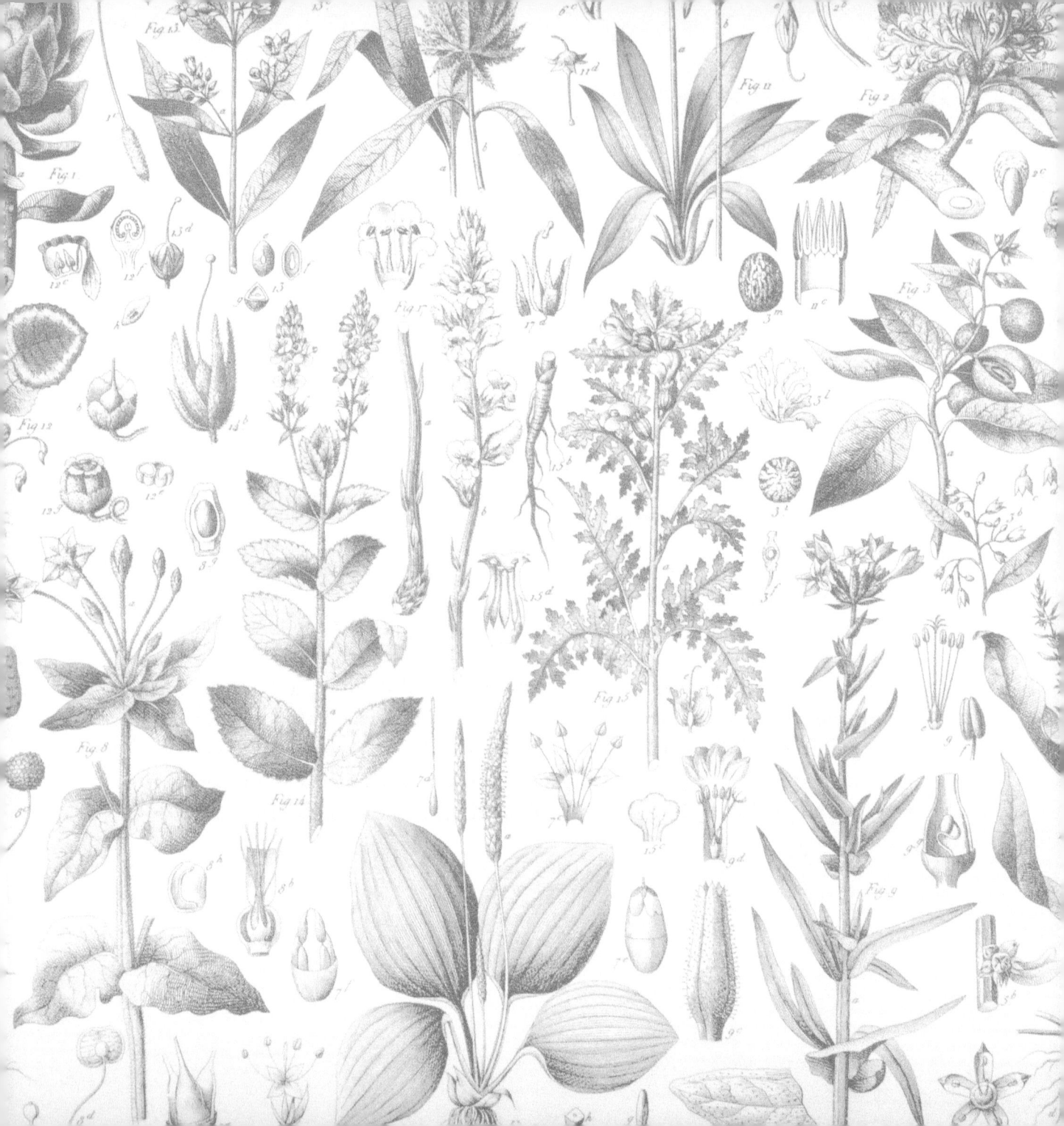

CHAPTER TEN

ACNE, WRINKLES, AND OTHER SKIN CARE

Acne 254	Oily Skin 266
Age Spots 256	Puffy Eyes 268
Body Odor 258	Razor Bumps 270
Cellulite 260	Rosacea 272
Dry Skin 262	Wrinkles 274
Ingrown Hair 264	

ACNE

Hormone fluctuations, clogged follicles, inflammation, bacteria, and a high-sugar/high-fat diet are some major contributors to acne. This condition shows up as inflamed skin, pimples, and clogged pores. Aromatherapy treatments work quickly and gently, leaving you with better-looking skin, naturally.

Anti-Acne "Spot Not" Mask
MAKES 1 TREATMENT

Acne breakouts can be annoying at best and disfiguring at worst. Commercial acne treatments are harsh and drying to the skin, and for people with sensitive skin they may present special problems. This simple facial treatment contains rosemary essential oil, which stimulates and regenerates cell growth, and thyme essential oil, which fights bacteria and infection that contribute to acne breakouts. The lactic acid in the yogurt serves as a mini treatment, peeling away dead skin that may contribute to blocked pores.

3 tablespoons plain full-fat yogurt
2 tablespoons organic raw honey
2 drops rosemary essential oil
2 drops thyme essential oil

1. In a small bowl, mix the yogurt, honey, and essential oils.
2. Using a fan brush, apply the mixture in a thin layer to the face and allow it to dry. Add a second layer to the first and allow it to dry. Continue applying layers and allowing them to dry until you have used all the mixture.
3. Leave the mask on for 15 minutes. Then rinse it away with warm water and remove any stubborn spots with a washcloth.
4. Pat your face dry with a clean towel.

SUBSTITUTION TIP: You can use other antibacterial agents in place of the rosemary and thyme, such as tea tree or lavender essential oils.

Cooling Cucumber Seed–Tea Tree Toner

MAKES ABOUT 4 FLUID OUNCES (½ CUP)

Cucumber seed essential oil is a natural astringent, while tea tree essential oil kills bacteria. Witch hazel offers a cool, non-drying tingle.

½ cup alcohol-free witch hazel
20 drops cucumber seed essential oil
4 drops tea tree essential oil

1. In a small bottle or jar with a lid, combine the witch hazel and essential oils, shake well to blend, and then shake again before each use.
2. Apply ¼ teaspoon of the toner to a cotton cosmetic pad and gently swipe it all over your freshly washed face.
3. Repeat morning and evening, before moisturizing.

Tea Tree Neat Treatment for Blemishes

MAKES 1 TREATMENT

Tea tree essential oil kills bacteria and shrinks blemishes quickly. Be sure to conduct a patch test before using this neat treatment.

1 drop tea tree essential oil

1. With a cotton swab, apply the essential oil to the blemish.
2. Repeat the treatment on any additional blemishes.
3. Repeat once or twice daily until blemishes are gone.

AGE SPOTS

Flat brown, gray, or black patches of skin caused by exposure to the sun, age spots vary in size and are common in adults over age 40. While age spots are harmless, they can look similar to skin cancer; to be on the safe side, have them checked out by your doctor before proceeding with aromatherapy treatments.

Lemon Mask

MAKES 1 TREATMENT

Lemon essential oil and yogurt encourage discolored skin to slough off quickly. Although this treatment is time-consuming, it is refreshing.

1 tablespoon plain full-fat yogurt
1 tablespoon oat flour
4 drops lemon essential oil

1. In a small bowl, combine the yogurt, flour, and essential oil. Whisk to blend thoroughly.
2. Wash and dry your face, and then apply the mask to your facial skin, being careful to avoid your eyes, as well as to any other areas where age spots are a concern. Leave the mask in place for 30 minutes and relax.
3. Rinse the mask off with cold water, and then apply your favorite moisturizer.
4. Repeat three times weekly, until age spots fade.

Sandalwood Neat Treatment

MAKES 1 TREATMENT

Sandalwood essential oil reduces the size and color of age spots, leaving fresh skin behind. Like other natural treatments, it takes several weeks to work. Be sure to conduct a patch test before using this neat treatment.

1 drop sandalwood essential oil

1. With a cotton swab, apply the sandalwood essential oil directly to the age spots. Add another drop if you need to cover a larger area.
2. Repeat once or twice daily, until age spots are gone.

Synergistic Age Spot Salve

MAKES ABOUT 1 OUNCE (2 TABLESPOONS)

Lavender, rose geranium, frankincense, and myrrh essential oils encourage the growth of healthy skin while helping fade age spots. Fractionated coconut oil helps prevent irritation by providing moisture.

2 tablespoons fractionated coconut oil
10 drops frankincense essential oil
10 drops lavender essential oil
10 drops myrrh essential oil
10 drops rose geranium essential oil

1. In a small bottle or jar with a lid, combine the coconut oil and essential oils. Shake well to blend.
2. With a cotton swab, apply 1 drop of the salve to each age spot.
3. Repeat two or three times daily, until age spots fade.

BODY ODOR

Body odor doesn't have to be a fact of life, even if you're avoiding commercial deodorants with harmful ingredients. Try these natural solutions for smelling fresh and clean, 24/7.

Lavender Body Powder

MAKES ABOUT 8 FLUID OUNCES (1 CUP)

Lavender essential oil offers antibacterial and antifungal properties, making it a good choice for dealing with body odor. If you prefer a citrus scent, replace the lavender with lemon eucalyptus essential oil.

¼ cup baking soda
40 drops lavender essential oil
½ cup non-GMO cornstarch
¼ cup rice flour
1 teaspoon uncooked rice (optional; for humidity control)

1. In a small bowl, combine the baking soda and essential oil. Stir well to combine.
2. Sift the mixture into a medium bowl, and then add the cornstarch and rice flour. Whisk to blend thoroughly. If you live in a humid climate, add the rice to keep the powder from clumping, and mix in well. Transfer the powder to a medium glass jar with a lid or a metal sugar shaker.
3. Sprinkle about ½ teaspoon of the powder onto the palm of your hand, and then apply to underarms and other body parts.

Minty Rosemary-Patchouli Body Spray

MAKES ABOUT 8 FLUID OUNCES (1 CUP)

Peppermint, rosemary, and patchouli essential oils combine to keep you smelling fresh and clean. As an added benefit, this spray is an all-natural insect repellent.

1 cup less 2 tablespoons distilled water
2 tablespoons alcohol-free witch hazel
12 drops patchouli essential oil
10 drops peppermint essential oil
5 drops rosemary essential oil

1. In a medium bottle with a fine-mist spray top, combine the water, witch hazel, and essential oils. Shake well to blend, and then shake again before each use.
2. Apply 1 spritz to each area of your body you'd like to address.

Rosewood Deodorant

MAKES ABOUT 4 FLUID OUNCES (½ CUP)

Fragrant rosewood essential oil combined with coconut oil and nourishing shea butter prevents fungal growth and stops odor. This deodorant offers gender-neutral appeal, thanks to its soft, woody aroma.

2 tablespoons coconut oil, melted
1 tablespoon arrowroot powder
1 tablespoon beeswax, melted
1 tablespoon food-grade diatomaceous earth
1 tablespoon shea butter
1 tablespoon sweet almond oil
25 drops rosewood essential oil
10 drops vitamin E oil

1. In a small bowl, combine the coconut oil, arrowroot, beeswax, diatomaceous earth, shea butter, almond oil, essential oil, and vitamin E oil. Whisk to blend thoroughly.
2. Pour the blend into a small jar with a lid and allow it to cool completely before capping.
3. With your fingertips, apply a pea-sized amount of the blend to each armpit, and massage the deodorant in, using light strokes, until absorbed.
4. Repeat once or twice daily as needed.

CELLULITE

Cellulite is harmless, but its lumpy, bumpy appearance can make you feel self-conscious. Aromatherapy helps improve the appearance of cellulite, and a sensible diet, daily exercise, and adequate hydration create the right environment for lasting improvement.

Anti-Cellulite Bath Salts

MAKES 8 TREATMENTS

Cypress, fennel seed, juniper berry, and grapefruit essential oils combine with Epsom salts to encourage your body to release toxins and get rid of the excess water weight that makes cellulite look so puffy.

2 tablespoons fractionated coconut oil
16 drops fennel seed essential oil
16 drops juniper berry essential oil
8 drops cypress essential oil
8 drops grapefruit essential oil
4 cups Epsom salts

1. In a large bowl, combine the coconut oil and essential oils. Add the Epsom salts and stir well to blend. Transfer the bath salts to a large jar with a lid.

2. Draw a hot bath and add ½ cup of the bath salts. Soak in the bath for at least 15 minutes.

3. Repeat at least twice weekly.

Synergistic Cellulite Massage Oil

MAKES ABOUT 2 FLUID OUNCES (¼ CUP)

A combination of grapefruit, cypress, juniper berry, and lavender essential oils flush out toxins and encourage stretched skin to firm up. Apply this massage oil after exercising, when circulation is at its best.

¼ cup jojoba oil
30 drops cypress essential oil
30 drops grapefruit essential oil
30 drops juniper berry essential oil
10 drops lavender essential oil

1. In a small bottle or jar with a lid, combine the jojoba oil and essential oils. Shake well to blend.
2. Apply 1 teaspoon of the massage oil to areas where cellulite is a concern, and massage the skin with firm, deep strokes.
3. Repeat once daily.

Synergistic Skin-Firming Lotion

MAKES ABOUT 8 FLUID OUNCES (1 CUP)

Lemon, cypress, rose geranium, and juniper essential oils encourage the body to release toxins while supporting lymphatic circulation and improving the appearance of cellulite.

7 fluid ounces (1 cup less 2 tablespoons) unscented body lotion or hand cream
2 tablespoons alcohol-free witch hazel
20 drops cypress essential oil
20 drops lemon essential oil
16 drops juniper essential oil
16 drops rose geranium essential oil

1. In a medium bowl, combine the lotion, witch hazel, and essential oils. Whisk to blend thoroughly, and then transfer the lotion to a medium jar with a lid, or back into the empty lotion container.
2. Apply 1 teaspoon of the lotion to areas where cellulite is a concern. Use a little more or less as needed, and feel free to apply the lotion to other body parts.
3. Use as often as you like throughout each day, especially after bathing or showering.

NOTE: Keep this lotion in a convenient location if you plan to use it all within 2 weeks; otherwise, store it in a glass bottle or jar in a cool, dark place.

DRY SKIN

Sun, wind, air-conditioning, and cold tend to leave skin feeling dry and itchy. Stay away from very hot water while working to repair it, and enjoy these nourishing aromatherapy remedies.

Moisturizing Chamomile Body Wash

MAKES 14 FLUID OUNCES (1½ CUPS)

Roman chamomile essential oil stimulates the skin's oil production, and it helps heal chapped and irritated areas.

1 cup plus 2 tablespoons unscented liquid castile soap

¼ cup fractionated coconut oil

20 drops Roman chamomile essential oil

1. In a large bowl, combine the soap, coconut oil, and essential oil. Whisk to blend thoroughly, and then pour the body wash into a large plastic squeeze bottle with a cap.
2. Apply 1 teaspoon of the body wash to a wet sponge or bath pouf, using a little more or less as needed. Lather briskly, and then rinse.
3. Pat yourself dry and follow up with Soothing Benzoin-Myrrh Body Lotion (page 263).

NOTE: Keep this body wash in the shower if you plan to use it all within 2 weeks; otherwise, store it in a glass bottle or jar in a cool, dark place.

Soothing Benzoin-Myrrh Body Lotion

MAKES ABOUT 8 FLUID OUNCES (1 CUP)

Benzoin, myrrh, and elemi essential oils help repair compromised skin while promoting deep moisture. The lotion forms a barrier between dry air and delicate skin.

8 fluid ounces (1 cup) unscented body lotion
20 drops myrrh essential oil
10 drops benzoin essential oil
10 drops elemi essential oil

1. In a medium bowl, combine the lotion and essential oils. Whisk to blend thoroughly, and then transfer the lotion to a medium jar with a lid or back into the empty lotion container.
2. Apply 1 teaspoon of the lotion to each area of dry skin, using a little more or less as needed.
3. Use as often as you like to keep skin moisturized.

NOTE: Keep this lotion in a convenient location if you plan to use it all within 2 weeks; otherwise, store it in a glass bottle or jar in a cool, dark place.

Sweet Orange–Rose Geranium Body Oil

MAKES ABOUT 8 FLUID OUNCES (1 CUP)

Sweet orange and rose geranium essential oils nourish and protect dry skin while helping compromised tissue repair itself. Body oil seals in moisture after a bath or shower, helping you stay comfortable longer.

½ cup jojoba oil
¼ cup sweet almond oil
¼ cup light sesame oil
30 drops rose geranium essential oil
20 drops sweet orange essential oil
10 drops prediluted jasmine essential oil (optional)

1. In a medium bowl, combine the jojoba, almond, and sesame oil. Stir in the essential oils. Whisk to blend thoroughly, and then pour the body oil into a medium plastic bottle with a pump top.
2. Shower or bathe as usual, but before drying off, stand on a towel and apply 1 teaspoon of body oil to your arms, legs, torso, hands, and feet, using a little more or less as needed.
3. Pat yourself dry, and then apply Soothing Benzoin-Myrrh Body Lotion.

NOTE: Keep this body oil near the shower if you plan to use it all within 2 weeks; otherwise, store it in a glass bottle or jar in a cool, dark place.

INGROWN HAIR

An ingrown hair sometimes looks like a little dark spot on your skin, but when bacteria get trapped below the surface, the skin around the hair swells and becomes inflamed. With a good scrub, it's easy to remove a hair that has grown back into the skin. Meanwhile, essential oils help prevent infection and calm inflammation.

Lavender Neat Treatment

MAKES 1 TREATMENT

If an ingrown hair is inflamed, lavender essential oil helps stop the pain and kill bacteria. You can use this treatment alongside a sugar scrub, or apply it after using tweezers to remove the hair and washing the area. Be sure to conduct a patch test before using this neat treatment.

1 drop lavender essential oil

1. Apply the lavender essential oil by dripping it directly onto the ingrown hair from the bottle, being careful not to touch the bottle to the skin.
2. Repeat once daily while irritation persists.

Peppermint Sugar Scrub

MAKES ABOUT 4 FLUID OUNCES (½ CUP)

Peppermint essential oil helps ease discomfort, while the sugar and coconut oil work together to free trapped hair. When the hair emerges, you can pluck it out, shave it off, or leave it.

½ cup brown sugar
¼ cup fractionated coconut oil
20 drops peppermint essential oil

1. In a small widemouth glass jar with a lid, combine the brown sugar, coconut oil, and essential oil. Stir well to blend.
2. After bathing or showering, apply 1 teaspoon of the sugar scrub to the ingrown hair, and massage the area, using firm circular strokes.
3. Rinse with warm water.
4. Repeat daily until the ingrown hair emerges.

Soothing Tea Tree Compress

MAKES 1 TREATMENT

Tea tree essential oil combines with soothing heat to ease pain and stop inflammation, while helping prevent infection.

½ teaspoon fractionated coconut oil
2 drops tea tree essential oil

1. In the palm of your hand, combine the coconut oil and essential oil.
2. Apply the blend to the site of the ingrown hair.
3. Relax and cover the area with a warm heating pad, following the manufacturer's instructions for safe use. Leave the heating pad in place for at least 15 minutes.
4. Repeat two or three times daily while working to free an inflamed ingrown hair.

OILY SKIN

Your skin produces oil to protect itself from outside elements, but the extra oil can feel heavy and uncomfortable while attracting impurities that can lead to acne. Aromatherapy helps bring your skin back into balance, leaving you feeling fresh and looking fantastic.

Cooling Spearmint-Strawberry Mask

MAKES 1 TREATMENT

Fresh strawberries and spearmint essential oil gently exfoliate and tone your skin without causing irritation. This treatment takes a little bit of time, but the result is worth it.

2 ripe strawberries, hulled and mashed
1 drop spearmint essential oil

1. In a small bowl, combine the strawberries and essential oil. Mash thoroughly with a fork to blend.
2. Spread the pulp on a facial mask sheet or a paper towel in which you've cut holes for your eyes and mouth.
3. Lie down comfortably and apply the mask to your face, pressing lightly to ensure that the pulp is in contact with your skin. Leave the mask in place for 15 minutes.
4. Rinse your face with water, pat dry, and then apply your favorite moisturizer.
5. Repeat up to three times weekly.

SUBSTITUTION TIP: If you dislike the idea of putting fruit on your face, you can blend the spearmint essential oil with 1 tablespoon of aloe vera gel instead.

Deep-Cleansing Lavender-Lemon Steam

MAKES 1 TREATMENT

Fragrant lavender and lemon essential oils work together to detoxify your skin without over-drying it. This luxurious steam is ideal for use before exfoliation.

2 cups near-boiling water
3 drops lavender essential oil
3 drops lemon essential oil

1. Pour the hot water into a large bowl and then add the essential oils.
2. Sit comfortably in front of the bowl and drape a towel over your head and the bowl, creating a tent that concentrates the steam and vapors. Emerge to breathe cool air as needed. Try to spend 10 minutes exposing your face to the treatment.
3. Repeat two or three times weekly.

Refreshing Peppermint–Cucumber Seed Toner

MAKES ABOUT 4 FLUID OUNCES (½ CUP)

Crisp, cool peppermint essential oil combines with refreshing cucumber seed essential oil and witch hazel to create a toner that removes excess oil without causing irritation.

½ cup alcohol-free witch hazel
12 drops cucumber seed essential oil
8 drops peppermint essential oil

1. In a small bottle with a narrow neck and a lid, combine the witch hazel and essential oils. Shake well to blend, and then shake again before each use.
2. Apply ¼ teaspoon of the toner to a cotton cosmetic pad and gently swipe it all over your freshly washed face.
3. Repeat twice daily, following up with oil-free moisturizer, if you like.

PUFFY EYES

Allergies, crying, overwork, or tiredness can lead to inflammation around the eyes. Puffiness goes away on its own after several hours, but you can use aromatherapy to help speed the process along.

Helichrysum–Cucumber Seed Compress

MAKES 1 TREATMENT

Refreshing cucumber seed and helichrysum essential oils combine with ice cubes to shrink swollen tissue and provide a feeling of refreshment.

½ teaspoon distilled water
1 drop helichrysum essential oil
1 drop cucumber seed essential oil
2 ice cubes

1. In a small bowl, combine the water and essential oils.
2. Soak 2 cotton cosmetic pads in the solution until saturated.
3. Lie down comfortably with your eyes closed, and gently place a pad over each eyelid. Top each pad with an ice cube. Leave the compress in place for 15 minutes.
4. Repeat two or three times daily, if needed.

Lavender Eye Massage

MAKES 1 TREATMENT

Soothing lavender essential oil and nourishing rosehip oil combine to stop swelling and heal delicate tissue. If the puffy areas around your eyes have a purple or blue tone, this is a good remedy to try.

2 drops lavender essential oil
2 drops rosehip oil

1. In the palm of your nondominant hand, combine the essential oil and rosehip oil.
2. With the ring finger of your dominant hand, gently dab a drop of the blend onto each swollen area. Using very light pressure, massage the area until the blend is fully absorbed.
3. Repeat daily.

Synergistic Eye Serum

MAKES 100 TREATMENTS

Soothing cypress, frankincense, and Roman chamomile essential oils combine to calm the inflammation that causes puffy eyes.

1 tablespoon sweet almond oil
8 drops cypress essential oil
8 drops frankincense essential oil
2 drops Roman chamomile essential oil

1. In a small bottle, preferably with a roll-on applicator, combine the almond oil and essential oils. Shake well to blend.
2. With your fingertips or the roller, apply 1 drop of the serum to each swollen area below your eye. Gently massage the serum in, taking care not to get it in your eye or on sensitive eye tissue.

NOTE: Keep in a convenient location if you plan to use it up within a few weeks; otherwise, store it in a cool, dark place for up to a year.

RAZOR BUMPS

Shaving leaves you hair free, but all too often with irritated red bumps left behind. These simple aromatherapy treatments address the swelling, itchiness, and discomfort, leaving your skin looking smooth and healthy.

Honey-Lavender Mask

MAKES 1 TREATMENT

Honey and lavender essential oil offer antibacterial properties, plus they soothe the itching, reduce redness, and help bring swelling down.

10 drops lavender essential oil
1 teaspoon plain honey

1. After completing a patch test, with your fingertips or a cotton swab, apply the lavender essential oil directly to the affected area. Use additional drops if treating a large area or reduce the number of drops if treating a small area.

2. With your fingertips, apply the honey over the lavender essential oil. Use a little more or less as needed to cover the affected area. Leave the treatment in place for 10 to 15 minutes.

3. Rinse the area with cool water and pat dry.

4. Repeat once or twice daily, as needed.

Lavender–Tea Tree Balm

MAKES ABOUT 1 FLUID OUNCE (2 TABLESPOONS)

Soothing lavender and tea tree essential oils combine with antibacterial coconut oil to help prevent razor bumps on freshly shaved skin.

2 tablespoons coconut oil, melted
24 drops tea tree essential oil
14 drops lavender essential oil

1. In a small bowl, combine the coconut oil and essential oils. Whisk to blend thoroughly, and then transfer the balm to a small jar with a lid.
2. After shaving, apply ½ teaspoon of the balm to the shaved area, and rub it in gently.
3. Repeat each time you shave to prevent razor bumps.

Tea Tree Gel

MAKES ABOUT 4 FLUID OUNCES (½ CUP)

Antiseptic tea tree essential oil combines with soothing aloe vera gel to stop infection and ease inflammation quickly.

½ cup aloe vera gel
20 drops tea tree essential oil

1. In a small bowl, combine the aloe vera and essential oil. Whisk to blend thoroughly, and then transfer the gel to a small jar with a lid.
2. Apply 1 teaspoon of the blend to the affected area, using a little more or less as needed.
3. Repeat two or three times daily, whenever razor bumps are a problem.

NOTE: If you like, you can keep this gel in the refrigerator for an intense cooling sensation upon application; otherwise, store in a cool, dark place.

ROSACEA

Rosacea causes redness on the cheeks, chin, forehead, and nose, often with accompanying bumps and pimples. Avoiding triggers is the best way to prevent flare-ups, but when a flare-up does occur, aromatherapy can help bring your skin back to normal.

Rosacea Treatment for Mature Skin

MAKES 1 FLUID OUNCE (2 TABLESPOONS)

Rosacea can become more pronounced with age, and what began as a healthy-looking flush to the cheeks as a teen can turn into something far more serious, including disfigurement. This blend uses jojoba oil, which is recommended for use with rosacea. The carrot seed essential oil provides vitamin A, which is good for aging skin. The bergamot and lavender essential oils soothe and reduce inflammation.

2 tablespoons jojoba oil
2 drops carrot seed essential oil
2 drops bergamot essential oil
2 drops lavender essential oil

1. In a small bottle with a lid, combine the jojoba oil and essential oils and shake to mix well.
2. Shake before each use. Smooth a few drops onto a clean, dry face once daily.

NOTE: Store in a tightly sealed container in a cool, dark place for up to a year.

Soothing Chamomile-Cypress Gel

MAKES 4 FLUID OUNCES (½ CUP)

German chamomile and cypress essential oils combine with peppermint essential oil to soothe inflammation, shrink swollen tissue, and promote cooling.

7 tablespoons aloe vera gel
1 tablespoon fractionated coconut oil
6 drops cypress essential oil
6 drops German chamomile essential oil
4 drops peppermint essential oil

1. In a small bowl, combine the aloe vera, coconut oil, and essential oils. Whisk to blend thoroughly, and then transfer the gel to a small jar with a lid.
2. Apply 1 teaspoon of the blend to the affected area, using a little more or less as needed.
3. Repeat two or three times daily, until the rosacea flare-up subsides.

NOTE: If you like, you can keep this gel in the refrigerator for an intense cooling sensation upon application; otherwise, store in a cool, dark place.

Synergistic Rosacea Blend

MAKES 4 FLUID OUNCES (½ CUP)

Sweet orange, fragrant geranium, and soothing helichrysum essential oils combine with grapefruit and cypress essential oils to shrink swelling and help irritated skin heal.

½ cup calendula oil
4 drops helichrysum essential oil
3 drops cypress essential oil
2 drops geranium or rose geranium essential oil
2 drops grapefruit essential oil
2 drops lavender essential oil
2 drops sweet orange essential oil

1. In a small bottle or jar with a lid, combine the calendula oil and essential oils. Shake well to blend.
2. With a cotton cosmetic pad, apply ½ teaspoon of the blend to your freshly washed face, targeting all areas where rosacea is present. Use a little more or less as needed.
3. Repeat twice daily.

WRINKLES

Wrinkles are a by-product of facial expressions, repetitive facial movements, and sun damage. Most people will develop wrinkles at some point. Aromatherapy can help firm skin and reduce the appearance of wrinkles and crow's-feet, especially if you make a point of taking preventive action.

Rosewood-Patchouli Toner

MAKES ABOUT 4 FLUID OUNCES (½ CUP)

Rosewood and patchouli essential oils nourish your skin and improve circulation, while the rosewater provides a skin-softening effect.

½ cup rosewater
10 drops rosewood essential oil
10 drops patchouli essential oil

1. In a small bottle or jar with a lid, combine the rosewater and essential oils. Shake well to blend, and then shake again before each use.
2. Apply ¼ teaspoon of the toner to a cotton cosmetic pad and gently swipe it all over your freshly washed face.
3. Repeat morning and evening, before moisturizing.

Synergistic Firming Serum

MAKES ABOUT 2 FLUID OUNCES (¼ CUP)

Refreshing cucumber seed essential oil joins forces with others to tighten, moisturize, balance, and even out your skin's appearance. Rosehip oil is a must-have for this treatment because it increases collagen production and encourages cell regeneration.

2 tablespoons sweet almond oil
2 tablespoons rosehip oil
10 drops cypress essential oil
10 drops geranium essential oil
7 drops frankincense essential oil
3 drops cucumber seed essential oil

1. In a small bottle with an orifice reducer, combine the almond and rosehip oil, and then stir in the essential oils. Shake well to blend.
2. With your fingertips, apply 2 to 3 drops of serum to your freshly washed face. Use a little more or less, so that the serum covers your entire face and absorbs completely.
3. Treat your neck and décolletage areas, if you like.
4. Repeat once or twice daily.

Synergistic Smoothing Blend

MAKES ABOUT 2 FLUID OUNCES (¼ CUP)

Rosehip oil delivers the potent elemi, lavender, and neroli essential oils deep into skin, helping reduce the appearance of fine lines and wrinkles.

¼ cup rosehip oil
10 drops elemi essential oil
10 drops lavender essential oil
10 drops neroli essential oil

1. In a small bottle with an orifice reducer, combine the rosehip oil and essential oils. Shake well to blend.
2. With your fingertips, apply 2 to 3 drops to your freshly washed face. Use a little more or less so that the blend covers your entire face and absorbs completely. Treat your neck and décolletage areas, if you like.
3. Repeat once or twice daily.

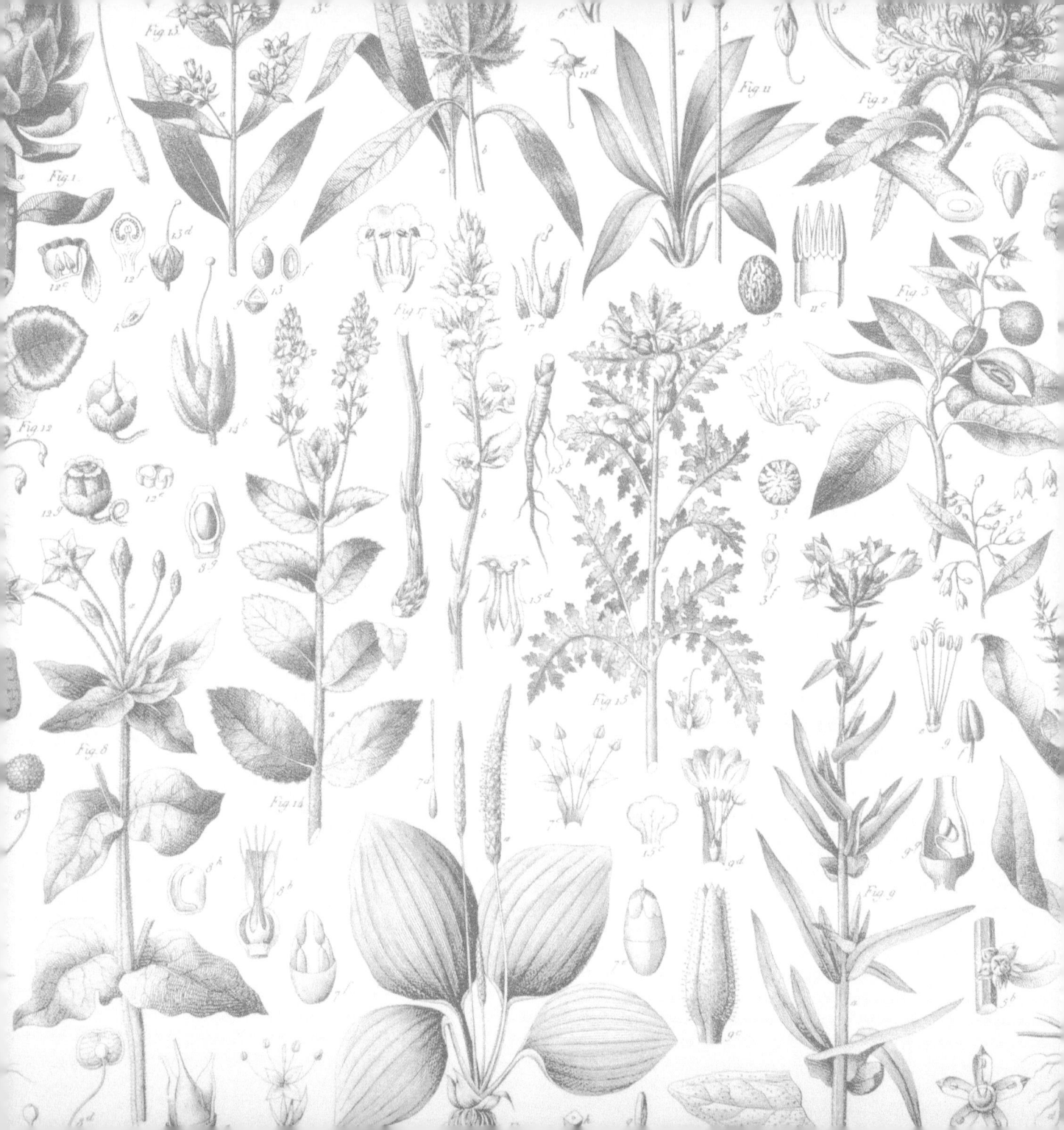

CHAPTER ELEVEN

MOISTURIZERS AND TONERS

Basic Body Butter

MAKES ABOUT 3 FLUID OUNCES (¾ CUP)

"Body butter" is a marketing term that basically means a heavy moisturizer intended to be used on the body rather than the face, where it might clog pores and cause acne. Body butters usually have a base that is a solid carrier oil, such as shea butter or coconut oil.

½ cup shea butter
2 tablespoons sweet almond oil
20 drops essential oil of choice

1. In a medium bowl, blend the shea butter and almond oil with a fork.
2. Add the essential oil and mix well. To make the texture creamier, whip the mixture with a hand mixer for 6 to 10 minutes to "fluff" it up.
3. Transfer the butter to a medium jar with a lid.
4. Smooth some of the butter liberally on dry skin once or twice a day.

NOTE: Store the tightly sealed jar in a cool, dark place for up to a year.

Citrus-Flower Body Butter

MAKES 8 FLUID OUNCES (1 CUP)

The sweet floral notes of the ylang-ylang essential oil pair well with the soft orange scent of neroli essential oil to create a light, fragrant, and nourishing body butter. Smooth it on all over the body after a bath when the skin more readily absorbs moisture from lotions and butters.

½ cup sweet almond oil
½ cup coconut oil, melted
6 drops neroli essential oil
4 drops ylang-ylang essential oil

1. In a medium bowl, mix the almond oil and coconut oil. Stir in the essential oils.
2. Using a hand mixer, beat the mixture for 6 to 10 minutes, until it's creamy and has increased in bulk. Transfer the mixture to a medium jar with a lid.
3. Smooth 1 teaspoon at a time of the body butter on dry skin after a bath.

NOTE: Store the tightly sealed jar in a cool, dark place for up to a year.

SUBSTITUTION TIP: Neroli essential oil can be pricey, so feel free to substitute sweet orange, mandarin, or any other low-cost citrus essential oil.

Citrus Serum for Combination Skin

MAKES 1 FLUID OUNCE (2 TABLESPOONS)

If you have combination skin, it's probably oily in the T-zone (forehead, nose, and chin) and dry on the cheeks. Sweet almond oil is a light carrier oil that moisturizes but won't clog pores. It will keep dry skin moisturized without making it oily.

2 tablespoons sweet almond oil
8 drops sweet orange essential oil
7 drops lemon essential oil

1. In a small bottle with a dropper top, combine the almond oil and essential oils. Shake to mix well.
2. Shake before each use. With your fingertips, pat a small amount onto the skin before moisturizing each night at bedtime.

NOTE: Store the tightly sealed bottle in a cool, dark location for up to a year.

Easy Whipped Moisturizer

MAKES 8 FLUID OUNCES (1 CUP)

With just two ingredients and 6 minutes of your time, you can create a lovely moisturizing blend. Use it as a facial moisturizer or a body butter. Geranium essential oil is known for its medicinal properties and has been used in cosmetics since ancient times to moisturize the skin and fight wrinkles.

1 cup coconut oil, melted
6 drops geranium essential oil

1. In a medium bowl, combine the coconut oil and essential oil. Using a hand mixer with the whisk attachment, whip the lotion for 6 to 10 minutes, until fluffy.
2. Transfer the mixture to a medium jar with a lid.
3. Use your fingertips to smooth a small amount of this lotion onto clean, dry skin.

NOTE: Store the tightly sealed jar in a cool, dark location for up to a year.

Frankincense and Commonsense Serum

MAKES ABOUT 2 FLUID OUNCES (¼ CUP)

Frankincense essential oil has been used since ancient times as a skin conditioner, and this richly fragrant serum is healing and restorative. The rosehip oil and vitamin E add to the antiaging properties of this serum, while the carrot seed and geranium essential oils boost the serum's antioxidants.

2½ tablespoons sweet almond oil
½ tablespoon jojoba oil
2 drops evening primrose oil
2 drops vitamin E oil
10 drops frankincense essential oil
10 drops geranium essential oil
10 drops cypress essential oil
2 drops carrot seed essential oil

1. In a small bottle with a lid, combine the almond, jojoba, and evening primrose oils, then add the vitamin E oil and the essential oils and stir to combine.
2. Use your fingertips to smooth the serum over the face and neck nightly before going to bed.

NOTE: Store, tightly sealed, in the refrigerator for up to 6 months. Discard the mixture if it smells odd or looks discolored.

Green Tea Toner

MAKES 8 FLUID OUNCES (1 CUP)

Green tea lends a strong herbal note to this toner. The tea and vinegar serve as astringents to close the pores and fight oil, while the thyme essential oil has disinfectant and antiseptic properties to clean and tone skin.

¾ cup brewed green tea, cooled
¼ cup apple cider vinegar
15 drops thyme essential oil

1. In a medium bowl, combine the tea and vinegar. Add the essential oil and stir to mix well.
2. Transfer the mixture to a medium spray bottle.
3. Spritz on your face after cleansing it thoroughly. Allow the toner to air-dry.

NOTE: Store the tightly sealed spray bottle in the refrigerator for up to 3 months.

SUBSTITUTION TIP: You can replace the thyme oil with rosemary essential oil for the same effects but with a different scent.

Nourishing Nighttime Lotion

MAKES 2 FLUID OUNCES (¼ CUP)

It is a common misconception that acne-prone skin doesn't need any more lubrication. Moisturizing can help open pores, which works to prevent blemishes from forming in the first place. Avoid using alcohol-based moisturizers, as they can cause inflammation. The combination of essential oils in this lotion has a clean, unisex scent, and the hazelnut oil is absorbed by the skin without leaving behind excess oil.

¼ cup hazelnut oil
4 drops borage seed oil
4 drops fennel essential oil
2 drops bergamot essential oil
2 drops carrot seed essential oil (optional)

1. In a small bottle with a lid, combine the hazelnut and borage seed oils, then add the essential oils and shake well.
2. Using your fingertips, gently pat the oil onto your face at bedtime.

NOTE: Store the tightly sealed bottle in the refrigerator for up to 6 months.

SUBSTITUTION TIP: Sweet almond oil is another light and noncomedogenic (doesn't clog pores) carrier oil that makes an excellent substitute here. To make this a wrinkle-fighting oil, try using rosehip oil in place of the borage oil.

Sandalwood Serum

MAKES 1 FLUID OUNCE (2 TABLESPOONS)

Next to exfoliation, the other secret to treating dry skin is keeping it hydrated and moisturized. Use this serum in addition to your regular moisturizers to boost the effectiveness of both in areas that need a little extra help.

1 tablespoon rosehip oil
1 tablespoon sweet almond oil
10 drops sandalwood essential oil
2 drops lemon essential oil

1. In a small bottle with a lid, combine the rosehip and almond oils, then add the essential oils and shake to blend.
2. Shake before using. Smooth 1 or 2 drops on your face at bedtime before moisturizing.
3. Allow the serum to settle into the skin for a minute or so before applying moisturizer.

NOTE: Rosehip oil spoils quickly, so make very small batches of this serum and keep it tightly sealed in the refrigerator for 3 to 6 months. If it develops an off smell, discard it.

SUBSTITUTION TIP: Either bergamot oil or the less-expensive orange essential oil work for this mix as well, as sandalwood essential oil blends well with a number of citrus oils. Note that the citrus oils are phototoxic, so stay out of the sun after applying this serum.

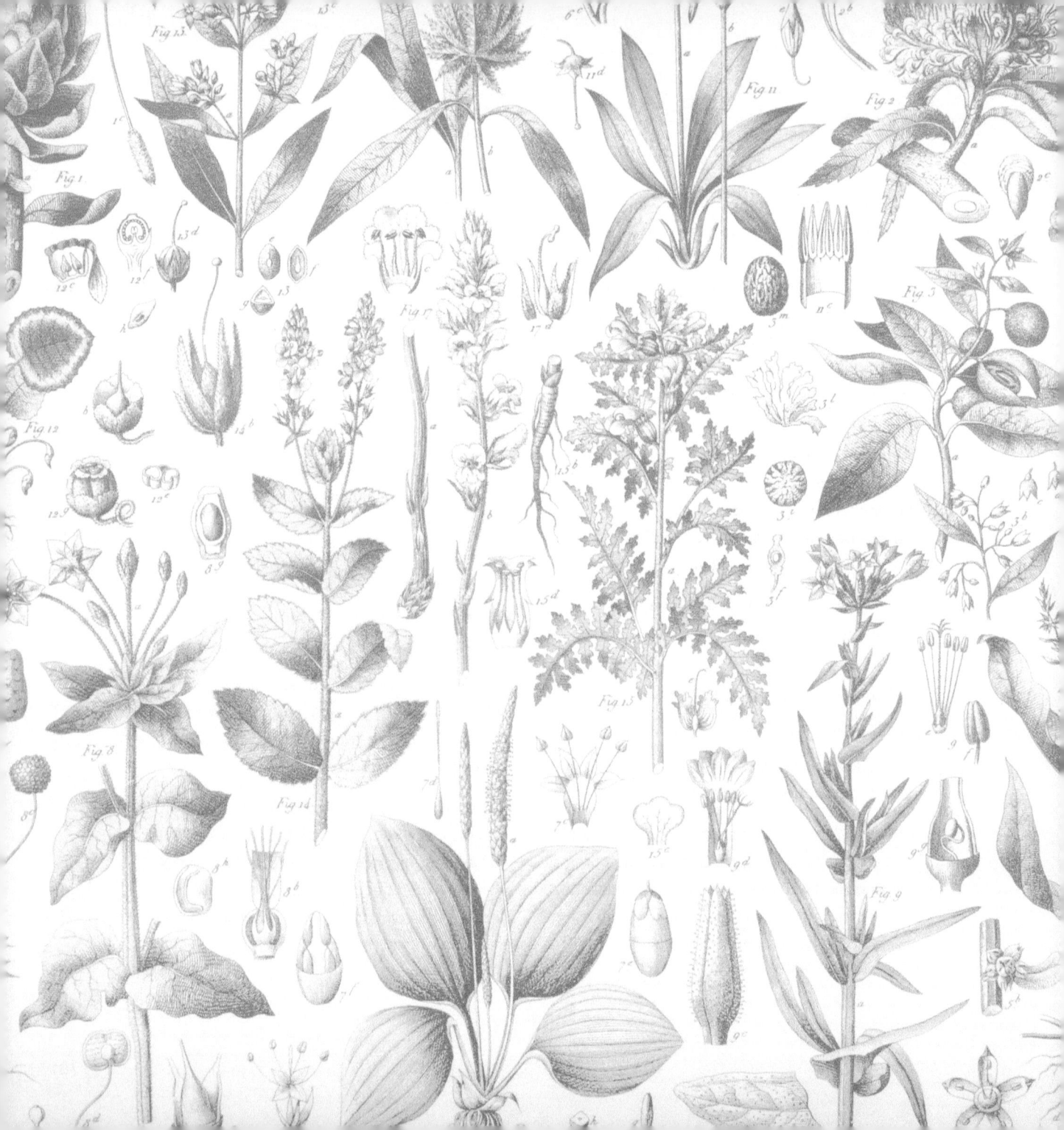

CHAPTER TWELVE

HEALTHY, STRONG HAIR

Dandruff 284

Dry Hair 286

Oily Hair 288

Split Ends 290

DANDRUFF

While many view dandruff as a cosmetic problem, it's also an itchy condition that can cause much discomfort. Because dandruff can worsen when you're sick or stressed, relaxing aromatherapy shampoos prove helpful on multiple fronts.

Peppermint-Rosemary Conditioner

MAKES ABOUT 8 FLUID OUNCES (1 CUP)

Peppermint, rosemary, and lavender essential oils soothe itching and help stop dandruff while also promoting healthy, shiny hair.

8 fluid ounces (1 cup) unscented conditioner
25 drops peppermint essential oil
20 drops lavender essential oil
10 drops rosemary essential oil

1. In a medium bowl, combine the conditioner and essential oils. Whisk to blend thoroughly, and then pour into a medium plastic squeeze bottle or back into the empty conditioner bottle.

2. After shampooing, apply 1 teaspoon of the conditioner to your hair, using a little more or less as needed. Massage it gently into your scalp, wait 1 minute, and then rinse with cool water.

3. Repeat every time you wash your hair.

NOTE: Keep this conditioner in the shower if you plan to use it all within 2 weeks; otherwise store it in a glass bottle or jar in a cool, dark place.

Synergistic Dandruff Shampoo

MAKES ABOUT 8 FLUID OUNCES (1 CUP)

Rosemary, lavender, and tea tree essential oils combine with a touch of refreshing peppermint essential oil to soothe itching and kill bacteria that contribute to dandruff. You can use this shampoo every time you wash your hair.

8 fluid ounces (1 cup) unscented shampoo
20 drops lavender essential oil
20 drops peppermint essential oil
10 drops tea tree essential oil
5 drops rosemary essential oil

1. In a medium bowl, combine the shampoo and essential oils. Whisk to blend thoroughly, and then pour into a medium plastic squeeze bottle or back into the empty shampoo bottle.
2. Wet your hair and apply 1 teaspoon of the shampoo to your hair, using a little more or less as needed. Lather briskly, and then rinse.
3. Follow up with the Peppermint-Rosemary Conditioner (page 284).

NOTE: Keep this shampoo in the shower if you plan to use it all within 2 weeks; otherwise, store it in a glass bottle or jar in a cool, dark place.

Tea Tree–Orange Dandruff Treatment

MAKES ABOUT 2 FLUID OUNCES (¼ CUP)

Tea tree essential oil is well known for its antidandruff properties. Here, orange essential oil sweetens the scent of this treatment, keeping it from becoming overly medicinal. The peppermint scent cools the scalp as you massage it, while the sweet almond oil moisturizes and exfoliates, removing the flakes.

3 tablespoons sweet almond oil
20 drops orange essential oil
10 drops tea tree essential oil
10 drops peppermint essential oil

1. In a small spray bottle, combine the almond oil and essential oils and shake to mix well.
2. Spray over dry hair, making sure the mixture gets down to the scalp. Use your fingers to massage it into your scalp. (You may have to section off your hair with a comb and clips.)
3. Leave the mixture on overnight. Then rinse out the next morning with just a small amount of shampoo.

NOTE: Store the tightly sealed bottle in a cool, dark place for up to a year.

DRY HAIR

Dry, damaged hair often has a dull appearance, and it is much less manageable than healthy hair. Moisturizing aromatherapy treatments help restore shine and smoothness. If possible, stop using heated styling tools and allow your hair to dry naturally.

Clary Sage–Sandalwood Conditioner

MAKES ABOUT 8 FLUID OUNCES (1 CUP)

Clary sage essential oil stimulates the scalp, encouraging healthy new hair growth, while sandalwood essential oil softens hair and leaves an intoxicating fragrance behind.

8 fluid ounces (1 cup) unscented hair conditioner
20 drops sandalwood essential oil
10 drops clary sage essential oil

1. In a medium bowl, combine the conditioner and essential oils. Whisk to blend thoroughly, and then pour into a medium plastic squeeze bottle or back into the empty conditioner bottle.

2. After shampooing, apply 1 teaspoon of the conditioner to your hair, using a little more or less as needed. Massage it gently into your scalp, wait 1 minute, and then rinse with cool water.

3. Repeat every time you wash your hair.

NOTE: Keep this conditioner in the shower if you plan to use it all within 2 weeks; otherwise, store it in a glass bottle or jar in a cool, dark place.

Moisturizing Chamomile Hair Mask

MAKES 1 TREATMENT

Chamomile essential oil soothes your scalp while lending softness and shine to your hair.

2 tablespoons olive oil, warmed
10 drops Roman chamomile essential oil

1. In a small bottle or bowl, combine the olive oil and essential oil. Shake or stir well to blend.
2. Apply the entire treatment to your hair, working it in. Wrap your head in a towel and leave the towel on for 10 minutes.
3. Wash and condition your hair as usual, and then allow it to air-dry before styling it.
4. Repeat three or four times weekly, as needed.

Moisturizing Geranium-Myrrh Shampoo

MAKES ABOUT 8 FLUID OUNCES (1 CUP)

Myrrh and geranium essential oils smell marvelous together, and they help strengthen hair. A touch of fractionated coconut oil provides softness and shine. You can use this shampoo every time you wash your hair.

7½ fluid ounces (1 cup less 1 tablespoon) unscented shampoo
1 tablespoon fractionated coconut oil
20 drops myrrh essential oil
20 drops geranium essential oil

1. In a medium bowl, combine the shampoo, coconut oil, and essential oils. Whisk to blend thoroughly, and then pour into a medium plastic squeeze bottle or back into the empty shampoo bottle.
2. Wet your hair and apply 1 teaspoon of the shampoo to your hair, using a little more or less as needed. Lather briskly, and then rinse. Follow up with Clary Sage–Sandalwood Conditioner (page 286).

NOTE: Keep this shampoo in the shower if you plan to use it all within 2 weeks; otherwise, store it in a glass bottle or jar in a cool, dark place.

OILY HAIR

Not only does excess oil weigh down your hair, but it may also be accompanied by dandruff. Aromatherapy helps by balancing oil production and removing excess oil from your scalp, minus the chemicals found in many commercial hair products.

Dry Shampoo

MAKES 8 OUNCES (1 CUP)

Dry shampoo absorbs excess oil and leaves hair looking fresh. Peppermint essential oil provides a pleasant tingle and leaves a delightful fragrance behind.

FOR LIGHT HAIR

1 cup arrowroot powder

20 drops peppermint essential oil

FOR DARK HAIR

½ cup arrowroot powder

20 drops peppermint essential oil

½ cup unsweetened cocoa powder

1. For either hair type: In a medium bowl, combine the arrowroot and essential oil; for dark hair, also stir in the cocoa powder. Whisk to blend thoroughly. Sift the mixture into a second bowl to remove any lumps, and then transfer to a medium jar with a lid.

2. Use a long-handled cosmetic brush to apply a very light dusting of the powder to your scalp, focusing on just the areas where oiliness is a problem.

3. Use a fine-toothed comb or brush to work the powder away from your scalp.

4. Repeat as needed.

PREFERENCE TIP: Though the peppermint essential oil imparts a fresh smell, you can substitute any preferred essential oil.

Lavender–Tea Tree Conditioner

MAKES ABOUT 8 FLUID OUNCES (1 CUP)

Lavender and tea tree essential oils condition your hair but leave no oily residue behind. If dandruff is an issue for you, as is often the case when hair is oily, you'll be glad to know that this conditioner helps stop flaking, as well.

8 fluid ounces (1 cup) unsecented oil-free hair conditioner
20 drops lavender essential oil
10 drops tea tree essential oil

1. In a medium bowl, combine the conditioner and essential oils. Whisk to blend thoroughly, and then pour into a medium plastic squeeze bottle or back into the empty conditioner bottle.

2. After shampooing, apply 1 teaspoon of the conditioner to your hair, using a little more or less as needed. Massage it gently into your scalp, wait 1 minute, and then rinse with cool water.

NOTE: Keep this conditioner in the shower if you plan to use it within 2 weeks; otherwise, store it in a glass bottle or jar in a cool, dark place.

Rosemary-Peppermint Shampoo

MAKES ABOUT 8 FLUID OUNCES (1 CUP)

Rosemary and peppermint essential oils make a fantastic-smelling combo; they also help eliminate excess oil from your scalp.

8 fluid ounces (1 cup) unscented shampoo
20 drops peppermint essential oil
20 drops rosemary essential oil

1. In a medium bowl, combine the shampoo and essential oils. Whisk to blend thoroughly, and then pour into a medium plastic squeeze bottle or back into the empty shampoo bottle.

2. Wet your hair and apply 1 teaspoon of the shampoo to your hair, using a little more or less as needed. Lather briskly, and then rinse.

3. Follow up with Lavender–Tea Tree Conditioner (see previous).

NOTE: Keep this shampoo in the shower if you plan to use it all within 2 weeks; otherwise, store it in a glass bottle or jar in a cool, dark place.

SPLIT ENDS

Heated styling tools and rough handling are two of the main causes of split ends. While the only true way to get rid of split ends is to trim them off, aromatherapy treatments can help improve your look by smoothing and softening your hair to make it more manageable.

Sandalwood Split-End Gel

MAKES 1 FLUID OUNCE (2 TABLESPOONS)

Sandalwood essential oil softens and strengthens hair, which helps prevent breakage and keeps your split ends from getting worse. Just a little bit of this gel goes a long way.

2 tablespoons aloe vera gel
10 drops sandalwood essential oil

1. In a small bowl, combine the aloe vera and essential oil. Whisk to blend thoroughly, and then transfer the gel to a small jar with a lid.
2. With your fingertips, apply 1 drop of the gel to each area where split ends are present.
3. Repeat the treatment two or three times daily, as needed.

Synergistic Split-End Conditioner

MAKES 2 FLUID OUNCES (¼ CUP)

Rosemary, peppermint, geranium, lavender, and clary sage essential oils combine with rich coconut oil and sweet almond oil to nourish and soften hair between cuts.

3 tablespoons coconut oil, melted
1 tablespoon sweet almond oil
2 drops geranium essential oil
2 drops lavender essential oil
2 drops peppermint essential oil
1 drop clary sage essential oil
1 drop rosemary essential oil

1. In a small bowl, combine the coconut and almond oils, then stir in the essential oils. Whisk to blend thoroughly, and then transfer to a small jar with a lid.

2. Before showering, apply the conditioner to the tips of your hair. Allow it to sit for 15 minutes, then wash and condition hair as usual.

Ultra-Rich Conditioning Mask

MAKES 1 TREATMENT

A combination of helichrysum, myrrh, and lavender essential oils in a base of rich olive oil delivers intense moisture to hair and helps improve the appearance of split ends.

¼ cup olive oil
4 drops lavender essential oil
2 drops helichrysum essential oil
2 drops myrrh essential oil

1. In a small bowl, combine the olive oil and essential oils. Whisk to blend thoroughly.

2. Before showering, apply the mask to your hair, completely saturating it. Allow it to sit for 15 minutes, then wash and condition hair as usual.

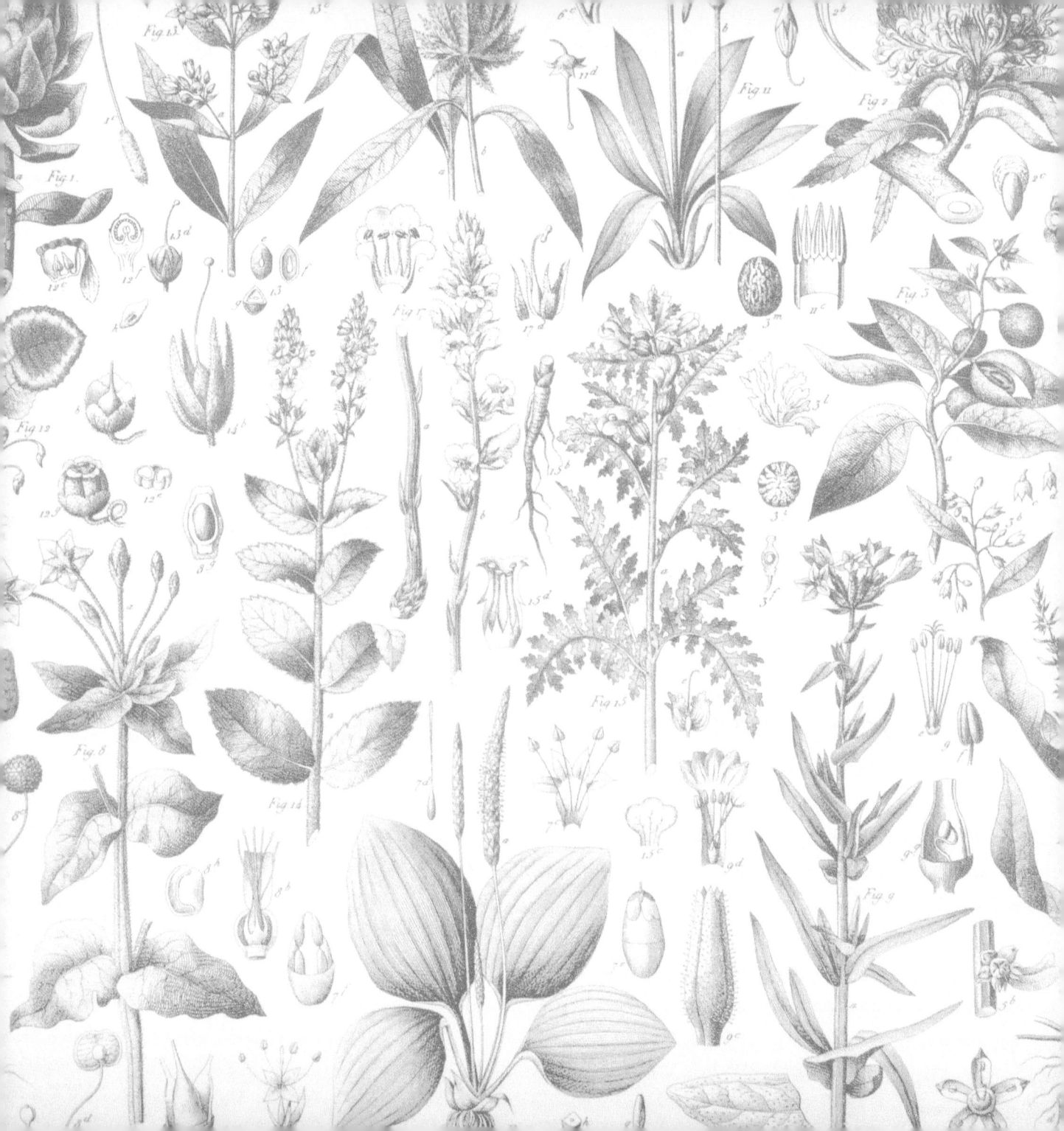

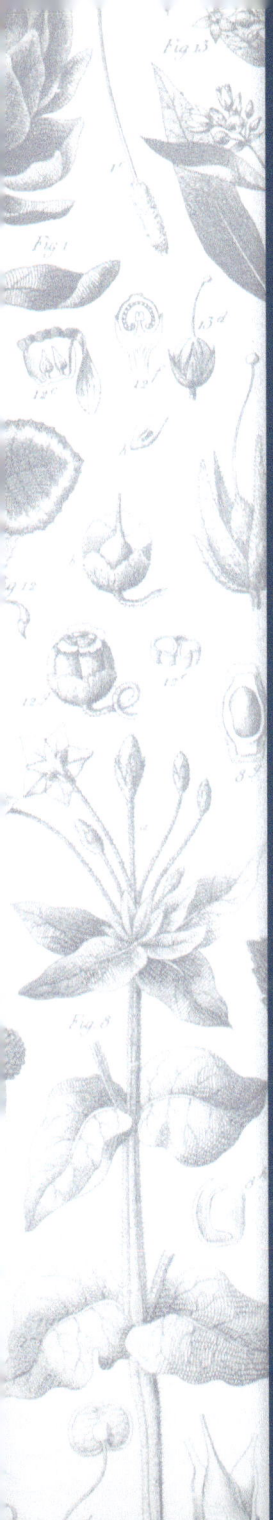

CHAPTER THIRTEEN

NURTURING THE HANDS AND FEET

Athlete's Foot 294

Brittle Nails 296

Bunions 298

Calluses 300

Cracked Heels 302

Dry Hands 304

Foot Odor 306

Ingrown Toenails 308

ATHLETE'S FOOT

Intense itching and scaly skin on your feet are signs you've got athlete's foot. This fungal infection responds very well to aromatherapy treatments, especially when you address symptoms as soon as you notice them.

Clove Bud Spray
MAKES ABOUT 4 FLUID OUNCES (½ CUP)

Clove bud is a potent antifungal essential oil that makes short work of athlete's foot. You can use this spicy-smelling spray on floors and shoes, too.

½ cup distilled water

40 drops clove bud essential oil

1. In a small bottle with a fine-mist spray top, combine the water and essential oil. Shake well to blend, and then shake again before each use.
2. Apply 1 spritz to each affected area once or twice daily.
3. Continue treatments for 1 week after symptoms subside.
4. Be sure to sanitize shoes and areas where you've walked barefoot.

May Chang Foot Powder

MAKES ABOUT 8 FLUID OUNCES (1 CUP)

May chang essential oil offers a fantastic fruity-spicy fragrance with strong lemon tones, and it also happens to be a strong antifungal agent. This powder is excellent for feet and shoes alike.

½ cup non-GMO cornstarch
½ cup baking soda
40 drops may chang essential oil

1. In a medium bowl, combine the cornstarch, baking soda, and essential oil. Whisk to blend thoroughly.
2. Sift the blend into a second bowl to remove any lumps, and then transfer the powder to a medium glass jar with a lid or a metal sugar shaker.
3. Apply a single shake of powder to each foot. Be sure to get between the toes.
4. Repeat once or twice daily to treat or prevent athlete's foot.

Tea Tree Neat Treatment

MAKES 1 TREATMENT

Tea tree is one of a few essential oils that can be applied neat, and it soothes itching while killing fungi. Be sure to conduct a patch test before using this neat treatment. If you have sensitive skin, apply a layer of carrier oil to each affected area before applying the tea tree.

1 drop tea tree essential oil

1. Wash and dry your feet. With a cotton swab, apply a drop of tea tree oil to each affected area.
2. Repeat once or twice daily, continuing treatment for 3 or 4 days after symptoms disappear.

BRITTLE NAILS

Weakness, chipping, and splitting layers are some signs that you have brittle nails. You don't have to live with the problem; just like your skin, nails respond very well to aromatherapy.

Frankincense Nail Balm

MAKES ABOUT 1 FLUID OUNCE (2 TABLESPOONS)

Frankincense essential oil promotes strong, healthy skin and nail tissue, while rich jojoba oil provides much-needed moisture.

2 tablespoons jojoba oil

50 drops frankincense essential oil

1. In a small bottle or jar with a lid, combine the jojoba oil and essential oil. Shake well to blend.
2. With a cotton swab, apply 1 drop of the balm to each of your nails. Gently massage the blend into your nails, cuticles, and the surrounding tissue.
3. Repeat three times weekly.

Lemon-Elemi Nail Soak

MAKES 1 TREATMENT

Brisk lemon and elemi essential oils kill any fungus that might be contributing to the problem, while warm water softens nails and prepares them to absorb the Frankincense Nail Balm (page 296) or the Synergistic Nail-Strengthening Blend (see next).

1 cup warm tap water
1 drop elemi essential oil
1 drop lemon essential oil

1. In a medium bowl, combine the water and essential oils.
2. Immerse your fingertips in the solution and soak your nails and cuticles for 5 minutes.
3. Pat your hands dry and immediately apply a moisturizing treatment.
4. Repeat as often as you like.

Synergistic Nail-Strengthening Blend

MAKES ABOUT 1 FLUID OUNCE (2 TABLESPOONS)

Lemon, peppermint, frankincense, and myrrh essential oils combine with nourishing vitamin E and wheat germ oils to moisturize and strengthen nails.

1½ tablespoons wheat germ oil
½ tablespoon vitamin E oil
30 drops frankincense essential oil
20 drops lemon essential oil
20 drops myrrh essential oil
5 drops peppermint essential oil

1. In a small bottle or jar with a lid, combine the wheat germ and vitamin E oil. Stir in the essential oils. Shake well to blend.
2. With a cotton swab, apply 1 drop of the blend to each of your nails. Gently massage it into your nails, cuticles, and the surrounding tissue.
3. Repeat once daily, preferably at bedtime.

BUNIONS

When the bones in the big toe are out of alignment, pain, inflammation, and even arthritis can result. Aromatherapy can help bring relief, especially when combined with ice, heat, and/or massage.

Copaiba-Peppermint Foot Cream

MAKES ABOUT 4 FLUID OUNCES (½ CUP)

Copaiba and peppermint essential oils combine with rich emollients to offer deep, penetrating pain relief and improve circulation while moisturizing feet.

¼ cup coconut oil, melted
2 tablespoons shea butter
1 tablespoon sweet almond oil
1 tablespoon beeswax, melted
12 drops copaiba essential oil
8 drops peppermint essential oil

1. In a small bowl, combine the coconut oil, shea butter, almond oil, beeswax, and essential oils. Whisk to blend thoroughly.
2. Pour the blend into a small jar with a lid and allow it to cool completely before capping.
3. Wash your feet, and then pat them dry.
4. Apply a dime-sized amount of the blend to each foot, and massage lightly. Repeat as needed.

Frankincense Cold Compress

MAKES 1 TREATMENT

Frankincense essential oil relieves discomfort by targeting inflammation, while a cold compress helps minimize swelling.

1 drop carrier oil of choice
1 drop frankincense essential oil

1. Elevate your foot. With your fingertips or a cotton ball, apply the carrier oil to the bunion, and then apply the essential oil.
2. Wrap an ice pack in a hand towel and lay it over the bunion. Leave the compress in place for 10 to 20 minutes, removing it periodically if your skin starts to feel uncomfortably numb.

Tagetes Bunion Balm

MAKES 1 FLUID OUNCE (2 TABLESPOONS)

Tagetes essential oil brings relief by targeting inflammation. This is a very powerful oil, and if you have sensitive skin, you should double the amount of carrier oil in the recipe.

2 tablespoons jojoba oil
8 drops tagetes essential oil

1. In a small bottle or jar with a lid, combine the jojoba oil and essential oil. Shake well to blend.
2. Apply 1 drop of the blend to each bunion, and gently massage the area, using circular strokes.
3. Also massage the arch of your foot, focusing on the forward portion. Repeat as needed.

CALLUSES

Hard, thick skin on your feet, hands, or fingers is caused by things like hard handiwork, walking barefoot on rough surfaces, and even poorly fitting shoes. While painless, calluses are unsightly. Aromatherapy solves the problem by promoting softer skin.

Lavender-Myrrh Massage

MAKES ABOUT 2 FLUID OUNCES (¼ CUP)

Fragrant benzoin, myrrh, and lavender essential oils combine with sweet almond oil to deliver lasting softness.

¼ cup sweet almond oil

8 drops lavender essential oil

4 drops myrrh essential oil

2 drops benzoin essential oil

1. In a small bottle or jar with a lid, combine the almond oil and essential oils. Shake well to blend.
2. With your fingertips, apply 3 drops of the blend to each callus. Gently massage it into the affected area and the surrounding tissue.
3. Repeat once daily, preferably at bedtime.

Rose Geranium Sugar Scrub

MAKES ABOUT 4 FLUID OUNCES (½ CUP)

Gritty brown sugar gently exfoliates the skin, while fractionated coconut oil and rose geranium essential oil smooth and heal it.

½ cup brown sugar
¼ cup fractionated coconut oil
20 drops rose geranium essential oil

1. In a small jar with a lid, combine the brown sugar, coconut oil, and essential oil. Stir well to combine.
2. After bathing or showering, apply 1 teaspoon of the sugar scrub to the affected area and massage the skin, using firm circular strokes.
3. Rinse with warm water, and then apply the moisturizer of your choice.
4. Repeat three or four times weekly.

Synergistic Callus Blend

MAKES ABOUT 2 FLUID OUNCES (¼ CUP)

This combination of rich carrot seed, palmarosa, myrrh, and benzoin essential oils, along with jojoba oil and vitamin E, softens thickened skin.

3 tablespoons jojoba oil
1 tablespoon vitamin E oil
10 drops carrot seed essential oil
10 drops patchouli essential oil
5 drops benzoin essential oil
5 drops lavender essential oil
5 drops myrrh essential oil
5 drops Roman chamomile essential oil
4 drops bergamot essential oil
4 drops palmarosa essential oil

1. In a small bottle or jar with a lid, combine the jojoba and vitamin E oils, then add the essential oils. Shake well to blend.
2. With your fingertips, apply 3 drops of the blend to each callus. Gently massage it into the affected area and the surrounding tissue.
3. Repeat two or three times daily, preferably applying the final treatment at bedtime.

CRACKED HEELS

Unsightly and often painful, cracked heels aren't just a cosmetic problem; they also expose your feet to bacteria that could lead to infection. Delightful aromatherapy treatments help reveal soft skin and improve the overall health of your feet.

Lemon-Lavender Foot Soak

MAKES 1 TREATMENT

Lavender and lemon essential oils smell marvelous together, but that's not all; they also eliminate bacteria and soften skin, especially when combined with soothing Epsom salts.

1 gallon warm tap water
⅓ cup Epsom salts
8 drops lavender essential oil
6 drops lemon essential oil

1. In a wide, large basin that will accommodate your feet, combine the water, Epsom salts, and essential oils. Soak your feet for 15 minutes while relaxing.

2. Use a scrub brush or pumice stone to exfoliate your heels, but don't dig deep into the cracks; concentrate just on the tough outer layer of skin.

3. Pat your feet dry and apply a moisturizer.

4. Repeat three or four times weekly, until cracked heels resolve.

Patchouli–Tea Tree Foot Balm

MAKES ABOUT 2 FLUID OUNCES (¼ CUP)

Patchouli, tea tree, and lavender essential oils make quick work of fungus and bacteria, while rich emollients can help make your feet feel as soft as a petal.

1 tablespoon coconut oil, melted
1 tablespoon olive oil
1 tablespoon sweet almond oil
1 tablespoon shea butter
16 drops lavender essential oil
12 drops patchouli essential oil
6 drops tea tree essential oil

1. In a small bowl, combine the coconut, olive, and almond oils, the shea butter, and the essential oils. Whisk to blend thoroughly, and then transfer the balm to a small jar with a lid.
2. Apply 1 teaspoon of the balm to each foot, and massage into cracked heels.
3. Repeat once or twice daily until cracked heels resolve.

Synergistic Overnight Foot Cream

MAKES ABOUT 8 FLUID OUNCES (1 CUP)

This synergistic blend includes benzoin, myrrh, and geranium essential oils; it addresses bacteria and fungi while helping sore and cracked heels feel better quickly. Consider wearing socks to bed to help keep the treatment on your feet overnight. In the morning, your feet will feel much softer and less painful.

1 cup shea butter
20 drops geranium essential oil
10 drops benzoin essential oil
10 drops myrrh essential oil
8 drops lavender essential oil
4 drops tea tree essential oil

1. In a medium bowl, combine the shea butter and essential oils. Whisk to blend thoroughly, and then transfer the cream to a medium jar with a lid.
2. Apply 1 teaspoon of the cream to each foot, concentrating on the heels, just before getting into bed. Put on a pair of socks and settle in for the night.
3. Repeat nightly until cracked heels resolve.

DRY HANDS

Arid indoor air, cold weather, and frequent hand washing can add up to dry, cracked skin on your hands. Moisturizing aromatherapy treatments can make a big difference, especially when used daily.

Lavender-Rosewood Hand Cream

MAKES ABOUT 4 FLUID OUNCES (½ CUP)

Lavender and rosewood essential oils moisturize the skin and repair cracked and chapped areas while providing you with a bit of protection from germs.

4 fluid ounces (½ cup) unscented hand cream
10 drops lavender essential oil
10 drops rosewood essential oil

1. In a small bowl, combine the hand cream and essential oils. Whisk to blend thoroughly, and then transfer the cream to a small jar with a lid or back into the empty hand cream jar.

2. Apply 1 teaspoon of the cream to your hands, using a little more or less as needed.

3. Use as often as you like, especially after washing your hands.

Skin-Softening Hand Soap
MAKES ABOUT 8 FLUID OUNCES (1 CUP)

Fragrant lavender, soothing coconut oil, and natural castile soap make a marvelous antibacterial blend that soothes dry skin while protecting you from germs.

⅓ cup unscented liquid castile soap
20 drops lavender essential oil
⅔ cup distilled water
1 teaspoon fractionated coconut oil

1. In a medium bottle or jar with a foaming pump, combine the soap and essential oil. Add the water and coconut oil, and stir with a thin utensil to blend.
2. Pump once for a dollop of foam and then wash your hands.
3. Use as often as needed.

Soothing Hand Balm
MAKES ABOUT 4 FLUID OUNCES (½ CUP)

Lavender and helichrysum essential oils soothe and heal chapped, cracked hands, while rich emollients moisturize deeply. For an unusual, but effective, nighttime deep-moisturizing treatment, put a pair of socks over your hands after applying the balm and leave the socks on overnight.

2 tablespoons coconut oil, melted
2 tablespoons shea butter
2 tablespoons sweet almond oil
1 tablespoon fractionated coconut oil
32 drops lavender essential oil
24 drops helichrysum essential oil

1. In a small bowl, combine the melted coconut oil, the shea butter, almond butter, other coconut oil, and essential oil. Whisk to blend thoroughly, and then transfer the balm to a small jar with a lid.
2. Apply 1 teaspoon of the balm to your hands and massage it in.
3. Repeat as needed.

FOOT ODOR

Just about everyone experiences foot odor sometimes. A combination of sweat and bacteria is to blame for the vinegary, cheesy, or ammonia-like stink; luckily, aromatherapy treatments handle the problem quickly and leave your tootsies smelling fresh.

Grapefruit-Spearmint Foot Spray

MAKES ABOUT 8 FLUID OUNCES (1 CUP)

Cheerful grapefruit and fresh spearmint essential oils combine with fungus-fighting tea tree essential oil to create a delightful fragrance for your feet.

1 cup less 2 tablespoons distilled water
2 tablespoons alcohol-free witch hazel
20 drops grapefruit essential oil
10 drops spearmint essential oil
5 drops tea tree essential oil

1. In a medium bottle with a fine-mist spray top, combine the water, witch hazel, and essential oils. Shake well to blend, and then shake again before each use.
2. Apply 1 spritz to each area you'd like to address.
3. Repeat two or three times a day, as needed.

Peppermint-Eucalyptus Pedicure Lotion

MAKES ABOUT 8 FLUID OUNCES (1 CUP)

Peppermint and eucalyptus essential oils kill bacteria. Plus, they provide a fresh, uplifting scent while imparting a cool, pleasant tingle.

- 8 fluid ounces (1 cup) unscented body lotion or hand cream
- 20 drops peppermint essential oil
- 10 drops lemon eucalyptus essential oil

1. In a medium bowl, combine the lotion and essential oils. Whisk to blend thoroughly, and then transfer the lotion to a medium jar with a lid or back into the empty lotion container.
2. Apply ½ teaspoon of the lotion to each foot. Use a little more or less as needed, and feel free to apply the lotion to your ankles and lower legs if you like.
3. Use once or twice daily to keep feet smelling fantastic.

NOTE: Keep this lotion in a convenient location if you plan to use it all within 2 weeks; otherwise, store it in a glass bottle or jar in a cool, dark place.

Rosemary-Lavender Foot Powder

MAKES 8 OUNCES (1 CUP)

Lavender and rosemary essential oils have antibacterial and antifungal properties, making them the natural choice for better-smelling feet.

- ¼ cup baking soda
- 40 drops lavender essential oil
- 10 drops rosemary essential oil
- ½ cup non-GMO cornstarch
- ¼ cup rice flour
- 1 teaspoon uncooked rice (optional; for humidity control)

1. In a small bowl, combine the baking soda and essential oils. Whisk to blend thoroughly.
2. Sift the mixture into a medium bowl, and then add the cornstarch and rice flour. Whisk again. If you are in a humid climate, add the rice to keep the powder from clumping, and mix in well. Transfer the powder to a medium jar with a lid or a metal sugar shaker.
3. Sprinkle about ½ teaspoon of the powder onto each foot. Be sure to get some powder between each of your toes, too.
4. Repeat two or three times daily.

INGROWN TOENAILS

Trimming your toenails too short and following the curvature of the toe rather than cutting straight across sets the stage for ingrown toenails. Aromatherapy treatments and proper trimming can help in minor cases, but serious ingrown toenails sometimes require medical intervention.

Healing Frankincense Balm

MAKES 1 FLUID OUNCE (2 TABLESPOONS)

Frankincense essential oil helps stop inflammation while helping skin heal. This balm is a good one to use after successfully trimming back an ingrown toenail.

2 tablespoons fractionated coconut oil
10 drops frankincense essential oil

1. In a small bottle or jar with a lid, combine the coconut oil and essential oil. Shake well to blend.

2. With a cotton swab, apply 2 drops of the balm to the affected toenail. Allow the treatment to absorb before putting on socks or shoes.

3. Repeat two or three times daily.

Lavender–Tea Tree Footbath

MAKES 1 TREATMENT

When combined with a softening footbath, lavender and tea tree essential oils help compromised skin heal while providing protection from infection.

1 gallon hot tap water
2 tablespoons Epsom salts
10 drops lavender essential oil
4 drops tea tree essential oil

1. In a large, shallow basin that's large enough to accommodate your foot, combine the hot water and Epsom salts.
2. Add the essential oils to the basin, and then put the affected foot into the water.
3. Soak your foot for 10 minutes, and then pat it dry. Apply an additional drop of lavender essential oil to the ingrown toenail.
4. If possible, trim the toenail back at a very slight angle to relieve the pressure. If you're not able to trim the toenail, gently slide a piece of waxed dental floss between the nail and the skin and try to trim again. If this doesn't work, repeat the footbath treatment every 2 to 4 hours until you are able to trim the toenail and relieve the pressure.

Lemon Eucalyptus–Clove Bud Compress

MAKES 1 TREATMENT

A cold compress made with lemon eucalyptus and clove bud essential oils helps stop infection, soothe pain, and soften skin so that you can trim an ingrown toenail more comfortably.

½ cup distilled water
2 ice cubes
4 drops clove bud essential oil
2 drops lemon eucalyptus essential oil

1. In a small bowl, pour the water over the ice cubes, and then add the essential oils.
2. Soak a folded washcloth in the solution, and then place it on the affected toe. Rest your foot on a towel and top the washcloth with a folded hand towel to catch any drips.
3. Leave the compress in place for 15 minutes. Allow your skin to air-dry after removal.
4. Repeat as needed until you are able to trim the ingrown toenail.

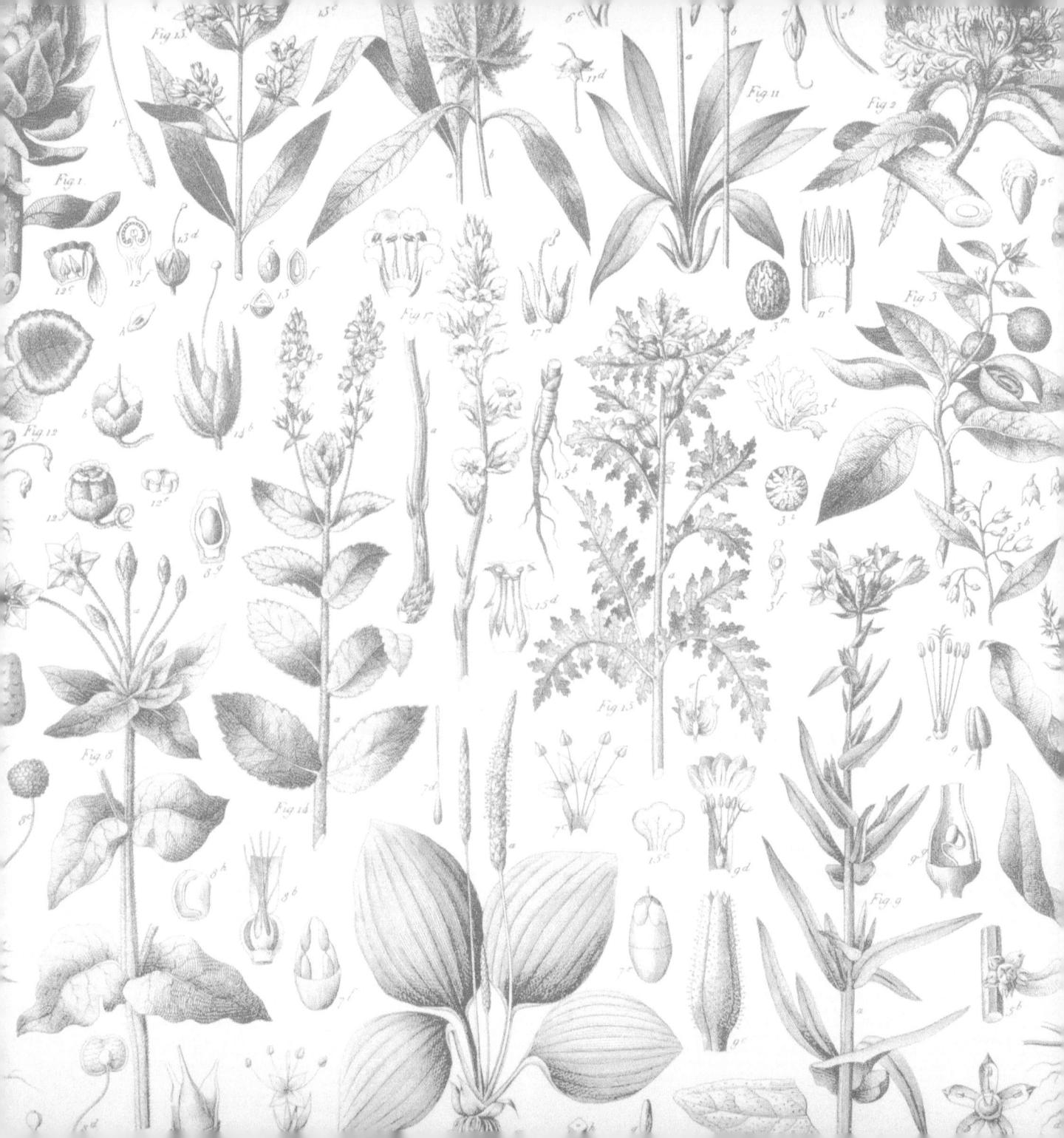

CHAPTER FOURTEEN

SCENTS AND PERFUMES

Eau de parfum is the most popular type of fragrance blend—a little bit goes a long way.

Eau de toilette is a more diluted, and thus weaker, fragrance formulation than *eau de parfum*.

Eau de cologne, or simply "cologne," is the most diluted form of perfume sold, and typically refers to a man's fragrance.

The term *splash* originally referred to any astringent, healing liquid applied (splashed on) after shaving to heal and tighten the skin.

Citrus and Spice Splash

MAKES 1 FLUID OUNCE (2 TABLESPOONS)

This blend of grapefruit and ginger essential oils is uplifting and energizing, so it's perfect to splash on after your morning shave and/or shower. The fragrance will linger without being overpowering.

2 tablespoons unflavored vodka
2 drops grapefruit essential oil
2 drops ginger essential oil
2 drops vetiver essential oil

1. In a small bottle, combine the vodka and essential oils, and shake to blend.
2. Shake before each use.
3. Splash 1 teaspoon of the blend on the face and as desired on the body, avoiding the eyes.

NOTE: Store the tightly sealed bottle in the refrigerator for up to a year.

SUBSTITUTION TIP: Lemon, sweet orange, or lime essential oil work well in this splash in place of the grapefruit.

Fleur Classique Parfum

EAU DE PARFUM
MAKES 5 FLUID OUNCES

If you love florals, this is the perfect fragrance for you. The heady perfume blend combines sweet ylang-ylang essential oil with citrus and other florals to create a sophisticated, layered scent that isn't too heavy. The vodka will help preserve and extend the fragrance, and it won't smell like you spilled a drink on yourself when you applied your perfume.

½ cup carrier oil of choice
2 tablespoons unflavored vodka
15 drops ylang-ylang essential oil
6 drops lavender essential oil
3 drops neroli essential oil

1. In a small atomizer bottle, combine the carrier oil and vodka, and shake to blend.
2. Add the essential oils and shake to blend all the ingredients.
3. Spritz lightly onto pulse points, or spray lightly in the air and walk through the fragrance cloud.

NOTE: Store in the tightly sealed atomizer in a cool, dark place for up to a year.

SUBSTITUTION TIP: Grapefruit or lemon essential oils will also work well in place of the bitter orange in this blend.

Garden in the Woods Eau de Toilette

EAU DE TOILETTE
MAKES 18 FLUID OUNCES (2¼ CUPS)

This light floral scent will transport you to a lovely woodland garden with its soothing aroma.

- 2 cups distilled water
- ¼ cup unflavored vodka
- 10 drops geranium essential oil
- 10 drops bergamot essential oil
- 5 drops sandalwood essential oil

1. In a large spray bottle, combine the water and vodka, and shake to blend.
2. Add the essential oils and shake again to mix all the ingredients.
3. Spritz onto pulse points.

NOTE: Store in the spray bottle in a cool, dark place for up to a year.

Lavender–Lemon Eau de Toilette

EAU DE TOILETTE
MAKES 2 FLUID OUNCES (¼ CUP)

Floral and citrus essential oils combine well, and this light scent won't overpower. Lemon and lavender create a classic combination that smells clean and fresh, perfect for a summer afternoon or a casual event. Dab it on your pulse points, and the light scent will surround you as you go about your day.

- 2 tablespoons unflavored vodka
- 2 tablespoons distilled water
- 5 drops lavender essential oil
- 5 drops lemon essential oil

1. In a small bottle, combine the vodka and water, and shake to mix.
2. Add the essential oils and shake again to mix.
3. Allow the perfume to mellow for 24 hours before using.
4. Shake before each use. Dab on pulse points.

NOTE: Store the tightly sealed bottle in a cool, dark place for up to a year.

Luxurious Solid Perfume

EAU DE PARFUM
MAKES 3 FLUID OUNCES

Because this sensuous blend contains benzoin essential oil, you shouldn't use it while you are pregnant. The perfume has a deep base resin note from the benzoin, with a floral middle and a top note coming from the lush fragrance of ylang-ylang essential oil. If you prefer, you can replace the benzoin with a few drops of frankincense essential oil.

3 tablespoons beeswax
3 tablespoons coconut oil
6 drops benzoin essential oil
6 drops ylang-ylang essential oil

1. Fill a small saucepan with a few inches of water and set it on the stove over low heat. Fit a small metal or glass bowl in the pan so that the bottom does not touch the water below.
2. Put the beeswax in the bowl; once it melts, stir in the coconut oil and whisk until melted.
3. Remove the bowl from the heat and add the essential oils.
4. Immediately transfer the mixture to a small jar or tin with a lid and allow it to cool and harden before putting on the lid.
5. Rub a small amount of the perfume onto pulse points.

NOTE: Store the tightly sealed container in a cool, dark place for up to a year.

Hungary Water

EAU DE COLOGNE
MAKES 8 FLUID OUNCES (1 CUP)

This summery cologne is based on the fabled "Hungary water" formula first crafted for Queen Elizabeth of Hungary in the fourteenth century. The light, citrus formula with floral middle notes and earthy bottom notes may boost mood. With such an intoxicating scent, it's a cologne fit for a queen.

1 cup unflavored vodka
30 to 35 drops bergamot essential oil
½ teaspoon lavender essential oil
¼ teaspoon neroli essential oil

1. In a medium bottle with an atomizer lid, combine the vodka and essential oils, and shake well to blend.
2. Store the mixture in the refrigerator for a week to "mellow" before using.
3. Shake before using. Spritz a little cologne on your pulse points, or spray some in the air and walk through the mist.

NOTE: Store the tightly sealed bottle in a cool, dark place for up to a year.

Healing Aftershave Splash

SPLASH
MAKES 1 FLUID OUNCE (2 TABLESPOONS)

This healing aftershave splash refreshes as it soothes irritated skin. The scents of cedarwood, cypress, and bergamot essential oils have a lovely woody character. Store it in the refrigerator so it cools even more.

2 tablespoons unflavored vodka
2 drops cedarwood essential oil
2 drops cypress essential oil
2 drops bergamot essential oil

1. In a small bottle, combine the vodka and essential oils, and shake to blend.
2. Shake before each use.
3. Splash a teaspoon or so of the aftershave on the face after shaving, avoiding the eyes.

NOTE: Store the tightly sealed bottle in the refrigerator for up to 3 months.

Winter Spice Cologne

EAU DE COLOGNE
MAKES 2 FLUID OUNCES (¼ CUP)

Traditionally, heavier perfumes are worn in winter, but this light fragrance will remind you of an evergreen forest dusted with snow. With cypress, pine, and peppermint essential oils, it's the perfect holiday fragrance, either to wear yourself or to give as a gift.

¼ cup unflavored vodka
3 drops cypress essential oil
2 drops pine essential oil
2 drops black pepper essential oil
2 drops peppermint essential oil
1 drop cardamom essential oil

1. In a small bottle, combine the vodka and essential oils, and shake to blend.
2. Shake before each use. Dab on pulse points.

NOTE: Store the tightly sealed bottle in a cool, dark place away from vibration.

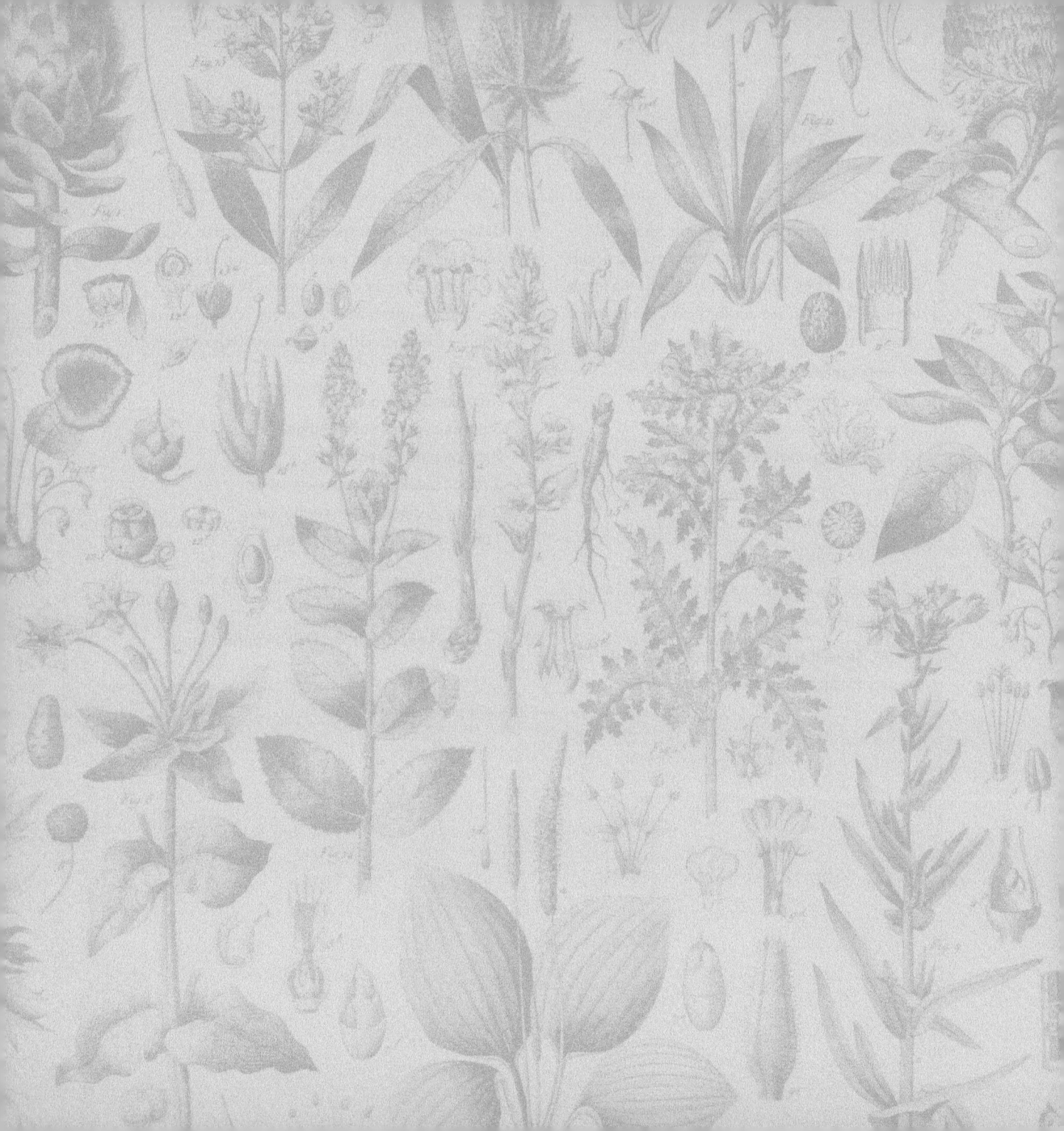

PART FIVE

Recipes, Remedies, and Applications for the Home and Outdoors

Store shelves are stocked with products designed to deliver cleanliness, freshen air, and more. While the number of natural, ecofriendly solutions is increasing, many products contain dangerous chemicals.

Instead of shelling out for products that have the potential to do more harm than good, why not make a few home products of your own? If you are interested in clearing your cupboards of toxins and making your home a healthier, more fragrant place to be, then this chapter was written with you in mind.

The following are easy recipes for everything from all-purpose cleaners to DIY laundry detergent that works just as well as the expensive stuff from the store. Insect repellent and pest solutions are found here, too. With simple ingredients and your favorite essential oils, you'll soon be enjoying a clean home.

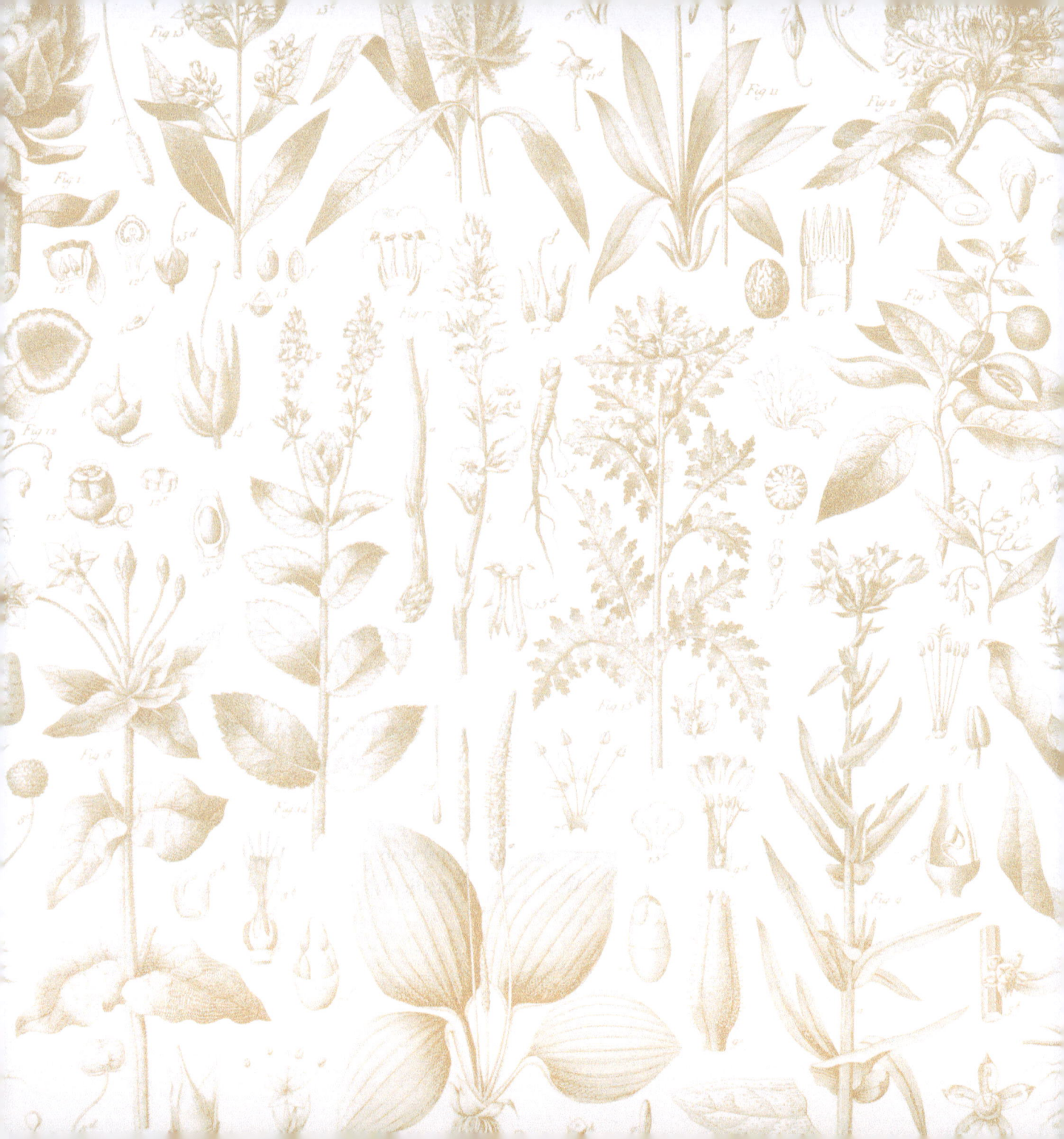

CHAPTER FIFTEEN

CLEANING AROUND THE HOME

Air Fresheners   320

Bathroom Cleansers   322

Floors   324

Glass and Mirrors   326

Kitchen Cleansers   328

Mold and Mildew   330

Refrigerator Cleansers   332

Stain Removers   334

AIR FRESHENERS

Commercial air fresheners may smell nice, but they often contain dangerous chemicals. Luckily, you can banish odors with aromatherapy and enjoy health benefits along the way. You can use these fun DIY air fresheners as inspiration for creating your own fragrant mists.

Fresh Summer Breeze Spray

MAKES ABOUT 4 FLUID OUNCES (½ CUP)

Pure, fresh floral notes blend with a touch of citrus to give your home a fresh, sunny scent while promoting positive emotions.

½ cup distilled water
40 drops geranium essential oil
40 drops mandarin essential oil
60 drops lavender essential oil
20 drops Roman chamomile essential oil

1. In a small bottle with a fine-mist spray top, combine the water and essential oils. Shake well to blend, and then shake again before each use.
2. Spritz the air a few times.
3. Repeat as needed.

PREFERENCE TIP: If you prefer a romantic floral scent, omit the mandarin essential oil and add 10 drops of ylang-ylang to the blend.

Plug-In Air Freshener Scent

FOR 1 DIFFUSER PAD

Plug-in air fresheners are convenient and smell nice, but most choices you'll find in your local stores contain toxins. Instead of one of these, consider freshening your home with a plug-in diffuser that's made specifically for use with aromatherapy.

5 to 7 drops essential oil or blend of choice
1 aromatherapy plug-in diffuser pad

Apply the essential oil or blend to the diffuser's pad, and then plug the unit in, following the manufacturer's instructions for safe use.

NOTE: If you don't already have one of these handy devices, look for a plug-in unit that's made specifically for use with aromatherapy. These units come with a set of diffuser pads, to which you add your favorite scents.

Spicy Autumn Room Deodorizer

MAKES 1 AIR FRESHENER

Bathrooms, baby-changing areas, and bedrooms are just a few places to put these simple, effective deodorizers. You can use them in your car, too.

10 drops clove bud essential oil
8 drops ginger essential oil
6 drops cinnamon leaf essential oil
5 drops sweet orange essential oil
2 drops lemon essential oil
1 drop anise essential oil
½ cup baking soda

1. In an 8-ounce glass canning jar, combine the essential oils and baking soda, using a fork to blend. Cover the jar opening with cheesecloth and secure with the ring, leaving the center lid off.

2. Place the jar in the area where odor control is needed, positioning it out of reach of small children and pets. Stir the powder every 2 or 3 days to revive the scent, and add more essential oil to refresh the fragrance.

3. Discard after refreshing two or three times.

SUBSTITUTION TIP: If you're missing one or two of these essential oils, increase the number of drops of one of the other oils to compensate. You can also make your own signature scent by using 30 to 40 drops of any essential oil or blend in this recipe.

BATHROOM CLEANSERS

Store-bought bathroom cleaners often have a strong antiseptic smell, but it doesn't have to be that way. Aromatherapy-based cleansers can transform your bathroom into a squeaky-clean spa-like environment. And as a bonus, there are no nasty chemicals.

All-Purpose Disinfectant Spray

MAKES ABOUT 8 FLUID OUNCES (1 CUP)

Lemon, sweet orange, and tea tree essential oils kill bacteria without the toxicity of regular cleaners. This fantastic all-purpose bathroom spray keeps surfaces sparkly and makes daily cleanups enjoyable. The spray is ideal for the bathtub, toilet, sink, tile, and hard-surface floors.

1 cup distilled water
1 teaspoon baking soda
1 tablespoon liquid castile soap
15 drops tea tree essential oil
10 drops sweet orange essential oil
5 drops lemon essential oil

1. In a medium bottle with a trigger spray top, combine the water and baking soda, and then shake to blend.
2. Add the soap and swirl the bottle to blend it in, then add the essential oils. Shake well to blend, and then shake again before each use.
3. Apply 1 spritz to each area you'd like to address, using more if needed. Wipe clean with a paper towel or cloth.
4. Use as often as needed.

Daily Tea Tree–Eucalyptus Shower Spray

MAKES ABOUT 32 FLUID OUNCES (4 CUPS)

Tea tree and eucalyptus essential oils inhibit mold growth, keeping your shower sanitary while preventing you from having to deep-clean it quite so often.

3½ cups distilled water
½ cup rubbing alcohol
20 drops tea tree essential oil
10 drops eucalyptus essential oil

1. In a large bottle with a trigger spray top, combine the water, alcohol, and essential oils. Shake well to blend, and then shake again before each use.
2. After every shower, mist the walls, floors, and shower curtain or door, making sure to coat all surfaces. Pay special attention to areas where water tends to collect.
3. Repeat daily.

PREFERENCE TIP: If you'd like a softer scent, try a combination of 20 drops of lavender essential oil and 10 drops of lemon, instead of the combo in this recipe.

Lemon Scouring Powder

MAKES ABOUT 8 OUNCES (1 CUP)

Lemon essential oil kills germs and combines with borax to gently scrub your toilet bowl clean without exposing you to harmful fumes found in traditional cleaners.

1 cup borax powder
12 drops lemon essential oil

1. In a metal sugar shaker, combine the borax with the essential oil, using a fork to stir.
2. Turn off the toilet's water supply, and then flush the toilet. Dust the bowl with a sprinkle of scouring powder, and then use a toilet brush to scrub thoroughly.
3. Turn the water supply back on. After the tank fills, flush the toilet.

FLOORS

With proper maintenance, your floors will look beautiful for many years. Instead of spending a fortune on expensive, toxic cleaning solutions, reach for these fragrant, all-natural floor cleaners.

Citrus Hardwood Floor Cleaner

MAKES 8 FLUID OUNCES (1 CUP)

With fragrant mandarin and grapefruit essential oils, this solution cuts through dirt, leaving hardwood floors sparkling while promoting a happy, carefree mood.

1 cup less 2 tablespoons distilled water
2 tablespoons distilled white vinegar
2 drops liquid dish detergent
4 drops grapefruit essential oil
2 drops mandarin essential oil

1. In a medium bottle with a fine-mist spray top, combine the water, vinegar, detergent, and essential oils. Shake well to blend, and then shake again before each use.

2. Apply a light mist of the solution to the floor, and then mop with a dry mop. Work in 2- to 4-foot sections to prevent the solution from evaporating before you arrive with the mop.

3. Repeat two or three times weekly, or as often as needed.

Lavender-Eucalyptus Mop Solution

MAKES 1 TREATMENT

Lavender and eucalyptus essential oils sanitize your floors, while the vinegar and baking soda combine with a little bit of liquid dish soap to remove dirt and leave surfaces clean and shiny. This solution is best for tile and linoleum floors.

2 gallons hot tap water
1 cup baking soda
1 cup distilled white vinegar
2 teaspoons liquid dish detergent
8 drops lavender essential oil
4 drops eucalyptus essential oil (any species)

1. In a mop bucket, combine the water, baking soda, vinegar, detergent, and essential oils. Swish the mop through the mixture to blend.
2. Mop the floor as usual, occasionally rinsing the dirt from your mop in a bucket of clear water before dipping it back into the solution.

SUBSTITUTION TIP: For laminate floors, combine 2 cups hot water, 1 tablespoon vinegar, 1 tablespoon baking soda, and 4 drops of your favorite essential oil in a medium spray bottle. Spritz the floors before using a dry mop or apply to a Swiffer-type pad.

Mandarin-Neroli Carpet Powder

MAKES ABOUT 8 OUNCES (1 CUP)

Mandarin and neroli essential oils combine with a hint of ginger essential oil and powerful baking soda to knock out odors and give your home a fresh, irresistible fragrance that's sure to boost your mood.

1 cup baking soda
20 drops mandarin essential oil
8 drops neroli essential oil
3 drops ginger essential oil
1 teaspoon uncooked rice (optional; for humidity control)

1. In a medium bowl, combine the baking soda and essential oils. Whisk to blend thoroughly. If you are in a humid climate, add the rice to keep the powder from clumping, and mix in well. Transfer the powder to a medium jar with a lid or a metal sugar shaker.
2. Sprinkle a light dusting of the powder onto your carpets and area rugs. Allow the blend to remain in place for 10 minutes to 1 hour, and then vacuum it up.
3. Repeat as often as you like.

PREFERENCE TIP: You can use any of your favorite aromatherapy blends to create a carpet powder that appeals to you, so feel free to experiment with different oils.

GLASS AND MIRRORS

Clean, sparkling windows and mirrors make your home a more pleasant place to be. Try these fragrant solutions instead of reaching for expensive sprays that might contain toxic ingredients.

Heavy-Duty Window Cleaner
MAKES ABOUT 16 FLUID OUNCES (2 CUPS)

Tea tree essential oil and simple ingredients like vinegar and dish detergent make a strong window cleaner that removes heavy layers of grime or pollen. This is ideal for the exterior side of the window, as well as for grimy glass doors.

1 cup distilled white vinegar
1 cup warm tap water
½ teaspoon liquid dish detergent
8 drops tea tree essential oil

1. In a large bottle with a trigger spray top, combine the vinegar, water, detergent, and essential oil. Shake well to blend, and then shake again before each use.
2. Spray the blend onto the window, and then wipe clean with a rag or a paper towel.
3. Repeat as needed.

Lemon Window Cleaner

MAKES ABOUT 16 FLUID OUNCES (2 CUPS)

A combination of lemon essential oil, rubbing alcohol, and vinegar removes smudges from windows quickly. It's also ideal for glass tabletops.

1 cup tap water
1 cup rubbing alcohol
1 tablespoon distilled white vinegar
6 drops lemon essential oil

1. In a large bottle with a trigger spray top, combine the water, alcohol, vinegar, and essential oil. Shake well to blend, and then shake again before each use.
2. Spray the blend onto the window, and then wipe clean with a rag or a paper towel.
3. Repeat as needed.

Streak-Free Glass and Mirror Cleaner

MAKES ABOUT 10 FLUID OUNCES (1¼ CUPS)

Lemon eucalyptus essential oil kills bacteria and imparts a light, fresh scent to this simple streak-free cleaner.

1 cup distilled water
2 tablespoons rubbing alcohol
2 tablespoons distilled white vinegar
1½ teaspoons non-GMO cornstarch
12 drops lemon eucalyptus essential oil

1. In a large bottle with a trigger spray top, combine the water, alcohol, vinegar, cornstarch, and essential oil. Shake well to blend, and then shake again before each use.
2. Spray the blend onto the window, and then wipe clean with a rag or a paper towel.
3. Repeat as needed.

KITCHEN CLEANSERS

Foodborne illness is a real threat, so it's important to keep your kitchen clean. Luckily, you can accomplish this task without relying on toxic commercial solutions.

Microwave Disinfectant

MAKES 1 TREATMENT

Clean and disinfect your microwave without spending any time scrubbing. Lemon essential oil provides a fresh, clean scent.

1 cup hot tap water
1 cup distilled white vinegar
1 drop lemon essential oil

1. In a microwave-safe large bowl, combine the water, vinegar, and essential oil. Place the bowl in the microwave and run on high power for 5 to 10 minutes.
2. With oven mitts, remove the bowl from the microwave and discard the solution. Wipe down the interior of the microwave with paper towels or a rag.
3. Repeat as needed.

Oven/Stovetop Gentle Scrubbing Soap

MAKES ABOUT 12 FLUID OUNCES (1½ CUPS)

Sweet orange and clove bud essential oils kill bacteria, and baking soda makes short work of grime. This blend is fantastic for ovens, stovetops, and sinks, and it's great for bathtubs and showers, too. It will keep your appliances looking sparkly inside and out.

1 cup baking soda
2 tablespoons liquid castile soap
2 tablespoons distilled water
12 drops sweet orange essential oil
4 drops clove bud essential oil
2 tablespoons distilled white vinegar

1. In a large bowl, combine the baking soda and soap. Stir well to blend. Add the water and essential oils, and stir again.
2. Add the vinegar slowly. It is normal for the mixture to produce bubbles. Stir again until well combined. If the mixture is thicker than desired, add a little more water, 1 teaspoon at a time. Transfer the scrubbing soap to a large plastic squeeze bottle.
3. Apply 1 teaspoon of the soft scrub to a sponge, moisten the area to be cleaned, and scrub. Rinse with water when finished.
4. Repeat as needed.

Quick Countertop Wipes

MAKES 80 TO 100 DISPOSABLE WIPES

Lemon, rosemary, and tea tree essential oils kill germs, while castile soap is gentle on delicate surfaces. These wipes are safe for all countertops, including granite and marble.

1 roll premium paper towels
1 cup distilled water
1 cup rubbing alcohol
1 tablespoon liquid castile soap
10 drops lemon essential oil
10 drops rosemary essential oil
10 drops tea tree essential oil

1. With a sharp plain-edged knife, cut the paper towel roll in half horizontally.
2. In a large bowl, combine the water, alcohol, soap, and essential oils. Stir well.
3. Place one half-roll of the toweling into the bowl, allowing the paper to absorb some of the liquid. Flip the half-roll over to ensure even absorption. Repeat the process with the other half-roll.
4. Pull the cardboard cores out of the center of each half-roll to allow you to pull wipes up from the center. Place each half-roll of wipes in a 1-gallon zip-top bag. (Plastic food storage containers also work well.)
5. Use the wipes as needed to clean up spills or just to spruce up your countertops.

MOLD AND MILDEW

Mold and mildew grow best in dark, damp places. Essential oils work wonders for prevention, as well as for cleanup. For major issues, it's best to contact a mold remediation expert.

Mold and Mildew Prevention Spray

MAKES ABOUT 10 FLUID OUNCES (1¼ CUPS)

Tea tree and lemon essential oils kill mold and mildew spores in areas where they tend to grow. This spray is ideal for kitchen and bath use.

¾ cup distilled white vinegar
⅔ cup distilled water
6 drops tea tree essential oil
4 drops lemon essential oil
2 drops clove bud essential oil

1. In a large bottle with a fine-mist spray top, combine the vinegar, water, and essential oils. Shake well to blend, and then shake again before each use.
2. Apply 1 or 2 spritzes to each area where mold and mildew tend to appear.
3. Allow the area to air-dry.
4. Repeat once weekly, and increase use to twice per week in warm, damp spaces or during periods of muggy weather.

Tea Tree Mold Remover
MAKES 1 FLUID OUNCE (2 TABLESPOONS)

Tea tree essential oil kills tough mold, like the kind that can show up on grout, wooden backsplashes, and other vulnerable areas.

1 tablespoon tea tree essential oil
1 tablespoon distilled water

1. In a small bottle with an orifice reducer, combine the essential oil and water. Shake well to blend, and then shake again before each use.
2. Apply 1 drop to each area of mold that you'd like to address, using a little more if needed and making sure to cover the entire moldy area.
3. Allow to air-dry.
4. Repeat as needed to stop moldy patches from forming.

Tea Tree Wall Mold Diffusion
MAKES 1 TREATMENT

Painted walls and bare wood often attract mold during muggy weather, even when the rest of your home is spotless. Diffusing tea tree essential oil next to the affected area kills the mold and prevents its return.

10 drops tea tree essential oil

1. Remove pets and children under 12 years from the room requiring treatment.
2. Add the essential oil to your diffuser according to the manufacturer's instructions.
3. Run the diffuser for 1 hour within a foot of the moldy area, positioning it so that the diffused oil will contact the affected surface.
4. Leave the moldy area alone for 24 hours, and then wipe the area with a paper towel, working from the mold's outer edge toward its center.
5. If any stubborn mold remains, repeat the process.

REFRIGERATOR CLEANSERS

Every so often, your refrigerator needs a good scrubbing, inside and out. In between deep cleanings, keep it looking and smelling fresh with these simple cleansers.

Lemon-Basil Sanitizing Spray

MAKES ABOUT 8 FLUID OUNCES (1 CUP)

Perky lemon and fragrant basil essential oils sanitize your refrigerator inside and out, and leave it smelling fresh and clean.

1 cup less 2 tablespoons distilled water
2 tablespoons unflavored vodka
15 drops lemon essential oil
10 drops basil essential oil

1. In a medium bottle with a fine-mist spray top, combine the water, vodka, and essential oils. Shake well to blend, and then shake again before each use.
2. Apply 1 spritz to each area of your refrigerator you'd like to address. Wipe clean with a soft cloth or a paper towel.
3. Repeat as needed.

Minty Fresh Fridge

MAKES 1 TREATMENT

Spearmint and grapefruit essential oils combine with baking soda to absorb odors and leave your refrigerator smelling fresh and clean.

1 cup baking soda
8 drops grapefruit essential oil
4 drops spearmint essential oil

1. In a medium bowl, combine the baking soda and essential oils. Whisk to blend thoroughly, and then transfer the mixture to a medium jar.
2. Place the uncovered jar in the back of the refrigerator where it will not be knocked over.
3. Replace the refrigerator treatment once a month or as often as needed.

Quick Spot Cleaner

MAKES 1 TREATMENT

Sweet orange essential oil and baking soda make short work of sticky spills that happen around jelly jars, juice pitchers, and other containers.

1 tablespoon tap water
½ tablespoon baking soda
2 drops sweet orange essential oil

1. In a small bowl, combine the water, baking soda, and essential oil. Whisk to blend thoroughly.
2. With a soft scrub brush, apply the cleaner to the sticky spot, and allow it to sit for 30 seconds to 1 minute.
3. With the brush, vigorously scrub the affected area. Once all soil has loosened, use a cloth or paper towel soaked in warm tap water to wipe up.
4. Repeat as needed.

STAIN REMOVERS

Despite efforts to stay tidy, life can be messy. Aromatherapy blends don't just smell good; many are ideal for removing tough stains.

Bodily Fluids and Pet Accident Cleaner

MAKES ABOUT 8 FLUID OUNCES (1 CUP)

Lavender essential oil and white vinegar neutralize odors and remove urine and vomit stains quickly.

Baking soda, as needed
1 cup less 2 tablespoons distilled white vinegar
2 tablespoons distilled water
20 drops lavender essential oil

1. Blot up any liquid with a paper towel and discard the towel. Cover the area with a layer of baking soda and allow it to sit for 20 minutes.

2. In a medium bottle with a fine-mist spray top, combine the vinegar, water, and essential oil. Shake well to blend, and then shake again before each use.

3. Use a paper towel to scoop up any liquid that the baking soda has absorbed and discard it. Apply 1 to 3 spritzes of the cleaner to the baking soda on top of the stain. Do not saturate the carpet with the cleaner; a light mist is all you need to get the mixture to bubble. When the bubbling action stops, wipe up the moisture and allow the area to dry.

4. Use a stiff brush to loosen any remaining baking powder, and then vacuum the area. Repeat the treatment for deep stains.

5. Use as often as needed.

Grass Stain Remover

MAKES 1 TREATMENT

Dirt, grass stains, and other organic materials, including fresh blood and red wine, come right out with the help of lemon essential oil and a few laundry room basics.

1 drop liquid castile soap
2 drops hydrogen peroxide
2 drops lemon essential oil

1. In a small bottle, combine the soap, peroxide, and essential oil. Shake well to blend. Apply the remover to the grass-stained area, working it in with your fingers or a scrub brush.
2. Let the treatment sit for 3 minutes. With a scrub brush and cold water, scrub the stain from its outer edge in, and then rinse.
3. Repeat as needed until the stain is gone.

Lemon Grease Treatment

MAKES 1 TREATMENT

Lemon essential oil cuts through grease stains on fabric or hard surfaces, making it easy to wash up. Even motor oil and black bicycle grease come out with lemon.

1 drop lemon essential oil

1. Apply the lemon essential oil straight from the bottle onto the grease spot. Use a little more for large spots.
2. On clothing, allow the essential oil to sit for 20 minutes, and then wash and dry the items as usual. On surfaces, allow the essential oil to sit for 20 minutes, and then use a soft scrub brush and some natural dish detergent to break up the stain. Rinse the area with hot water when finished.
3. Repeat as needed.

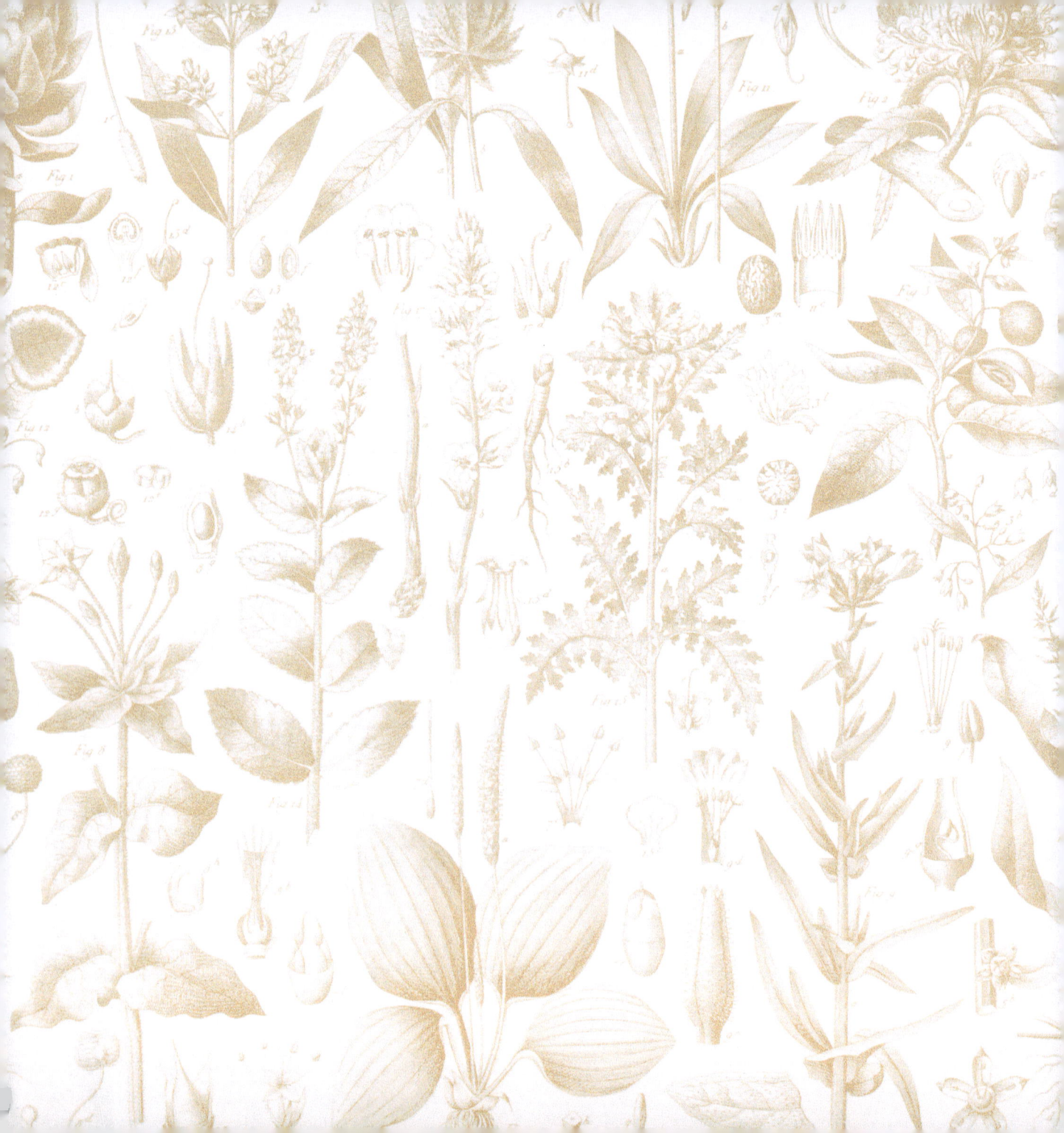

CHAPTER SIXTEEN

PROTECTING PETS AND BANISHING PESTS

Ant Repellent   338

Fleas   340

Mosquitoes   342

Moths   344

Spiders   346

ANT REPELLENT

No one likes to discover that ants have infested an area of their home, and so may be quick to reach for dangerous pesticides. Fortunately, aromatherapy offers a fragrant, nontoxic solution to ant problems.

Ant-Eliminating Lavender Neat Treatment

MAKES 1 TREATMENT

Lavender essential oil is an ant irritant, so if ants find it along their route, they'll look elsewhere. This treatment works best when you first notice just a few ants. Use Peppermint–Tea Tree Ant Spray (page 339) or Peppermint Ant Killer (page 339) for more serious infestations.

3 drops lavender essential oil (per entry point)

1. Watch the ants as they make their way from one place to the next, but don't disturb them. If you follow their path, you'll find their entry point; it's usually along a doorframe or within a windowsill.

2. Look outside in that area to see if you can find a corresponding trail of ants entering your home. If so, treat both the inside and outside entry points.

3. At night, after the ants have gone back to their nest, apply the lavender essential oil to each entry point.

4. Repeat twice daily until the ants stop looking for a way inside your home.

Peppermint Ant Killer

MAKES ABOUT 6 FLUID OUNCES (¾ CUP)

Peppermint essential oil combines with old-fashioned blue dish soap to kill and repel ants.

¼ cup blue dish soap, such as Dawn
½ cup distilled water
30 drops peppermint essential oil

1. In a small bottle with a trigger spray top, combine the soap, water, and essential oil. Shake well to blend, and then shake again before each use.
2. Spray any ants you see with the solution; they will die immediately. Wipe up dead ants with a paper towel and discard it.
3. Spray the spaces of your home where the ants are entering, but do not wipe it up. Check every few hours for dead ants and wipe them up.
4. Repeat the treatment two or three times daily, until ant activity stops.

Peppermint–Tea Tree Ant Spray

MAKES ABOUT 4 FLUID OUNCES (½ CUP)

Peppermint, tea tree, and lavender essential oils are natural ant repellants. While this spray won't kill them, it can prevent them from staying in your home. For best results, treat countertops, sinks, garbage cans, windowsills, and doorframes with this spray.

¼ cup distilled water
¼ cup rubbing alcohol
20 drops peppermint essential oil
15 drops tea tree essential oil
8 drops lavender essential oil

1. In a small bottle with a fine-mist spray top, combine the water, alcohol, and essential oils. Shake well to blend, and then shake again before each use.
2. Spray a fine mist onto areas where ant activity has been noticed.
3. Repeat two or three times daily until ant activity stops.

FLEAS

Dogs and cats enrich our lives, but when they attract fleas—or, worse, become infested—discomfort and even disease can result. Before reaching for chemical flea treatments, give these simple, all-natural solutions a try.

Indoor Flea Powder
MAKES 16 OUNCES (2 CUPS)

Lavender essential oil, borax, and salt combine to kill fleas and their eggs inside your home. For outdoor use, replace the salt with diatomaceous earth to avoid harming plants. This remedy is not for use on your pets.

1½ cups borax powder

½ cup table salt

8 drops lavender essential oil

1 teaspoon uncooked rice (optional; for humidity control)

1. In a large bowl, combine the borax, salt, and essential oil. Whisk to blend thoroughly. If you are in a humid climate, add the rice to keep the powder from clumping, and mix in well. Transfer the powder to a pint jar with a lid.

2. Sprinkle the powder liberally throughout your home. Use a stiff broom to work the powder deep into carpeting or area rugs. On uncarpeted floors, use the broom to work the powder into all the crevices. Leave the treatment in place for 2 days.

3. After 2 days, wash all your pet's bedding in very hot, soapy water to kill any fleas that may be hiding there. Then, thoroughly vacuum all areas throughout your home.

4. Repeat this treatment once weekly during a heavy infestation; for a light infestation, one treatment should be enough.

Lavender Flea Powder

MAKES 8 OUNCES (1 CUP)

Lavender essential oil is safe for cats and dogs, and it repels fleas. Baking soda damages the exoskeletons of the fleas and kills them, plus it soothes your pet's itchy skin. Use this remedy in conjunction with the Indoor Flea Powder (page 340), and wash your pet's bedding in hot, soapy water before applying the flea powder. Use the essential oil especially prepared for dogs or cats.

1 cup baking soda
12 drops lavender essential oil for dogs, or
 1 drop lavender essential oil for cats

1. Place the baking soda in a medium bowl. Using a fork, stir in the lavender essential oil. Sift the blend into another bowl to remove any lumps, and then transfer it to a medium glass jar with a lid or a metal sugar shaker.

2. To use on dogs, apply a light dusting of powder along the dog's back and then work it into the fur or hair with your fingers. Have your dog roll over and repeat the process on the underside.

3. To use on cats, sprinkle about ½ teaspoon of the powder onto the palm of your hand, and then gently stroke your cat's fur, being sure to avoid the eye area.

4. Wait 3 or 4 hours, and then use a flea comb to remove dead and dying fleas.

5. Repeat weekly during flea season.

Synergistic Dog Flea-Collar Blend

MAKES 1 FLUID OUNCE (2 TABLESPOONS)

A powerful combination of citronella, cedar, rosemary, and peppermint essential oils kills and repels fleas for up to a month. This blend is only safe for dogs; do not use this blend or any of these essential oils on cats or other small animals. Also, be sure to check your dog for sensitivity 1 hour after applying the collar and 24 hours later. If you notice irritation, remove the collar and try the Lavender Flea Powder (see previous) instead.

2 teaspoons citronella essential oil
2 teaspoons rosemary essential oil
1 teaspoon Atlas cedarwood essential oil
1 teaspoon peppermint essential oil
1 all-cotton dog collar in your dog's size

1. In a small bottle with an orifice reducer, combine the essential oils. Shake well to blend, and allow the blend to rest for 24 hours before use.

2. Apply the blend directly to the underside of the collar, which will come into contact with your dog's skin. For dogs weighing less than 30 pounds, use 6 drops; for dogs weighing more than 30 pounds, use 10 drops.

3. Remove the collar each time the dog bathes or swims.

4. Reapply the blend to the collar every 1 to 4 weeks.

MOSQUITOES

Mosquitoes, gnats, chiggers, and other insects can rapidly ruin your outdoor fun. Fragrant aromatherapy treatments keep biting insects at bay and eliminate the need for toxic insect repellents.

Mason Jar Luminaries

MAKES 3 LUMINARIES

Rosemary, lemon, cedarwood, and lavender essential oils combine with citronella essential oil to keep bugs from spoiling alfresco dining experiences. Add fresh herbs and citrus slices to create beautiful, natural decorations for your table.

3 (8-ounce/1 cup) mason jars
30 drops cedarwood essential oil
30 drops citronella essential oil
30 drops lavender essential oil
30 drops lemon essential oil
30 drops rosemary essential oil
6 sprigs fresh rosemary, lavender, or basil
1 lemon, thinly sliced
1 lime, thinly sliced
2 to 3 cups tap water, as needed
3 floating tea lights

1. Into the bottom of each jar, place 10 drops each of the essential oils.
2. Insert 2 herb sprigs into each jar, bending the stems as needed to keep the tops from poking out.
3. Divide the lemon and lime slices among the jars and layer them on top of the herbs.
4. Fill each jar with the water to just below its neck, and then float a tea light on top of the water.
5. Arrange the luminaries on the table and light the candles. Enjoy!
6. Discard the contents after a day or so.

Mosquito Repellent Spray

MAKES ABOUT 8 FLUID OUNCES (1 CUP)

Mosquitoes can't stand citronella or eucalyptus essential oil, and lemon essential oil is a strong deterrent as well.

½ cup distilled water
½ cup unflavored vodka
40 drops citronella essential oil
20 drops *Eucalyptus radiata* essential oil
10 drops lemon essential oil

1. In a medium bottle with a fine-mist spray top, combine the water, vodka, and essential oils. Shake well to blend, and then shake again before each use.
2. Apply 1 spritz to each area of exposed skin. When insect activity is high, use the spray on clothing, hats, and other items such as outdoor canopies and camping tents.

SUBSTITUTION TIP: If you don't have *Eucalyptus radiata*, feel free to use *Eucalyptus globulus* or lemon eucalyptus in its place.

Patchouli-Spearmint Repellent Lotion

MAKES ABOUT 8 FLUID OUNCES (1 CUP)

Patchouli, spearmint, and lavender essential oils repel biting bugs, while the lotion leaves skin feeling smooth and soft.

8 fluid ounces (1 cup) unscented body lotion or hand cream
20 drops patchouli essential oil
10 drops lavender essential oil
10 drops spearmint essential oil

1. In a medium bowl, combine the lotion and essential oils. Whisk to blend thoroughly, and then transfer the lotion to a medium jar with a lid or back into the empty lotion container.
2. Apply 1 teaspoon of the lotion to exposed skin. Use a little more or less as needed, and feel free to apply the lotion to body parts that are covered. The more fragrant you are, the less biting bugs will like you!
3. Repeat as needed.

NOTE: Keep this lotion in a convenient location if you plan to use it all within 2 weeks; otherwise, store it in a glass bottle or jar in a cool, dark place.

MOTHS

Given the opportunity, moths will get into linen closets, cupboards, and pantries, where they feed and reproduce. These preventives are safe, all-natural alternatives to toxic mothballs and insecticides.

Citronella-Lavender Mothballs
MAKES 20 MOTHBALLS

Citronella and lavender essential oils discourage wool moths from entering their favorite hiding spaces. These simple mothballs are nontoxic and leave your home smelling fresh.

20 cotton balls
40 drops citronella essential oil, or more as needed
40 drops lavender essential oil, or more as needed

1. On each cotton ball apply 2 drops of citronella and 2 drops of lavender essential oil.
2. Place the mothballs in cabinets, drawers, and other areas where moth activity has been a problem.
3. Refresh the mothballs with more essential oil every 2 to 4 weeks, or when you notice the scent has faded.

Pantry Moth Repellent

MAKES ABOUT 4 FLUID OUNCES (½ CUP)

Bay laurel and lavender essential oils combine with lemon, eucalyptus, and peppermint essential oils to keep pantry moths from invading dry foodstuffs. Remember to seal dried goods in airtight containers if pantry moths are a problem in your area.

½ cup distilled white vinegar
40 drops bay laurel essential oil
40 drops *Eucalyptus globulus* essential oil
20 drops lavender essential oil
20 drops lemon essential oil
10 drops peppermint essential oil

1. In a medium bottle with a fine-mist spray top, combine the vinegar and essential oils. Shake well to blend, and then shake again before each use.
2. Clear the pantry of all food and wash the shelves with soap and water. Allow the area to air-dry, and then apply a fine mist of the spray to shelves and walls, paying special attention to cracks and crevices. The solution will prevent any moth eggs from hatching.
3. Repeat every 2 or 3 months to prevent reinfestation.

Patchouli–Palo Santo Potpourri

MAKES 4 SMALL JARS

Patchouli and palo santo essential oils repel wool moths and combine beautifully with cedar chips. A jar of potpourri adds fragrance to your closet while deterring the pesky bugs.

4 cups cedar chips
40 drops palo santo essential oil, or more as needed
40 drops patchouli essential oil, or more as needed
4 (8-ounce/1 cup) mason jars

1. Place the cedar chips in a large bowl. Add the essential oils 4 or 5 drops at a time, stirring with a spatula between additions. Divide the potpourri among the 4 jars.
2. Place the jars, uncovered, in the back corners of closets or wardrobes.
3. Refresh the potpourri with more essential oils when the scent fades.

SPIDERS

Spiders play an important role in maintaining nature's balance, but you probably don't want them inside your house. These simple repellents keep them away while helping keep your home smelling its best.

Indoor Spider Repellent Spray

MAKES ABOUT 8 FLUID OUNCES (1 CUP)

Spiders hate peppermint and will go out of their way to avoid it. This spray is a quick, easy way to keep them out.

½ cup distilled water
½ cup rubbing alcohol
25 drops peppermint essential oil

1. In a medium bottle with a fine-mist spray top, combine the water, alcohol, and essential oil. Shake well to blend, and then shake again before each use.
2. Apply 1 spritz to each area where spiders may be gaining access to your home, especially around ducts, vents, windows, and doors.
3. Repeat as needed.

Lemon-Mint Spider Repellent Powder

MAKES 16 OUNCES (2 CUPS)

Peppermint and lemon essential oils deter spiders from making their way into your home. Spread this powder around the foundation to keep them out.

2 cups diatomaceous earth
16 drops peppermint essential oil
16 drops lemon essential oil

1. In a large bowl, combine the earth and essential oils. Stir well, and then transfer the blend to a pint jar with a lid.
2. Apply a dusting of repellent to the entire perimeter of your home. Pay special attention to areas near vents, windows, and doors. If it rains, reapply the outdoor treatment once the ground dries up.
3. Repeat as needed.

Synergistic Spider Spray

MAKES ABOUT 8 FLUID OUNCES (1 CUP)

Peppermint, eucalyptus, and tea tree essential oils combine to stop spiders in their tracks. This spray repels moths, silverfish, and cockroaches, too.

½ cup distilled water
½ cup rubbing alcohol
18 drops eucalyptus essential oil (any species)
12 drops peppermint essential oil
12 drops tea tree essential oil

1. In a medium bottle with a fine-mist spray top, combine the water, alcohol, and essential oils. Shake well to blend, and then shake again before each use.
2. Apply 1 spritz to each area where spiders may be gaining access to your home, especially around ducts, vents, windows, and doors.
3. Repeat as needed.

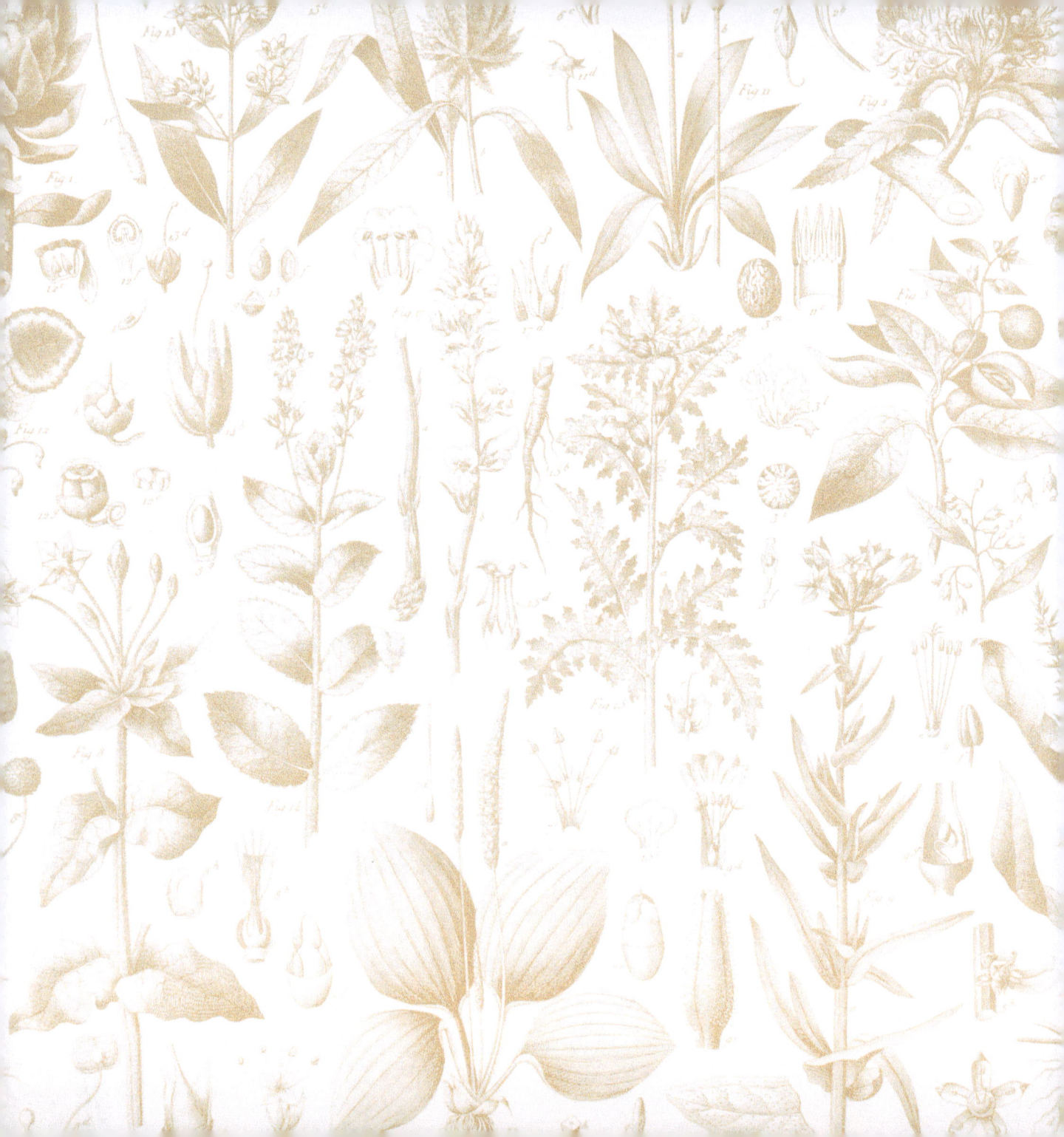

CHAPTER SEVENTEEN

TENDING TO THE OUTDOORS AND TREATING OUTDOOR CONCERNS

Hay Fever and Allergies   350

Insect Bites and Bee Stings   352

Lawn and Garden   354

Poison Ivy   356

Sunburn   358

HAY FEVER AND ALLERGIES

Sneezing, watery eyes, and a familiar itchy feeling in your airway tell you that hay fever or allergies are at work. Some aromatherapy treatments help block the histamines that cause your symptoms, while others address discomfort directly.

Breathe-Easy Synergistic Blend

MAKES 150 TREATMENTS

Refreshing eucalyptus, peppermint, and copaiba essential oils come together with crisp cypress essential oil to clear your head and relieve respiratory symptoms.

1 tablespoon fractionated coconut oil
12 drops copaiba essential oil
12 drops cypress essential oil
10 drops *Eucalyptus globulus* essential oil
8 drops peppermint essential oil

1. In a small bottle, preferably with a roll-on applicator, combine the coconut oil and essential oils. Shake well to blend.
2. With your fingertips or the roller, apply 1 drop to the pulse point behind each of your ears and gently massage the areas, drawing the blend toward the front of your throat.
3. Apply 1 drop of the blend to the base of your throat and gently massage the area.
4. Repeat every 2 hours, as needed.

NOTE: Keep in a convenient location if you plan to use it up within a few weeks; otherwise, store in a cool, dark place for up to a year.

Melissa-Chamomile Diffusion

MAKES 1 TREATMENT

Melissa and Roman chamomile essential oils offer antihistamine properties that lessen the impact allergens have on your body.

2 drops Roman chamomile essential oil
1 drop melissa essential oil

1. Add the essential oils to your diffuser according to the manufacturer's instructions. Run the diffuser nearby.
2. Repeat as needed throughout the day.

SUBSTITUTION TIP: If you are allergic to daisies, Roman chamomile may make your symptoms worse rather than better; omit the chamomile and diffuse 3 drops of melissa instead.

Niaouli Inhaler

MAKES 1 TREATMENT

Niaouli essential oil is an excellent decongestant that clears your head while improving your mood and giving your immune system a boost.

20 drops niaouli essential oil

1. Apply the essential oil to the cotton wick of the aromatherapy inhaler.
2. Hold the inhaler beneath your nose, and inhale slowly through both nostrils to a count of five. Hold your breath for another count of five, and then exhale slowly.
3. Repeat as needed to prevent and soothe symptoms.

SUBSTITUTION TIP: If you don't have an inhaler, you can transfer the blend to a small, dark glass bottle and inhale directly from the bottle, or place 3 drops of the niaouli in your diffuser.

INSECT BITES AND BEE STINGS

Some insects take tiny bites that can cause an irritating itch, while bees and wasps deliver a much more powerful punch. Aromatherapy treatments bring quick, reliable relief. If you are allergic to bees, seek medical attention immediately.

Chamomile-Lavender Gel

MAKES 1 FLUID OUNCE (2 TABLESPOONS)

This soothing chamomile-lavender essential oil combo provides relief from itchy bug bites while helping diminish swelling and inflammation. Aloe vera helps quicken skin healing, too.

2 tablespoons aloe vera gel

6 drops lavender essential oil

6 drops Roman or German chamomile essential oil

1. In a small bowl, combine the aloe vera and the essential oils. Whisk to blend thoroughly, and then transfer the gel to a small jar with a lid.
2. With a cotton swab, apply 1 drop of the blend to each insect bite.
3. Repeat two or three times daily, until the swelling and itching have subsided.

Lavender-Eucalyptus Bee Sting Relief

MAKES 1 TREATMENT

Lavender and eucalyptus essential oils provide pain relief and help prevent infection after a nasty bee sting. An ice pack on top reduces the swelling.

2 drops carrier oil of choice
1 drop lavender essential oil
1 drop eucalyptus essential oil (any species)

1. If the bee left behind a stinger, remove it with a pair of tweezers, and then wash and dry the affected area.
2. Apply 1 drop of the carrier oil to the sting site, and then apply the lavender essential oil.
3. Wait for 1 minute, and then apply the eucalyptus essential oil. Immediately top it with another drop of the carrier oil.
4. Cover the treatment with a soft cloth, and then apply an ice pack. Leave the ice pack in place for 15 minutes.
5. Repeat the treatment every 2 or 3 hours until pain subsides.

Lavender-Peppermint Anti-Itch Spray

MAKES ABOUT 4 FLUID OUNCES (½ CUP)

Lavender and peppermint essential oils combine with apple cider vinegar to provide rapid relief from the itching caused by mosquito, gnat, and chigger bites.

½ cup organic apple cider vinegar
24 drops lavender essential oil
16 drops peppermint essential oil

1. In a small bottle with a fine-mist spray top, combine the vinegar and essential oils. Shake well to blend, and then shake again before each use.
2. Apply 1 spritz to each itchy area every 1 or 2 hours, as needed.

NOTE: If you like, you can keep this spray in the refrigerator for an intense cooling sensation upon application; otherwise, store in a cool, dark place.

LAWN AND GARDEN

Chemical herbicides and pesticides are expensive, and they aren't the best choices for the planet or your homegrown vegetables. Try these gentle, earth-friendly options instead.

Cinnamon Leaf Weedkiller

MAKES ABOUT 8 FLUID OUNCES (1 CUP)

Cinnamon leaf essential oil contains a chemical called eugenol, which is a strong natural weedkiller. This remedy works best on young weeds; however, you can chop the tops off older weeds and apply it to the freshly cut area.

½ cup sunflower oil
½ cup distilled white vinegar
40 drops cinnamon leaf essential oil

1. In a medium bottle with a trigger spray top, combine the oil, vinegar, and essential oil. Shake well to blend, and then shake again before each use.
2. Choose a calm, sunny day to apply the weedkiller, and head out to the garden as soon as any dew dries so that the oil will have all day to work.
3. Spray the center growing tip and leaves of each weed you want to kill.
4. Repeat whenever weeds reemerge.

SUBSTITUTION TIP: If you don't have cinnamon leaf essential oil, you can try pine, clove bud, or thyme essential oil instead.

Slug and Snail Repellent

MAKES ABOUT 8 FLUID OUNCES (1 CUP)

Slugs and snails are sensitive creatures, and pine essential oil drives them away from tender plants.

1 cup tap water
20 drops pine essential oil, or more as needed
16 jar lids or small, flat containers

1. In a medium bottle, combine the water and essential oil. Cover and shake well to blend.
2. Pour 1 tablespoon of the blend into each jar lid and set them around your garden, especially near plants that tend to attract slugs and snails.
3. Check the lids periodically to ensure that they still smell like pine. Replace the repellent when the scent fades.
4. Repeat the process as needed.

Tea Tree Antifungal Plant Treatment

MAKES 128 FLUID OUNCES (1 GALLON)

Tea tree essential oil is a powerful antifungal agent that prevents fungi from attacking and killing your plants. Powdery mildew, blight, rust, and other common garden fungi are no match for it. Choose a mild, preferably overcast day for the treatment, or treat the plants in the evening to prevent sunburn.

1 gallon tap water
12 drops tea tree essential oil

1. In a clean garden pump sprayer that has never held herbicide, combine the water and essential oil. Cover and shake vigorously to blend.
2. Insert the pump, cover, and operate the sprayer according to the manufacturer's instructions. Apply a fine mist to all affected plants, as well as any that might be susceptible to fungus.
3. Transfer any remaining plant treatment to a gallon storage container with a lid. When ready to use, pour back into the sprayer, topping off with additional water and essential oil, as needed.

POISON IVY

Poison ivy, as well as poison oak and poison sumac, contains a compound called urushiol, which causes a burning, blistered rash that spreads like wildfire if you scratch it. Aromatherapy treatments help, especially when combined with traditional remedies like calamine lotion, aloe vera gel, and baking soda.

Lavender-Frankincense Bath

MAKES 8 TREATMENTS

Lavender and frankincense essential oils combine with baking soda to soothe inflammation and stop itching. Follow up with the Peppermint-Myrrh Lotion (page 357) or the Synergistic Itch-Relief Spray (page 357) for even more relief.

4 cups baking soda
24 drops lavender essential oil
16 drops frankincense essential oil

1. In a large bowl, combine the baking soda and essential oils. Whisk to blend thoroughly, and then transfer the resulting bath salts to a large jar with a lid.

2. Draw a lukewarm bath and add ½ cup of the bath salts. Soak in the bath for at least 15 minutes.

3. Repeat once or twice daily until the rash is gone.

Peppermint-Myrrh Lotion

MAKES ABOUT 8 FLUID OUNCES (1 CUP)

Soothing calamine lotion is a popular go-to when poison ivy strikes, but you can make it even more potent by adding peppermint and myrrh essential oils, both of which help relieve the itching.

8 fluid ounces (1 cup) calamine lotion
40 drops peppermint essential oil
20 drops myrrh essential oil

1. In a medium bowl, combine the calamine and essential oils. Whisk to blend thoroughly, and then transfer the lotion to a medium jar with a lid or back into the empty calamine bottle.

2. Use a cotton ball to gently apply a pea-sized amount of the blend to each affected area, working from the outer edge of the rash to the inside. Use a little more or less as needed and prevent cross contamination by using a new cotton ball to treat each affected area.

3. Repeat every 2 hours, until the rash is gone.

NOTE: Keep this lotion in a convenient location if you plan to use it all within 2 weeks; otherwise, store it in a glass bottle or jar in a cool, dark place.

Synergistic Itch-Relief Spray

MAKES ABOUT 8 FLUID OUNCES (1 CUP)

Lavender, helichrysum, geranium, cypress, chamomile, and peppermint essential oils combine with witch hazel and Epsom salts to deliver rapid relief from itching and burning.

½ cup distilled water
½ cup alcohol-free witch hazel
1 teaspoon Epsom salts
12 drops cypress essential oil
12 drops geranium essential oil
12 drops helichrysum essential oil
12 drops lavender essential oil
12 drops Roman chamomile essential oil
4 drops peppermint essential oil

1. In a medium bottle with a fine-mist spray top, combine the water, witch hazel, Epsom salts, and essential oils. Shake very well to dissolve the Epsom salts, and then shake again before each use.

2. Apply 1 spritz to each affected area.

3. Repeat every 1 or 2 hours, until the rash is gone.

SUNBURN

While prevention is the best medicine, sunburns can and do happen. Aromatherapy treatments help by easing the pain and promoting faster healing. When applied immediately, they sometimes prevent the skin from peeling.

Geranium-Lavender Sunburn Gel

MAKES ABOUT 1 CUP

Geranium and lavender essential oils combine with cool aloe vera gel to ease sunburn pain and help skin heal a bit faster. If you can get this gel onto your skin as soon as you notice a burn forming, you may be able to prevent peeling.

¾ cup aloe vera gel

2 tablespoons fractionated coconut oil

20 drops lavender essential oil

12 drops geranium essential oil

1. In a small bowl, combine the aloe vera, coconut oil, and essential oils. Whisk to blend thoroughly, and then transfer the gel to a small jar with a lid.

2. Apply 1 teaspoon of the blend to the affected area, using a little more or less as needed.

3. Repeat two or three times daily, until the skin is healed.

NOTE: If you like, you can keep this gel in the refrigerator for an intense cooling sensation upon application; otherwise, store in a cool, dark place.

Helichrysum Milk Bath

MAKES 4 TREATMENTS

Helichrysum essential oil combines with comforting, protein-rich powdered goat milk to soothe burning and help compromised skin heal.

2 cups powdered goat milk
20 drops helichrysum essential oil

1. In a large bowl, combine the powdered milk and essential oil. Whisk to blend thoroughly.
2. Sift the powder into another bowl to break up any lumps, and then transfer the blend to a pint jar with a lid.
3. Draw a lukewarm bath and add ½ cup of the blend to the tub, using your hand to stir it in. Soak in the bath for 15 to 20 minutes.
4. Repeat once daily to encourage your skin to heal.

Lavender–Cucumber Seed Spray

MAKES ABOUT 14 FLUID OUNCES (1¾ CUPS)

Alongside aloe vera, soothing lavender and cucumber seed essential oils help take the sting out of sunburned skin while promoting faster healing. Meanwhile, witch hazel offers a welcome cooling sensation.

¾ cup distilled water
¾ cup alcohol-free witch hazel
¼ cup aloe vera gel
40 drops lavender essential oil
20 drops cucumber seed essential oil

1. In a medium bottle with a fine-mist spray top, combine the water, witch hazel, aloe vera, and essential oils. Shake well to blend, and then shake again before each use.
2. Apply 1 spritz to each burned area, using more as needed and ensuring that you cover the entire sunburn.
3. Repeat hourly as needed.

NOTE: If you like, you can keep this spray in the refrigerator for an intense cooling sensation upon application; otherwise, store it in a cool, dark place.

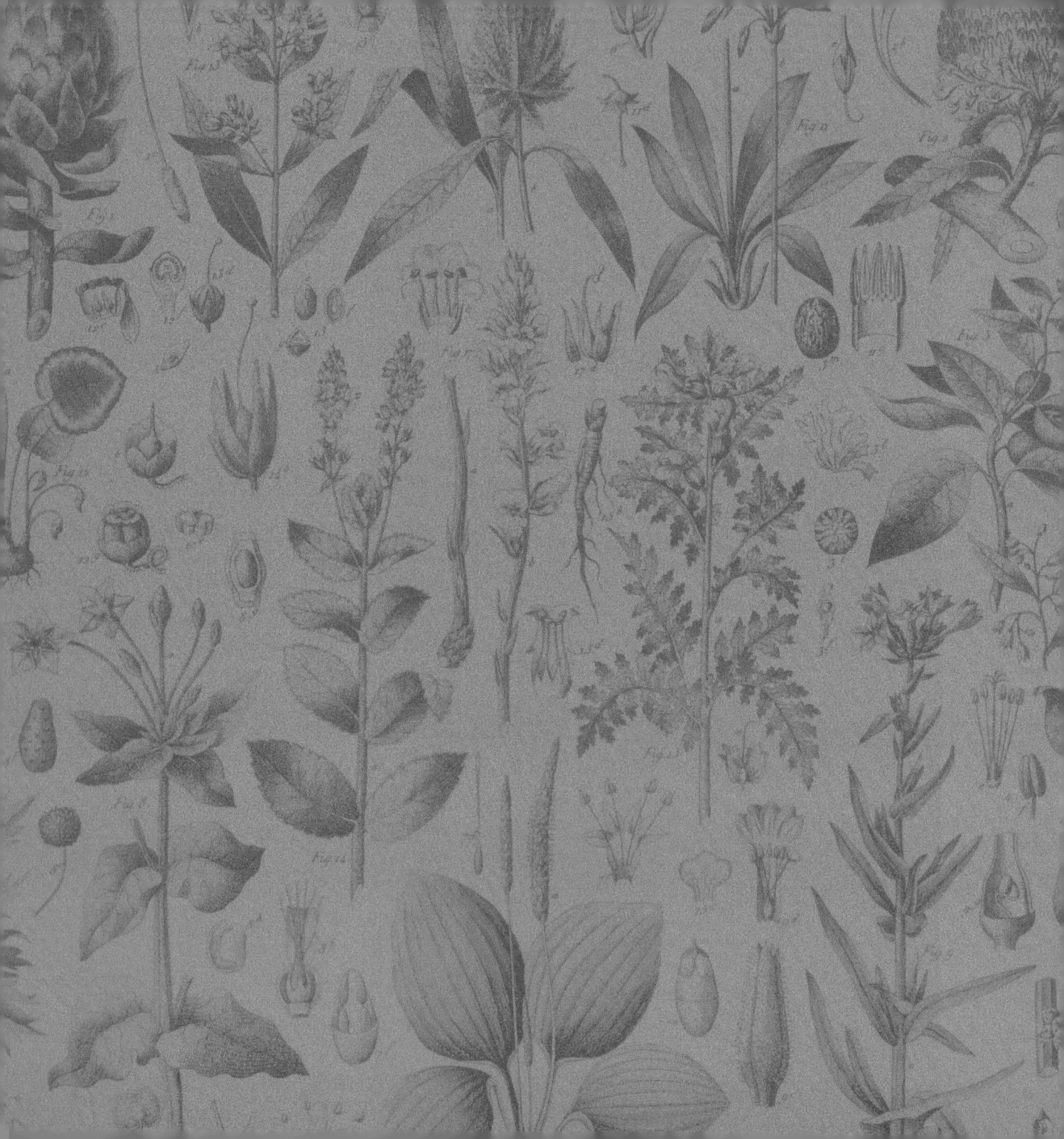

MEASUREMENT CONVERSIONS

Owing to differences in utensils, variation in drop size, and differences in user judgment, these measurement conversions are approximate. You will find some of these measurements in this book; others are found in other aromatherapy resources.

1 milliliter = 20 drops = 0.03 fluid ounce = 0.27 dram

15 milliliters = 0.5 fluid ounce = ½ fluid ounce

1 teaspoon = 100 drops = ⅙ fl oz = 5 milliliters

3 teaspoons = 1 tablespoon

2 tablespoons = 1 fluid ounce

4 tablespoons = 2 fluid ounces = ¼ cup

8 tablespoons = 4 fluid ounces = ½ cup

16 tablespoons = 8 fluid ounces = 1 cup

2 cups = 1 pint

4 cups = 1 quart

4 quarts = 1 gallon

GLOSSARY

adulterate: to mix pure essential oils with less-expensive substances, but advertise the product as 100 percent pure essential oil.

analgesic: a substance that relieves or deadens pain.

anaphrodisiac: a substance that reduces sexual desire.

anesthetic: a substance that relieves pain via loss of sensation.

anti-allergenic: a substance that reduces allergy symptoms.

antibacterial: a substance that fights bacterial growth.

antibiotic: a substance that fights infections by destroying bacteria in the body, or by preventing bacterial growth within the body.

antidepressant: a substance that elevates the mood and counteracts depression.

anti-emetic: a substance that reduces the severity or frequency of vomiting.

antifungal: a substance that prevents fungal growth.

anti-inflammatory: a substance that reduces or prevents inflammation.

antimicrobial: a substance that reduces microbial growth.

antioxidant: a substance that inhibits molecular oxidization.

antiseborrheic: a substance that helps control the oily secretions produced by the sebaceous glands.

antiseptic: a substance that helps control infection.

antispasmodic: a substance that helps prevent and relieve muscle spasms and cramping.

antitussive: a substance that relieves coughing.

antiviral: a substance that combats viral infections.

aperient: a substance that relieves constipation.

aperitive: a substance that stimulates appetite.

aphrodisiac: a substance that enhances sexual libido and improves sexual functioning.

astringent: a substance that causes tissues to contract.

bactericide: a substance that kills bacteria.

calmative: a substance that acts as a mild sedative.

carminative: a substance that relieves flatulence and facilitates the digestive process.

cholagogue: a substance that stimulates the secretion of bile.

cicatrizant: a substance that promotes healing by encouraging the formation of scar tissue.

cordial: a substance that offers comfort while promoting healing.

cytophylactic: a substance that enhances the body's defense against infection by increasing white blood cell activity.

decongestant: a substance that relieves congestion.

deodorant: a substance that combats body odor.

depurative: a substance that facilitates the removal of toxins from the body and bloodstream.

diaphoretic: a substance that promotes perspiration.

digestive: a substance that promotes normal digestion.

disinfectant: a substance that destroys germs.

diuretic: a substance that removes excess water from the body by promoting urination.

emmenagogue: a substance that induces menstruation.

emollient: a substance that softens and soothes skin.

eugenol: an oxygenated chemical compound.

euphoriant: a substance that promotes an intense feeling of happiness.

expectorant: a substance that facilitates the expulsion of mucus from the lungs.

febrifuge: a substance that may reduce fever.

fungicide: a substance that kills fungi.

galactagogue: a substance that increases lactation in nursing mothers.

hemostatic: a substance that helps stop bleeding.

hypertensive: a substance that can elevate blood pressure.

hypnotic: a substance that induces sleep.

hypotensive: a substance that can reduce blood pressure.

insect repellent: a substance that repels insects.

insecticide: a substance that kills insects.

laxative: a substance that induces bowel movements.

nervine: a substance that strengthens and tones the nervous system.

parturient: able to assist in labor and delivery.

phototoxic: a substance that can increase the risk of sunburn when exposed to direct sunlight after being applied to skin.

relaxant: a substance that encourages relaxation.

rubefacient: a substance that can cause skin to turn red.

sedative: a substance that promotes feelings of tranquillity, and that may induce sleep.

stimulant: a substance that enhances alertness.

stomachic: a substance that both enhances appetite and improves digestion.

styptic: a substance that stops external bleeding.

sudorific: a substance that causes sweating.

tonic: a substance that enhances overall well-being.

vasoconstrictor: a substance that can cause blood vessel walls to contract.

vermifuge: a substance that expels intestinal worms.

vulnerary: a substance that helps wounds to heal.

RESOURCES

Books

The Art of Aromatherapy: The Healing and Beautifying Properties of the Essential Oils of Flowers and Herbs by Robert B. Tisserand (Rochester, VT: Healing Arts Press, 1977)

The Complete Book of Essential Oils and Aromatherapy by Valerie Ann Worwood (Novato, CA: New World Library, 2016)

The Illustrated Encyclopedia of Essential Oils by Julia Lawless (Rockport, MA: Element Books, 1995)

Websites

Base Formula Aromatherapy

Offers a wide range of aromatherapy products, tools, and supplies. baseformula.com

BioSource Naturals

Carries a full line of aromatherapy supplies and more. biosourcenaturals.com

Nature's Gift

Offers a wide variety of essential oils, aromatherapy products and tools, books, and more. naturesgift.com

Plant Therapy

Provides daily and monthly specials. The company distinguishes itself with KidSafe, their proprietary line of essential oils and blends for children. Articles, recipes, and other resources for learning are available. planttherapy.com

Somatherapy: Dreaming Earth Botanicals

Offers an extensive selection of aromatherapy supplies, plus articles and recipes. dreamingearth.com

CONTINUING EDUCATION

Alliance of International Aromatherapists

alliance-aromatherapists.org

Aromahead Institute

aromahead.com

Flora Medica

floramedica.com

National Association for Holistic Aromatherapy

naha.org

AILMENTS AND OILS QUICK REFERENCE

Allergies

chamomile, melissa, peppermint

Congestion

cajuput, eucalyptus (all species), marjoram

Constipation

black pepper, fennel seed, peppermint

Cuts and Scrapes

Eucalyptus radiata, lavender

Dental Pain

clove bud, lemon, peppermint

Digestive Complaints

peppermint, ginger, Roman chamomile

Exhaustion

basil, grapefruit, mandarin

Hangover

ginger, lemon, peppermint

Headache

basil, lavender, melissa

Heartburn

ginger, fennel seed, spearmint

Insect Bites and Bee Stings

basil, lavender, niaouli

Insect Repellent

citronella, lemongrass, patchouli

Insomnia

clary sage, lavender, valerian

Laryngitis

lavender, naiouli

Menopause

clary sage, geranium, vitex berry

Menstrual Problems

clary sage, calendula, vitex berry

Nosebleed

cypress, lavender, lemon

Sinusitis

eucalyptus (all species), spearmint, tea tree

Sunburn

cucumber seed, geranium, lavender

REFERENCES

Abbas, Abul K., Andrew H. Lichtman, and Shiv Pillai. *Basic Immunology: Functions and Disorders of the Immune System.* 4th ed. Philadelphia: Saunders, 2012.

Appleton, Jeremy, ND. "Lavender Oil for Anxiety and Depression: Review of the Literature on the Safety and Efficacy of Lavender." *Natural Medicine Journal* 4, no. 2 (February 2012). Accessed August 18, 2017. naturalmedicinejournal.com/journal/2012-02/lavender-oil-anxiety-and-depression-0.

Aromahead Institute. *Component Database.* Aromahead.com. Accessed March 18, 2016. components.aromahead.com.

Ballard, Clive G., John T. O'Brien, Katharina Reichelt, and Elaine K. Perry. "Aromatherapy as a Safe and Effective Treatment for the Management of Agitation in Severe Dementia." *Journal of Clinical Psychiatry* 63, no. 7 (2002): 553–58.

Bartsch, Jennifer, Erik Uhde, and Tunga Salthammer. "Analysis of Odour Compounds from Scented Consumer Products Using Gas Chromatography-Mass Spectrometry and Gas Chromatography-Olfactometry." *Analytica Chimica Acta* 904 (January 2016): 98–106. doi.org/10.1016/j.aca.2015.11.031.

Basketter, David A., Sylvie Lemoine, and John P. McFadden. "Skin Sensitisation to Fragrance Ingredients: Is There a Role for Household Cleaning/Maintenance Products?" *European Journal of Dermatology* 25, no. 1 (January–February 2015): 7–13. ncbi.nlm.nih.gov/pubmed/25547642.

Bouchez, Colette. "Fragrance Allergies: A Sensory Assault." Allergies Health Center, WebMD. Accessed March 17, 2016. webmd.com/allergies/features/fragrance-allergies-a-sensory-assault.

Boukhatem, Mohamed Nadjib, Mohamed Amine Ferhat, Abdelkrim Kameli, Fairouz Saidi, and Hadjer Tchoketch Kebir. "Lemongrass (*Cymbopogon citratus*) Essential Oil as a Potent Anti-Inflammatory and Antifungal Drug." *Libyan Journal of Medicine* 9 (2014). doi.org/10.3402/ljm.v9.25431.

Branham, Erin. "The Scent of Love: Ancient Perfumes." *The Getty Iris* (blog), May 1, 2012. blogs.getty.edu/iris/the-scent-of-love-ancient-perfumes.

Brunei Times. "Pouches: A Class of Their Own." bt.com, September 21, 2010. Accessed March 17, 2016. bt.com.bn/art-culture/2010/09/21/pouches-class-their-own.

California College of Ayurveda. "Ayurveda and Aromatherapy: Alternative Medicine for Healing Body-Mind-Spirit," August 6, 2014. Accessed March 17, 2016. ayurvedacollege.com/blog/ayurveda-and-aromatherapy-alternative-medicine-healing-body-mind-spirit.

Central Nervous System: Visual Perspectives. "The Thalamus." Accessed March 18, 2016. cnsvp.stanford.edu/atlas/thalamus.html.

Chee, Hee Youn, and Min Hee Lee. "Antifungal Activity of Clove Essential Oil and its Volatile Vapour Against Dermatophytic Fungi." *Mycobiology* 35, no. 4 (December 2007): 241–43. ncbi.nlm.nih.gov/pmc/articles/PMC3763181.

Chopra Center. "Ayurveda: The Science of Life." Accessed March 17, 2016. chopra.com/our-services/ayurveda.

Cooksley, Valerie Gennari. *Aromatherapy: A Lifetime Guide to Healing with Essential Oils*. Englewood Cliffs, NJ: Prentice-Hall, 1996.

Cunningham, Scott. *The Complete Book of Incense, Oils & Brews*. Woodbury, MN: Llewellyn Publications, 2014.

de Groot, A. C. "Contact Allergy for Perfume Ingredients in Cosmetics and Toilet Articles." *Tijdschrift voor Geneeskunde* 141, no. 12 (March 1997): 571–74. ncbi.nlm.nih.gov/pubmed/9190522.

de Sousa, A. A., P. M. Soares, A. N. de Almeida, A. R. Maia, E. P. de Souza, and A. M. Assreuy. "Antispasmodic Effect of *Mentha piperita* Essential Oil on Tracheal Smooth Muscle of Rats." *Journal of Ethnopharmacology* 130, no. 2 (July 20, 2010): 433–36. doi.org/10.1016/j.jep.2010.05.012. Epub May 19, 2010.

Dioscorides. "The Herbal of Dioscorides the Greek. Book One: Aromatics." CancerLynx. Accessed March 17, 2016. cancerlynx.com/BOOKONEAROMATICS.PDF.

Edwards, Victoria H. *The Aromatherapy Companion: Medicinal Uses/Ayurvedic Healing/Body-Care Blends/Perfumes & Scents/Emotional Health & Well-Being*. North Adams, MA: Storey Publishing, 1999.

Encyclopedia Britannica. "Avicenna: Persian Philosopher and Scientist." Accessed March 17, 2016. britannica.com/biography/Avicenna.

———. "Enkephalin: Biochemistry." Accessed March 18, 2016. britannica.com/science/enkephalin.

———. "Olfactory Bulb: Anatomy." Accessed March 18, 2016. britannica.com/science/olfactory-bulb.

Essential Oils Academy. "History of Essential Oils." Accessed March 17, 2016. essentialoilsacademy.com/history.

Essential Oils for Beginners: the Guide to Get Started with Essential Oils and Aromatherapy. Berkeley, CA: Althea Press, 2013.

Essential Oils Pocket Reference. 6th edition. Lehi, UT: Life Science Publishing, 2014.

Flaxman, D., and P. Griffiths. "Is Tea Tree Oil Effective at Eradicating MRSA Colonization? A Review." *British Journal of Community Nursing* 10, no. 3 (November 2005): 123–26. PubMed NCBI. Accessed May 8, 2015. ncbi.nlm.nih.gov/pubmed/15824699.

Fordham University. "The Life and Works of Hildegard von Bingen (1098–1179)." Accessed March 17, 2016. sourcebooks.fordham.edu/med/hildegarde.asp.

Friedmann, Terry S., MD, ABHM. "Attention Deficit And Hyperactivity Disorder (ADHD)." Meetup.com. Accessed April 3, 2016. files.meetup.com/1481956/ADHD%20Research%20by%20Dr.%20Terry%20Friedmann.pdf.

Gattefossé, René-Maurice. *Gattefossé's Aromatherapy: The First Book on Aromatherapy*. Saffron Walden, UK: C. W. Daniel, 1993.

Gibson, Emma Alvarez. "Best Bets for Beating Gas." Digestive Disorders Health Center, WebMD. Accessed March 25, 2016. webmd.com/digestive-disorders/features/embarrassing-conditions.

Haddad R, A. Medhanie, Y. Roth, D. Harel, N. Sobel. "Predicting Odor Pleasantness with an Electronic Nose." *PLoS Computational Biology* 6, no. 4 (2010): e1000740. doi.org/10.1371/journal.pcbi.1000740.

Harman, Ann. "Harvest to Hydrosol: Distill Your Own Exquisite Hydrosols at Home." Fruitland, WA: botANNicals, 2015.

Hay, I. C., M. Jamieson, and A. D. Ormerod. "Randomized Trial of Aromatherapy. Successful Treatment for Alopecia Areata." *Archives of Dermatology* 134, no. 11 (November 1998): 1349–52. pubmed.ncbi.nlm.nih.gov/9828867.

Healthy Hildegard. "Traditional German Herbal Medicine." healthyhildegard.com. Accessed March 17, 2016. healthyhildegard.com/traditional-german-herbal-medicine.

History of Medicine Division, U.S. National Library of Medicine, National Institutes of Health. "Greek Medicine: 'I Swear by Apollo Physician . . .': Greek Medicine from the Gods to Galen." Accessed March 17 and April 5, 2016. nlm.nih.gov/hmd/greek/greek_galen.html.

———. "Islamic Culture and the Medical Arts: Al-Razi, the Clinician." Accessed March 17, 2016. nlm.nih.gov/exhibition/islamic_medical/islamic_06.html.

Hongratanaworakit, T. "Stimulating Effect of Aromatherapy Massage with Jasmine Oil." *Natural Product Communications* 5, no. 1 (January 2010): 157–62. ncbi.nlm.nih.gov/pubmed/20184043.

Howdyshell, C. "Complementary Therapy: Aromatherapy with Massage for Geriatric and Hospice Care—a Call for an Holistic Approach." *The Hospice Journal* 13, no. 3 (1998): 69–75. Accessed May 12, 2015. ncbi.nlm.nih.gov/pubmed/9677958.

Jepson R. G., G. Williams, and J. C. Craig. "Cranberries for Preventing Urinary Tract Infections." *Cochrane Database System Review* 10 (October 2012). ncbi.nlm.nih.gov/pmc/articles/PMC7027998.

Juergens, U. R., M. Stöber, and H. Vetter. "The Anti-Inflammatory Activity of L-menthol Compared to Mint Oil in Human Monocytes in Vitro: A Novel Perspective for Its Therapeutic Use in Inflammatory Diseases." *European Journal of Medical Research* 3, no. 12 (December 16, 1998): 539–45.

Keville, Kathi, and Mindy Green. *Aromatherapy: A Complete Guide to the Healing Art*. New York: Crossing Press, 2009.

Kianpour, M., A. Mansouri, T. Mehrabi, and G. Asghari. "Effect of Lavender Scent Inhalation on Prevention of Stress, Anxiety, and Depression in the Postpartum Period." *Iranian Journal of Nursing and Midwifery Research* 21, no. 2 (March–April 2016): 197–201. doi.org/10.4103/1735-9066.178248.

Largo, Michael. *The Big, Bad Book of Botany: The World's Most Fascinating Flora*. New York: William Morrow, 2014.

Lawless, Julia. *The Illustrated Encyclopedia of Essential Oils: The Complete Guide to the Use of Oils in Aromatherapy and Herbalism*. Rockport, MA: Element Books, 1995.

Laws, Bill. *Fifty Plants that Changed the Course of History*. Ontario, Canada: Firefly Books, 2011.

Levine, Jeffrey M., MD. "Wound Odor: The View from Ancient Greece." jmlevinemd.com. Revised May 10, 2021. Accessed March 17, 2016. jmlevinemd.com/wound-odor-the-view-from-ancient-greece.

Lillehei, Angela Smith, Linda L. Halcón, Kay Savik, and Reilly Reis. "Effect of Inhaled Lavender and Sleep Hygiene on Self-Reported Issues: A Randomized Controlled Trial." *Journal of Alternative and Complementary Medicine* 21, no. 7 (July 2015): 430–38. doi.org/10.1089/acm.2014.0327.

Lis-Balchin, Maria. *Aromatherapy Science: A Guide for Healthcare Professionals*. Grayslake, IL: Pharmaceutical Press, 2006.

Lobo, V., A. Patil, A. Phatak, and N. Chandra. "Free Radicals, Antioxidants, and Functional Foods: Impact on Human Health." *Pharmacognosy Reviews* 4, no. 8 (July–December 2010): 118–26. ncbi.nlm.nih.gov/pmc/articles/PMC3249911.

Mahler, V. "Contact Allergies in the Elderly." *Der Hautarzt* 66, no. 9 (September 2015): 665–73. doi.org/10.1007/s00105-015-3668-z.

Manniche, Lise. *Sacred Luxuries: Fragrance, Aromatherapy, and Cosmetics in Ancient Egypt*. Ithaca, NY: Cornell University Press, 1999.

The Middle Ages.net. "The Black Death: Bubonic Plague." Accessed March 17, 2016. themiddleages.net/plague.html.

Miller, Light, and Bryan Miller. *Ayurveda & Aromatherapy: The Earth Essential Guide to Ancient Wisdom and Modern Healing*. Delhi, India: Motilal Banarsidass, 1998.

Moss, Mark, and Lorraine Oliver. "Plasma 1,8-Cineole Correlates with Cognitive Performance Following Exposure to Rosemary Essential Aroma." *Therapeutic Advances in Psychopharmacology* 2, no. 3 (June 2012): 103–13. ncbi.nlm.nih.gov/pmc/articles/PMC3736918.

National Association for Holistic Aromatherapy. "How Are Essential Oils Extracted?" NAHA.org. Accessed March 18, 2016. naha.org/explore-aromatherapy/about-aromatherapy/how-are-essential-oils-extracted.

———. "Safety Information." Accessed July 6, 2022. naha.org/explore-aromatherapy/safety.

———. "What Are Essential Oils?" NAHA. Accessed June 3, 2015. naha.org/explore-aromatherapy/about-aromatherapy/what-are-essential-oils.

———. "What Is Aromatherapy?" NAHA. Accessed June 3, 2015. naha.org/explore-aromatherapy/about-aromatherapy/what-is-aromatherapy.

National Center for Complementary and Integrative Health. "Aromatherapy." Accessed March 17, 2016. nccih.nih.gov/health/aromatherapy.

NHR Organic Oils. "New Legislation Concerning Allergens in Essential Oils and Toiletry Products." Accessed March 18, 2016. nhrorganicoils.com/frame.php?page=info_21.

Norman, Jeremy. "At Sibudu Cave, the Oldest Known Early Bedding and Use of Medicinal Plants (Circa 75000 BCE)." historyofinformation.com. Accessed March 17, 2016. historyofinformation.com/expanded.php?id=3465.

———. "The Vienna Dioscorides, Probably the Most Beautiful of the Earliest Surviving Scientific Codices (Circa 512 CE)." historyofinformation.com. Accessed March 17, 2016. historyofinformation.com/expanded.php?id=1647.

Oils and Plants. "Jean Valnet." Accessed March 17, 2016. oilsandplants.com/valnet.htm.

———. "René-Maurice Gattefossé." Accessed March 15, 2016. oilsandplants.com/gattefosse.htm.

Osborn, David K. "Galen: Greatest Physician of the Roman Empire." greekmedicine.net. Accessed March 17, 2016. greekmedicine.net/whos_who/Galen.html.

Pazyar, N., R. Yaghoobi, N. Bagherani, and A. Kazerouni. "A Review of Applications of Tea Tree Oil in Dermatology." *International Journal of Dermatology* 52, no. 7 (July 2013): 784–90. doi.org/10.1111/j.1365-4632.2012.05654.x.

PDQ Integrative, Alternative, and Complementary Therapies Editorial Board. "Aromatherapy and Essential Oils (PDQ) Health Professional Version." National Institutes of Health, U.S. National Library of Medicine. Accessed March 17, 2016. ncbi.nlm.nih.gov/pubmedhealth/PMH0032645.

———. "Aromatherapy and Essential Oils (PDQ), Patient Version." National Institutes of Health, U.S. National Library of Medicine. Accessed March 17, 2016. ncbi.nlm.nih.gov/pubmedhealth/PMH0032518.

Perchon, Nerys, and Lora Cantele. *The Complete Aromatherapy and Essential Oils Handbook for Everyday Wellness*. Toronto, Canada: Robert Rose, 2014.

Pinto, Eugénia, Luís Vale-Silva, Carlos Cavaleiro, and Lígia Salgueiro. "Antifungal Activity of the Clove Essential Oil from *Syzygium aromaticum* on *Candida*, *Aspergillus*, and Dermatophyte Species." *Journal of Medical Microbiology* 58, no. 11 (November 2009): 1454–62. doi.org/10.1099/jmm.0.010538-0.

Pollan, Michael. *The Botany of Desire: A Plant's-Eye View of the World*. New York: Random House, 2002.

Price, Shirley. *Aromatherapy Workbook: A Complete Guide to Understanding and Using Essential Oils*. London: Thorsons, 1999.

Redwood, Daniel. "Interviews with People Who Make a Difference: Alternative and Complementary Medicine: Interview with Marc Micozzi, MD." 1995. healthy.net. healthy.net/scr/interview.aspx?Id=239.

Roach, John. "Oldest Perfumes Found on 'Aphrodite's Island.'" *National Geographic News*, March 29, 2007. Accessed March 15, 2016. news.nationalgeographic.com/news/2007/03/070329-oldest-perfumes.html.

Robinson Library. "Galen." Accessed March 17, 2016. robinsonlibrary.com/medicine/medicine/history/galen.htm.

Rupp, Rebecca. *How Carrots Won the Trojan War: Curious (but True) Stories of Common Vegetables*. North Adams, MA: Storey Publishing, 2011.

Sallamander Concepts. "The Chemistry of Essential Oils, and Their Chemical Components." essentialoils.co.za. Accessed March 18, 2016. essentialoils.co.za/components.htm.

Sasannejad, P., M. Saeedi, A. Shoeibi, A. Gorji, M. Abbasi, and M. Foroughipour. "Lavender Essential Oil in the Treatment of Migraine Headache: A Placebo-Controlled Clinical Trial." *European Neurology* 67, no. 5 (2012): 288–91. doi:10.1159/000335249.

Schiller, Carol, and David Schiller. *500 Formulas for Aromatherapy: Mixing Essential Oils for Every Use*. New York: Sterling Publishing, 1994.

Schnaubelt, Kurt. *Medical Aromatherapy: Healing with Essential Oils*. Berkeley, CA: Frog Books, 1999.

Secret of Thieves. "Four Thieves Vinegar: Evolution of a Medieval Medicine." Accessed March 17, 2016. secretofthieves.com/four-thieves-vinegar.cfm.

Shea, Stephen D., Lawrence C. Katz, and Richard Mooney. "Noradrenergic Induction of Odor-Specific Neural Habituation and Olfactory Memories." *Journal of Neuroscience* 28, no. 42 (October 2008): 10711–19. doi:10.1523/JNEUROSCI.3853-08.2008.

Shehad, Meg. "Rosewood, Lavender, and Clary Sage: What's the Connection?" Gritman Essential Oils, September 9, 2013. Accessed August 10, 2017. gritman.com/blog/rosewood-lavender-and-clary-sage-whats-the-connection.

Stewart, Amy. *The Drunken Botanist: The Plants That Create the World's Great Drinks*. New York: Algonquin Books, 2013.

———. *Wicked Plants: The Weed That Killed Lincoln's Mother and Other Botanical Atrocities*. New York: Algonquin Books, 2009.

Thorpe, J. R. "The Ancient History of Perfume." *Bustle*, July 31, 2015. Accessed March 17, 2016. bustle.com/articles/101182-the-strange-history-of-perfume-from-ancient-roman-foot-fragrance-to-napoleons-cologne.

Tisserand Institute. "Dilution Guidelines for Essential Oils." 2015. Accessed August 26,

2017. tisserandinstitute.org/wp-content/uploads/2015/01/EO-dilution.pdf.

Tisserand, Robert B. *The Art of Aromatherapy: The Healing and Beautifying Properties of the Essential Oils of Flowers and Herbs.* Rochester, VT: Healing Arts Press, 1977.

———. "Safety." roberttisserand.com. Accessed March 21, 2016. roberttisserand.com/category/safety.

Tisserand, Robert, and Rodney Young. *Essential Oil Safety: A Guide for Health Care Professionals.* 2nd ed. London: Churchill Livingstone, 2013.

Tisserand, Robert, and Tony Balacs. *Essential Oil Safety: A Guide for Health Care Professionals.* London: Churchill Livingstone, 1995.

Tourles, Stephanie L. *Hands-On Healing Remedies: 150 Recipes for Herbal Balms, Salves, Oils, Liniments & Other Topical Therapies.* North Adams, MA: Storey Publishing, 2012.

U.S. Department of Health and Human Services, National Institutes of Health, National Center for Complementary and Integrative Health. "Peppermint Oil." Accessed August 13, 2017. nccih.nih.gov/health/peppermintoil.

University of Maryland Medical Center. "Aromatherapy." Accessed March 16, 2016. umm.edu/health/medical/altmed/treatment/aromatherapy.

———. "Lavender." Last modified January 1, 2015. umm.edu/health/medical/altmed/herb/lavender#ixzz3aH5KoHl0.

Veal, Lowana. "Headlice and Essential Oils." Aromatherapy Global Online Research Archives. August 17, 2011. Accessed March 26, 2016. wingedseed.com/Agora/Lice_page.htm.

Verot, Olivier. "The Scent of Opportunity: How China's Fragrance Market Can Reach Its Potential." *Jing Daily*, October 2, 2014. Accessed April 5, 2016. jingdaily.com/the-scent-of-opportunity-how-chinas-fragrance-market-can-reach-its-potential.

Warad, Shivaraj B., Sahana S. Kolar, Veena Kalburgi, and Nagaraj B. Kalburgi. "Lemongrass Essential Oil Gel as a Local Drug Delivery Agent for the Treatment of Periodontitis." *Ancient Science of Life* 32, no. 4 (April 2013): 205–11. doi.org/10.4103/0257-7941.131973.

WebMD. "Frankincense." Accessed July 6, 2022. webmd.com/vitamins/ai/ingredientmono-448/frankincense.

———. "Understanding Cold Sores Basics." Accessed June 3, 2015. webmd.com/skin-problems-and-treatments/guide/understanding-cold-sores-basics.

White, Gregory Lee. *Essential Oils and Aromatherapy: How to Use Essential Oils for Beauty, Health, and Spirituality.* Detroit: White Willow Books, 2013.

Worwood, Valerie Ann. *The Complete Book of Essential Oils and Aromatherapy, Revised and Expanded: Over 800 Natural, Nontoxic, and Fragrant Recipes to Create Health, Beauty, and Safe Home and Work Environments.* Novato, CA: New World Library, 2016.

———. *The Fragrant Mind: Aromatherapy for Personality, Mind, Mood, and Emotion.* Novato, CA: New World Library, 1996.

OILS INDEX

A

Allspice
  about, 42
  Allspice–Sweet Orange Diffusion, 134
Anise
  about, 43
  Anise–Caraway Seed Vapor, 135
  Spicy Autumn Room Deodorizer, 321
  Synergistic Heartburn Blend, 231
Atlas cedarwood
  about, 44
  Synergistic Dog Flea-Collar Blend, 341

B

Balsam of Peru, 45
Basil
  about, 46
  Basil, Rosemary, and Cypress Diffusion, 208
  Basil-Geranium Shower Steam, 210
  Lavender, Marjoram, and Basil Balm for Tension Headaches, 162
  Lavender-Basil Bath Salts for Restless Legs Syndrome, 219
  Lemon-Basil Sanitizing Spray, 332
  Peppermint-Basil Travel Gel, 167
  Restorative Shower Melts, 161
  Rosemary, Basil, and Mint Shower Melts for General Headaches, 163
  Synergistic Bath Blend, 227
  Synergistic Pain-Relief Blend, 173
  Uplifting Citrus-Basil Diffusion, 211
Bay laurel
  about, 47
  Bay Laurel–Lavender Diffusion, 138
  Pantry Moth Repellent, 345
Benzoin
  about, 48
  Benzoin Balm, 164
  Benzoin-Bergamot Lotion, 220
  Benzoin–Black Pepper Muscle Balm, 170
  Cinnamon Leaf–Ginger Salve, 157
  Lavender-Benzoin Bath Salts, 157
  Lavender-Myrrh Massage, 300
  Luxurious Solid Perfume, 314
  Soothing Benzoin-Myrrh Body Lotion, 263
  Synergistic Callus Blend, 301
  Synergistic Overnight Foot Cream, 303
Bergamot
  about, 49
  Benzoin-Bergamot Lotion, 220
  Cajuput-Bergamot Diffusion, 132
  Garden in the Woods Eau de Toilette, 313
  German Chamomile Bath Salts, 199
  Healing Aftershave Splash, 315
  Hungary Water, 314
  Nourishing Nighttime Lotion, 281

Bergamot (*continued*)
   Rosacea Treatment for Mature Skin, 272
   Soothing Bergamot-Lavender Neck Wrap, 149
   Synergistic Antibacterial Massage Blend, 247
   Synergistic Antiseptic Bath Salts, 247
   Synergistic Callus Blend, 301
Black pepper
   about, 50
   Benzoin–Black Pepper Muscle Balm, 170
   Ginger–Black Pepper Digestive Massage, 225
   Soothing Massage Oil, 169
   Synergistic Bath Blend, 227
   Winter Spice Cologne, 315

C

Cajuput
   about, 51
   Cajuput-Bergamot Diffusion, 132
   Cajuput–Cucumber Seed Gel, 198
   Synergistic Antiseptic Bath Salts, 247
Calendula
   about, 52
   Synergistic Rosacea Blend, 273
Caraway seed
   about, 53
   Anise–Caraway Seed Vapor, 135
   Caraway–Clove Bud Chest Rub, 139
   Caraway Seed–May Chang Shower Steam, 140
   Synergistic Heartburn Blend, 231
Cardamom
   about, 54
   Cardamom Balm, 234
   Cardamom-Mandarin Temple Rub, 221
   Winter Spice Cologne, 315
Carrot seed
   about, 55
   Frankincense and Commonsense Serum, 280
   Nourishing Nighttime Lotion, 281
   Rosacea Treatment for Mature Skin, 272
   Synergistic Callus Blend, 301
Cedarwood. *See also* Atlas cedarwood
   about, 56
   Cedarwood Massage Oil, 156
   Healing Aftershave Splash, 315
   Mason Jar Luminaries, 342
   Synergistic Sinusitis Inhaler, 153
   Valerian-Cedarwood Bedtime Balm, 213
Chamomile. *See* German chamomile; Roman chamomile
Cinnamon leaf
   about, 57
   Cinnamon Leaf–Fennel Seed Balm, 224
   Cinnamon Leaf–Ginger Salve, 157
   Cinnamon Leaf Weedkiller, 354
   Soothing Massage Oil, 169
   Spicy Autumn Room Deodorizer, 321
   Synergistic Pain-Relief Compress, 171
   Triple-Spice Massage Blend, 229
Citronella
   about, 58
   Citronella-Lavender Mothballs, 344
   Mason Jar Luminaries, 342
   Mosquito Repellent Spray, 343
   Synergistic Dog Flea-Collar Blend, 341

Clary sage
  about, 59
  Clary Sage–Citrus Diffusion, 217
  Clary Sage–Sandalwood Conditioner, 286
  Clary Sage Shower Melts, 243
  Relaxing Clary Sage–Lavender Chest Rub, 133
  Synergistic Blend for Irregular Cycles, 245
  Synergistic Relaxation Diffusion, 219
  Synergistic Split-End Conditioner, 291
Clove bud
  about, 5, 60
  Caraway–Clove Bud Chest Rub, 139
  Citrus–Clove Bud Breath Drops, 146
  Clove Bud Neat Treatment, 179
  Clove Bud Spray, 294
  Comforting Clove Bud Compress, 235
  Lemon Eucalyptus–Clove Bud Compress, 309
  Mold and Mildew Prevention Spray, 330
  Oven/Stovetop Gentle Scrubbing Soap, 329
  Spicy Autumn Room Deodorizer, 321
  Spicy Frankincense-Helichrysum Balm, 145
  Synergistic Antiseptic Bath Salts, 247
  Synergistic Toothache Blend, 179
  Triple-Spice Massage Blend, 229
Copaiba
  about, 61
  Breathe-Easy Synergistic Blend, 350
  Copaiba-Chamomile Compress, 236
  Copaiba-Coriander Compress, 228
  Copaiba-Peppermint Foot Cream, 298
  Copaiba–Spanish Sage Vapor, 141

Coriander
  about, 62
  Copaiba-Coriander Compress, 228
  Synergistic Heartburn Blend, 231
Cucumber seed
  about, 63
  Cajuput–Cucumber Seed Gel, 198
  Cooling Cucumber Seed–Tea Tree Toner, 255
  Cooling Oregano–Cucumber Seed Spray, 194
  Helichrysum–Cucumber Seed Compress, 268
  Lavender–Cucumber Seed Spray, 359
  Refreshing Peppermint–Cucumber Seed Toner, 267
  Synergistic Firming Serum, 275
Cypress
  about, 64
  Anti-Cellulite Bath Salts, 260
  Basil, Rosemary, and Cypress Diffusion, 208
  Breathe-Easy Synergistic Blend, 350
  Cypress–German Chamomile Compress for Menstrual Cramps, 244
  Cypress Nasal Compress, 174
  Frankincense and Commonsense Serum, 280
  Healing Aftershave Splash, 315
  Lemon-Cypress Compress, 232
  Minty Lavender-Cypress Gel, 169
  Soothing Chamomile-Cypress Gel, 273
  Synergistic Antibacterial Massage Blend, 247
  Synergistic Cellulite Massage Oil, 261

Cypress (*continued*)
  Synergistic Eye Serum, 269
  Synergistic Firming Serum, 275
  Synergistic Itch-Relief Spray, 357
  Synergistic Pain-Relief Blend, 173
  Synergistic Pinkeye Blend, 151
  Synergistic Rosacea Blend, 273
  Synergistic Skin-Firming Lotion, 261
  Winter Spice Cologne, 315

D

Davana
  about, 65
  Rose-Davana Perfume, 241
Dill seed
  about, 66
  Dill Seed Balm, 136

E

Elemi
  about, 67
  Lemon-Elemi Nail Soak, 297
  Soothing Benzoin-Myrrh Body Lotion, 263
  Synergistic Smoothing Blend, 275
Eucalyptus. See also *Eucalyptus globulus*; *Eucalyptus radiata*; Lemon eucalyptus
  Aromatic Eucalyptus Sponge Bath, 142
  Daily Tea Tree–Eucalyptus Shower Spray, 323
  Eucalyptus, Juniper, and Geranium Lotion, 144
  Eucalyptus-Spearmint Vapor, 152
  Lavender-Eucalyptus Bee Sting Relief, 353
  Lavender-Eucalyptus Mop Solution, 325
  Minty Fennel Seed–Eucalyptus Lotion, 230
  Rosemary-Eucalyptus Vapor for Sinus Headaches, 163
  Streak-Free Glass and Mirror Cleaner, 327
  Synergistic Asthma Inhaler, 133
  Synergistic Sinusitis Shower Melts, 153
  Synergistic Sinusitis Inhaler, 153
  Synergistic Spider Spray, 347
Eucalyptus globulus
  about, 68
  Breathe-Easy Synergistic Blend, 350
  Pantry Moth Repellent, 345
  Synergistic Antiseptic Bath Salts, 247
  Synergistic Pinkeye Blend, 151
Eucalyptus radiata
  about, 69
  Mosquito Repellent Spray, 343
  Synergistic Abdominal Massage Blend, 229

F

Fennel seed
  about, 70
  Anti-Cellulite Bath Salts, 260
  Cinnamon Leaf–Fennel Seed Balm, 224
  Fennel Seed–Grapefruit Massage for Bloating, 245
  Minty Fennel Seed–Eucalyptus Lotion, 230
  Nourishing Nighttime Lotion, 281
  Peppermint–Fennel Seed Location, 226

Synergistic Antibacterial Massage Blend, 247
Synergistic Blend for Irregular Cycles, 245
Synergistic Heartburn Blend, 231

Fir needle
  about, 71
  Fir Needle Gel, 171
  Marjoram–Fir Needle Compress, 173

Frankincense
  about, 72
  Frankincense and Commonsense Serum, 280
  Frankincense Cold Compress, 299
  Frankincense-Myrrh Barrier Cream, 192
  Frankincense Nail Balm, 296
  Healing Frankincense Balm, 308
  Lavender-Frankincense Bath, 356
  Spicy Frankincense-Helichrysum Balm, 145
  Synergistic Age Spot Salve, 257
  Synergistic Asthma Inhaler, 133
  Synergistic Eye Serum, 269
  Synergistic Firming Serum, 275
  Synergistic Nail-Strengthening Blend, 297
  Synergistic Pinkeye Blend, 151

G

Galbanum
  about, 73
  Galbanum Cream, 200

Geranium. *See also* Rose geranium
  about, 74
  Basil-Geranium Shower Steam, 210
  Clary Sage Shower Melts, 243
  Cypress–German Chamomile Compress for Menstrual Cramps, 244
  Easy Whipped Moisturizer, 279
  Eucalyptus, Juniper, and Geranium Lotion, 144
  Frankincense and Commonsense Serum, 280
  Fresh Summer Breeze Spray, 320
  Garden in the Woods Eau de Toilette, 313
  Geranium-Lavender Balm, 195
  Geranium-Lavender Sunburn Gel, 358
  Geranium-Neroli Cream, 201
  Moisturizing Geranium-Myrrh Shampoo, 287
  Synergistic Antifungal Douche, 249
  Synergistic Blend for Irregular Cycles, 245
  Synergistic Firming Serum, 275
  Synergistic Itch-Relief Spray, 357
  Synergistic Overnight Foot Cream, 303
  Synergistic Relaxation Diffusion, 219
  Synergistic Rosacea Blend, 273
  Synergistic Split-End Conditioner, 291

German chamomile
  about, 75
  Chamomile-Helichrysum Gel, 184
  Chamomile-Lavender Gel, 352
  Chamomile–Tea Tree Balm, 186
  Cool Chamomile Compress, 150
  Copaiba-Chamomile Compress, 236
  German Chamomile Bath Salts, 199
  Lavender-Geranium Compress, 187
  Lemon, Rosemary, and Chamomile Diffusion, 214
  Minty Helichrysum-Chamomile Compress, 176

German chamomile (*continued*)
  Minty Orange-Chamomile Lotion, 225
  Peppermint-Pine Liniment, 165
  Soothing Chamomile-Cypress Gel, 273
  substitutions, 38
  Synergistic Hot Compress, 185
  Synergistic Pain-Relief Compress, 171
  Synergistic Toothache Blend, 179
Ginger
  about, 76
  Cinnamon Leaf–Ginger Salve, 157
  Citrus and Spice Splash, 312
  Ginger–Black Pepper Digestive Massage, 225
  Ginger Inhaler, 166
  Mandarin-Neroli Carpet Powder, 325
  Minty Fennel Seed–Eucalyptus Lotion, 230
  Sensual Massage Oil, 241
  Soothing Massage Oil, 169
  Spicy Autumn Room Deodorizer, 321
  Synergistic First-Aid Gel and Sprain Compress, 177
  Synergistic Heartburn Blend, 231
  Synergistic Pain-Relief Compress, 171
  Synergistic Sinusitis Shower Melts, 153
  Synergistic Traveler's Body Lotion, 167
  Triple-Spice Massage Blend, 229
Grapefruit
  about, 77
  Anti-Cellulite Bath Salts, 260
  Citrus and Spice Splash, 312
  Citrus–Clove Bud Breath Drops, 146
  Citrus Hardwood Floor Cleaner, 324
  Everyday Citrus-Sandalwood Spritzer, 218
  Fennel Seed–Grapefruit Massage for Bloating, 245
  Grapefruit-Spearmint Foot Spray, 306
  Grapefruit-Spearmint Spritz, 209
  Grapefruit–Ylang-Ylang Diffusion, 221
  Minty Fresh Fridge, 333
  Synergistic Cellulite Massage Oil, 261
  Synergistic Rosacea Blend, 273
  Uplifting Citrus-Basil Diffusion, 211

H

Helichrysum
  about, 78
  Chamomile-Helichrysum Gel, 184
  Helichrysum–Cucumber Seed Compress, 268
  Helichrysum Milk Bath, 359
  Helichrysum Spray, 199
  Minty Helichrysum-Chamomile Compress, 176
  Myrrh-Helichrysum Compress, 183
  Soothing Hand Balm, 305
  Spicy Frankincense-Helichrysum Balm, 145
  substitutions, 38
  Synergistic First-Aid Gel and Sprain Compress, 177
  Synergistic Itch-Relief Spray, 357
  Synergistic Pinkeye Blend, 151
  Synergistic Rosacea Blend, 273
  Ultra-Rich Conditioning Mask, 291

Hops flower
    about, 79
    Soothing Niaouli-Hops Balm, 191
Hyssop
    about, 80
    Soothing Spearmint-Hyssop Gargle, 135
    substitutions, 38

J

Jasmine
    about, 81
    Clary Sage–Citrus Diffusion, 217
    Jasmine Linen Spray, 240
    substitutions, 38
    Sweet Orange–Rose Geranium Body Oil, 263
Juniper berry
    about, 82
    Anti-Cellulite Bath Salts, 260
    Eucalyptus, Juniper, and Geranium Lotion, 144
    Juniper-Peppermint Gel, 172
    Synergistic Antibacterial Massage Blend, 247
    Synergistic Antiseptic Bath Salts, 247
    Synergistic Cellulite Massage Oil, 261
    Synergistic Hot Compress, 185
    Synergistic Skin-Firming Lotion, 261

L

Lavandin, 83
Lavender
    about, 84
    Ant-Eliminating Lavender Neat Treatment, 338
    Bay Laurel–Lavender Diffusion, 138
    Bodily Fluids and Pet Accident Cleaner, 334
    Calming Temple Rub, 206
    Chamomile-Lavender Gel, 352
    Citronella-Lavender Mothballs, 344
    Clary Sage Shower Melts, 243
    Deep-Cleansing Lavender-Lemon Steam, 267
    Detoxifying Massage Oil, 161
    Fleur Classique Parfum, 312
    Fresh Summer Breeze Spray, 320
    Geranium-Lavender Balm, 195
    Geranium-Lavender Sunburn Gel, 358
    German Chamomile Bath Salts, 199
    Honey-Lavender Mask, 270
    Hungary Water, 314
    Indoor Flea Powder, 340
    Lavender, Marjoram, and Basil Balm for Tension Headaches, 162
    Lavender-Basil Bath Salts for Restless Legs Syndrome, 219
    Lavender-Benzoin Bath Salts, 157
    Lavender Body Powder, 258
    Lavender-Chamomile Nighttime Shower Melts, 212
    Lavender–Cucumber Seed Spray, 359
    Lavender-Eucalyptus Bee Sting Relief, 353
    Lavender-Eucalyptus Mop Solution, 325
    Lavender Eye Massage, 269
    Lavender Flea Powder, 341
    Lavender-Frankincense Bath, 356
    Lavender-Geranium Compress, 187

Lavender (*continued*)
   Lavender-Lemon Eau de Toilette, 313
   Lavender-Lemon Gargle, 149
   Lavender-Marjoram Compress, 168
   Lavender-Marjoram Sore Throat Spray, 148
   Lavender Mouthwash, 147
   Lavender-Myrrh Massage, 300
   Lavender Nasal Salve, 175
   Lavender Neat Treatment, 158, 182, 187, 264
   Lavender Neat Treatment for Post-Wart Removal, 202
   Lavender-Neroli Baby Powder, 193
   Lavender-Peppermint Anti-Itch Spray, 353
   Lavender-Peppermint Lip Salve, 189
   Lavender Rinse, 246
   Lavender–Roman Chamomile Cleansing Wipes, 193
   Lavender-Rosewood Hand Cream, 304
   Lavender-Spearmint Breath Spray, 147
   Lavender–Tea Tree Balm, 271
   Lavender–Tea Tree Compress, 151
   Lavender–Tea Tree Conditioner, 289
   Lavender–Tea Tree Footbath, 309
   Lavender–Tea Tree Tampon, 248
   Lemon-Lavender Foot Soak, 302
   Lemon-Lavender Lip Balm, 189
   Lemon-Lavender Nasal Compress, 175
   Mason Jar Luminaries, 342
   Minty Lavender-Cypress Gel, 169
   Minty Lemon-Lavender Temple Rub, 145
   Pantry Moth Repellent, 345

Patchouli-Spearmint Repellent Lotion, 343
Patchouli–Tea Tree Foot Balm, 303
Peppermint-Basil Travel Gel, 167
Peppermint-Rosemary Conditioner, 284
Peppermint–Tea Tree Ant Spray, 339
Relaxing Clary Sage–Lavender Chest Rub, 133
Relaxing Lavender-Vetiver-Rose Bedtime Lotion, 207
Restorative Shower Melts, 161
Roman Chamomile–Lavender Spritz, 197
Rosacea Treatment for Mature Skin, 272
Rosemary-Lavender Foot Powder, 307
Skin-Softening Hand Soap, 305
Soothing Bergamot-Lavender Neck Wrap, 149
Soothing Hand Balm, 305
Soothing Palmarosa-Lavender Bath Salts, 195
Synergistic Abdominal Massage Blend, 229
Synergistic Age Spot Salve, 257
Synergistic Antifungal Douche, 249
Synergistic Callus Blend, 301
Synergistic Cellulite Massage Oil, 261
Synergistic Cold Sore Ointment, 191
Synergistic Dandruff Shampoo, 285
Synergistic First-Aid Gel and Sprain Compress, 177
Synergistic Healing Balm, 177
Synergistic Hot Compress, 185
Synergistic Itch-Relief Spray, 357
Synergistic Overnight Foot Cream, 303
Synergistic Pain-Relief Blend, 173
Synergistic Pinkeye Blend, 151

Synergistic Relaxation Diffusion, 219
Synergistic Rosacea Blend, 273
Synergistic Smoothing Blend, 275
Synergistic Split-End Conditioner, 291
Tangerine-Lavender Lotion, 215
Ultra-Rich Conditioning Mask, 291

Lemon
  about, 85
  All-Purpose Disinfectant Spray, 322
  Citrus-Mint Diffusion, 160
  Citrus Serum for Combination Skin, 279
  Clary Sage–Citrus Diffusion, 217
  Deep-Cleansing Lavender-Lemon Steam, 267
  Detoxifying Massage Oil, 161
  Everyday Citrus-Sandalwood Spritzer, 218
  Grass Stain Remover, 335
  Lavender-Lemon Eau de Toilette, 313
  Lavender-Lemon Gargle, 149
  Lemon, Rosemary, and Chamomile Diffusion, 214
  Lemon-Basil Sanitizing Spray, 332
  Lemon-Cypress Compress, 232
  Lemon-Elemi Nail Soak, 297
  Lemon Grease Treatment, 335
  Lemon-Lavender Foot Soak, 302
  Lemon-Lavender Lip Balm, 189
  Lemon-Lavender Nasal Compress, 175
  Lemon Mask, 256
  Lemon-Mint Spider Repellent Powder, 347
  Lemon Salve, 249
  Lemon Scouring Powder, 323
  Lemon Window Cleaner, 327
  Mason Jar Luminaries, 342
  May Chang–Lemon Lotion, 139
  Microwave Disinfectant, 328
  Minty Lemon-Lavender Temple Rub, 145
  Mold and Mildew Prevention Spray, 330
  Mosquito Repellent Spray, 343
  Pantry Moth Repellent, 345
  Quick Countertop Wipes, 329
  Restorative Shower Melts, 161
  Rosemary-Lemon Hand Cream, 209
  Rosemary-Peppermint Temple Rub, 211
  Sandalwood Serum, 281
  Spicy Autumn Room Deodorizer, 321
  Synergistic Bath Blend, 227
  Synergistic Cold Sore Ointment, 191
  Synergistic Nail-Strengthening Blend, 297
  Synergistic Pinkeye Blend, 151
  Synergistic Skin-Firming Lotion, 261
  Synergistic Toothache Blend, 179
  Synergistic Traveler's Body Lotion, 167
  Uplifting Citrus-Basil Diffusion, 211

Lemon eucalyptus
  about, 86
  Lemon Eucalyptus–Clove Bud Compress, 309
  Peppermint-Eucalyptus Pedicure Lotion, 307

Lemongrass, 88

Lemon verbena, 87

Lime
　about, 89
　Everyday Citrus-Sandalwood Spritzer, 218

M

Mandarin
　about, 90
　Cardamom-Mandarin Temple Rub, 221
　Citrus Hardwood Floor Cleaner, 324
　Clary Sage–Citrus Diffusion, 217
　Detoxifying Massage Oil, 161
　Fresh Summer Breeze Spray, 320
　Mandarin-Neroli Carpet Powder, 325
　Rose-Davana Perfume, 241
　Sensual Massage Oil, 241
　Uplifting Citrus-Basil Diffusion, 211
Marjoram
　about, 91
　Lavender, Marjoram, and Basil Balm for Tension Headaches, 162
　Lavender-Marjoram Compress, 168
　Lavender-Marjoram Sore Throat Spray, 148
　Marjoram–Fir Needle Compress, 173
　Synergistic Abdominal Massage Blend, 229
　Synergistic Healing Balm, 177
　Synergistic Pain-Relief Blend, 173
　Synergistic Relaxation Diffusion, 219
May chang
　about, 92
　Balancing Vitex Berry Lotion, 242
　Caraway Seed–May Chang Shower Steam, 140
　May Chang Foot Powder, 295
　May Chang–Lemon Lotion, 139
Melissa
　about, 93
　Melissa-Chamomile Diffusion, 351
　Melissa Neat Treatment, 190
　Melissa-Spearmint Bath Salts, 237
　substitutions, 38
Mint. *See* Peppermint; Spearmint
Myrrh
　about, 94
　Frankincense-Myrrh Barrier Cream, 192
　Lavender-Myrrh Massage, 300
　Moisturizing Geranium-Myrrh Shampoo, 287
　Myrrh-Helichrysum Compress, 183
　Neroli-Myrrh Wipes, 233
　Patchouli-Myrrh Antiseptic Gel, 159
　Peppermint-Myrrh Lotion, 357
　Post-Pregnancy Stretch Mark Slather, 201
　Soothing Benzoin-Myrrh Body Lotion, 263
　Soothing Myrrh Bath, 197
　substitutions, 39
　Synergistic Age Spot Salve, 257
　Synergistic Asthma Inhaler, 133
　Synergistic Callus Blend, 301
　Synergistic Nail-Strengthening Blend, 297
　Synergistic Overnight Foot Cream, 303
　Ultra-Rich Conditioning Mask, 291
Myrtle, 95

N

Neroli
  about, 96
  Calming Chamomile-Neroli Steam, 216
  Citrus-Flower Body Butter, 278
  Fleur Classique Parfum, 312
  Geranium-Neroli Cream, 201
  Hungary Water, 314
  Lavender-Neroli Baby Powder, 193
  Mandarin-Neroli Carpet Powder, 325
  Neroli-Myrrh Wipes, 233
  Post-Pregnancy Stretch Mark Slather, 201
  Synergistic Smoothing Blend, 275
Niaouli
  about, 97
  Niaouli Inhaler, 351
  Soothing Niaouli-Hops Balm, 191
  Synergistic Sinusitis Inhaler, 153

O

Orange. *See also* Sweet orange
  about, 98
  Tea Tree–Orange Dandruff Treatment, 285
Oregano
  about, 99
  Cooling Oregano–Cucumber Seed Spray, 194
  Oregano Neat Treatment, 203
  Oregano Salve and Compress, 137
  Synergistic Sinusitis Inhaler, 153

P

Palmarosa
  about, 100
  Soothing Palmarosa-Lavender Bath Salts, 195
  Synergistic Callus Blend, 301
Palo santo
  about, 101
  Patchouli–Palo Santo Potpourri, 345
  substitutions, 39
Patchouli
  about, 102
  Minty Rosemary-Patchouli Body Spray, 259
  Patchouli-Myrrh Antiseptic Gel, 159
  Patchouli–Palo Santo Potpourri, 345
  Patchouli-Petitgrain Spritz, 217
  Patchouli-Spearmint Repellent Lotion, 343
  Patchouli–Tea Tree Foot Balm, 303
  Post-Pregnancy Stretch Mark Slather, 201
  Restorative Shower Melts, 161
  Rosewood-Patchouli Toner, 274
  Sensual Massage Oil, 241
  Synergistic Callus Blend, 301
Peppermint
  about, 103
  Breathe-Easy Synergistic Blend, 350
  Chamomile-Peppermint Compress, 178
  Citrus-Mint Diffusion, 160
  Cooling Peppermint Body Wrap, 143
  Copaiba-Peppermint Foot Cream, 298
  Detoxifying Massage Oil, 161
  Dry Shampoo, 288

Peppermint (*continued*)
  Indoor Spider Repellent Spray, 346
  Juniper-Peppermint Gel, 172
  Lavender-Peppermint Anti-Itch Spray, 353
  Lavender-Peppermint Lip Salve, 189
  Lemon-Mint Spider Repellent Powder, 347
  Minty Helichrysum-Chamomile Compress, 176
  Minty Lavender-Cypress Gel, 169
  Minty Lemon-Lavender Temple Rub, 145
  Minty Orange-Chamomile Lotion, 225
  Minty Rosemary-Patchouli Body Spray, 259
  Pantry Moth Repellent, 345
  Peppermint Ant Killer, 339
  Peppermint-Basil Travel Gel, 167
  Peppermint-Eucalyptus Pedicure Lotion, 307
  Peppermint–Fennel Seed Location, 226
  Peppermint Massage, 235
  Peppermint-Myrrh Lotion, 357
  Peppermint-Pine Liniment, 165
  Peppermint–Rose Geranium Gel for Hot Flashes, 243
  Peppermint-Rosemary Conditioner, 284
  Peppermint Sugar Scrub, 265
  Peppermint–Tea Tree Ant Spray, 339
  Refreshing Peppermint–Cucumber Seed Toner, 267
  Restorative Shower Melts, 161
  Rosemary, Basil, and Mint Shower Melts for General Headaches, 163
  Rosemary-Peppermint Shampoo, 289
  Rosemary-Peppermint Temple Rub, 211
  Soothing Chamomile-Cypress Gel, 273
  Synergistic Cold Sore Ointment, 191
  Synergistic Dandruff Shampoo, 285
  Synergistic Dog Flea-Collar Blend, 341
  Synergistic Healing Balm, 177
  Synergistic Heartburn Blend, 231
  Synergistic Itch-Relief Spray, 357
  Synergistic Nail-Strengthening Blend, 297
  Synergistic Pain-Relief Blend, 173
  Synergistic Spider Spray, 347
  Synergistic Split-End Conditioner, 291
  Synergistic Traveler's Body Lotion, 167
  Tea Tree–Orange Dandruff Treatment, 285
  Winter Spice Cologne, 315
Petitgrain
  about, 104
  Patchouli-Petitgrain Spritz, 217
Pine
  about, 105
  Peppermint-Pine Liniment, 165
  Slug and Snail Repellent, 355
  Synergistic Asthma Inhaler, 133
  Winter Spice Cologne, 315

R

Ravensara leaf
  about, 106
  Synergistic Abdominal Massage Blend, 229
Ravintsara
  about, 107
  Calming Ravintsara Balm, 196

Roman chamomile
  about, 108
  Calming Chamomile-Neroli Steam, 216
  Chamomile-Helichrysum Gel, 184
  Chamomile-Lavender Gel, 352
  Chamomile-Peppermint Compress, 178
  Chamomile–Tea Tree Balm, 186
  Clary Sage Shower Melts, 243
  Cool Chamomile Compress, 150
  Fresh Summer Breeze Spray, 320
  Grapefruit–Ylang-Ylang Diffusion, 221
  Lavender-Chamomile Nighttime Shower Melts, 212
  Lavender–Roman Chamomile Cleansing Wipes, 193
  Lemon, Rosemary, and Chamomile Diffusion, 214
  Melissa-Chamomile Diffusion, 351
  Minty Helichrysum-Chamomile Compress, 176
  Minty Orange-Chamomile Lotion, 225
  Moisturizing Chamomile Body Wash, 262
  Moisturizing Chamomile Hair Mask, 287
  Peppermint-Pine Liniment, 165
  Roman Chamomile–Lavender Spritz, 197
  Roman Chamomile Salve for Bleeding Hemorrhoids, 233
  Roman Chamomile–Tea Tree Balm, 183
  Synergistic Blend for Irregular Cycles, 245
  Synergistic Callus Blend, 301
  Synergistic Eye Serum, 269
  Synergistic Hot Compress, 185
  Synergistic Itch-Relief Spray, 357
  Synergistic Relaxation Diffusion, 219
  Synergistic Traveler's Body Lotion, 167
Rose
  about, 109
  Menopause, 242
  Relaxing Lavender-Vetiver-Rose Bedtime Lotion, 207
  Rose-Davana Perfume, 241
  Spikenard-Rose Bath Salts, 213
  substitutions, 39
Rose geranium
  about, 110
  Calming Temple Rub, 206
  Geranium-Neroli Cream, 201
  Peppermint–Rose Geranium Gel for Hot Flashes, 243
  Rose Geranium Sugar Scrub, 301
  Sweet Orange–Rose Geranium Body Oil, 263
  Synergistic Age Spot Salve, 257
  Synergistic Relaxation Diffusion, 219
  Synergistic Rosacea Blend, 273
  Synergistic Skin-Firming Lotion, 261
Rosemary
  about, 111
  Anti-Acne "Spot Not" Mask, 254
  Basil, Rosemary, and Cypress Diffusion, 208
  Lemon, Rosemary, and Chamomile Diffusion, 214
  Mason Jar Luminaries, 342
  Minty Rosemary-Patchouli Body Spray, 259
  Peppermint-Rosemary Conditioner, 284

Rosemary (*continued*)
   Quick Countertop Wipes, 329
   Rosemary, Basil, and Mint Shower Melts for General Headaches, 163
   Rosemary-Eucalyptus Vapor for Sinus Headaches, 163
   Rosemary-Lavender Foot Powder, 307
   Rosemary-Lemon Hand Cream, 209
   Rosemary-Peppermint Shampoo, 289
   Rosemary-Peppermint Temple Rub, 211
   Rosemary–Sweet Orange Compress, 227
   Synergistic Antifungal Douche, 249
   Synergistic Dandruff Shampoo, 285
   Synergistic Dog Flea-Collar Blend, 341
   Synergistic Split-End Conditioner, 291

Rosewood
   about, 112
   Lavender-Rosewood Hand Cream, 304
   Rosewood Deodorant, 259
   Rosewood-Patchouli Toner, 274
   Synergistic Relaxation Diffusion, 219
   Tagetes-Rosewood Balm, 159

S

Sage. *See* Clary sage; Spanish sage

Sandalwood
   about, 113
   Calming Temple Rub, 206
   Clary Sage–Sandalwood Conditioner, 286
   Everyday Citrus-Sandalwood Spritzer, 218
   Garden in the Woods Eau de Toilette, 313
   Sandalwood Neat Treatment, 257
   Sandalwood Serum, 281
   Sandalwood Split-End Gel, 290
   Sandalwood-Vetiver Spray, 215
   Sensual Massage Oil, 241
   Soothing Sandalwood Lotion, 237
   substitutions, 39

Spanish sage
   about, 114
   Copaiba–Spanish Sage Vapor, 141

Spearmint
   about, 115
   Cooling Spearmint-Strawberry Mask, 266
   Cool Spearmint Compress, 143
   Eucalyptus-Spearmint Vapor, 152
   Grapefruit-Spearmint Foot Spray, 306
   Grapefruit-Spearmint Spritz, 209
   Lavender-Spearmint Breath Spray, 147
   Melissa-Spearmint Bath Salts, 237
   Minty Fennel Seed–Eucalyptus Lotion, 230
   Minty Fresh Fridge, 333
   Patchouli-Spearmint Repellent Lotion, 343
   Soothing Spearmint-Hyssop Gargle, 135
   Spearmint Compress, 231

Spikenard
   about, 116
   Spikenard-Rose Bath Salts, 213
   substitutions, 39

Spruce
   about, 117
   Soothing Spruce-Yuzu Massage, 141
   Spruce Compress, 165

Sweet orange
  about, 118
  All-Purpose Disinfectant Spray, 322
  Allspice–Sweet Orange Diffusion, 134
  Citrus–Clove Bud Breath Drops, 146
  Citrus-Mint Diffusion, 160
  Citrus Serum for Combination Skin, 279
  Everyday Citrus-Sandalwood Spritzer, 218
  Minty Orange-Chamomile Lotion, 225
  Oven/Stovetop Gentle Scrubbing Soap, 329
  Quick Spot Cleaner, 333
  Rosemary–Sweet Orange Compress, 227
  Spicy Autumn Room Deodorizer, 321
  Sweet Orange–Rose Geranium Body Oil, 263
  Synergistic Rosacea Blend, 273

T

Tagetes
  about, 119
  Tagetes Bunion Balm, 299
  Tagetes-Rosewood Balm, 159
Tangerine
  about, 120
  Tangerine-Lavender Lotion, 215
Tea tree
  about, 121
  All-Purpose Disinfectant Spray, 322
  Chamomile–Tea Tree Balm, 186
  Cooling Cucumber Seed–Tea Tree Toner, 255
  Daily Tea Tree–Eucalyptus Shower Spray, 323
  Grapefruit-Spearmint Foot Spray, 306
  Heavy-Duty Window Cleaner, 326
  Lavender–Tea Tree Balm, 271
  Lavender–Tea Tree Compress, 151
  Lavender–Tea Tree Conditioner, 289
  Lavender–Tea Tree Footbath, 309
  Lavender–Tea Tree Tampon, 248
  Mold and Mildew Prevention Spray, 330
  Patchouli–Tea Tree Foot Balm, 303
  Peppermint–Tea Tree Ant Spray, 339
  Quick Countertop Wipes, 329
  Roman Chamomile Salve for Bleeding Hemorrhoids, 233
  Roman Chamomile–Tea Tree Balm, 183
  Soothing Bergamot-Lavender Neck Wrap, 149
  Soothing Tea Tree Compress, 265
  Synergistic Antibacterial Massage Blend, 247
  Synergistic Antifungal Douche, 249
  Synergistic Asthma Inhaler, 133
  Synergistic Cold Sore Ointment, 191
  Synergistic Dandruff Shampoo, 285
  Synergistic Hot Compress, 185
  Synergistic Overnight Foot Cream, 303
  Synergistic Pinkeye Blend, 151
  Synergistic Sinusitis Shower Melts, 153
  Synergistic Spider Spray, 347
  Tea Tree Antifungal Plant Treatment, 355
  Tea Tree Gel, 271
  Tea Tree Mold Remover, 331
  Tea Tree Neat Treatment, 203, 295
  Tea Tree Neat Treatment for Blemishes, 255
  Tea Tree–Orange Dandruff Treatment, 285

Tea tree (*continued*)
 Tea Tree Rinse, 137
 Tea Tree Steam Treatment, 185
 Tea Tree Wall Mold Diffusion, 331
Thyme
 about, 122
 Anti-Acne "Spot Not" Mask, 254
 Green Tea Toner, 280
 Synergistic Asthma Inhaler, 133
 Synergistic Sinusitis Shower Melts, 153

V

Valerian
 about, 123
 Valerian-Cedarwood Bedtime Balm, 213
Vetiver
 about, 124
 Citrus and Spice Splash, 312
 Relaxing Lavender-Vetiver-Rose Bedtime Lotion, 207
 Sandalwood-Vetiver Spray, 215
 substitutions, 39

Vitex berry
 about, 125
 Menopause, 242
 substitutions, 39
 Synergistic Blend for Irregular Cycles, 245

Y

Ylang-ylang
 about, 126
 Calming Temple Rub, 206
 Citrus-Flower Body Butter, 278
 Fleur Classique Parfum, 312
 Grapefruit–Ylang-Ylang Diffusion, 221
 Luxurious Solid Perfume, 314
 Sensual Massage Oil, 241
 Synergistic Relaxation Diffusion, 219
 Yuzu–Ylang-Ylang Diffusion, 207
Yuzu
 about, 127
 Soothing Spruce-Yuzu Massage, 141
 substitutions, 39
 Yuzu–Ylang-Ylang Diffusion, 207

GENERAL INDEX

A

Absolute oils, 19
Acne
  Anti-Acne "Spot Not" Mask, 254
  Cooling Cucumber Seed–Tea Tree Toner, 255
  Tea Tree Neat Treatment for Blemishes, 255
Age spots
  Lemon Mask, 256
  Sandalwood Neat Treatment, 257
  Synergistic Age Spot Salve, 257
Air fresheners
  Fresh Summer Breeze Spray, 320
  Plug-In Air Freshener Scent, 321
  Spicy Autumn Room Deodorizer, 321
Alcohols, 13
Allergies, 29
  Breathe-Easy Synergistic Blend, 350
  Melissa-Chamomile Diffusion, 351
  Niaouli Inhaler, 351
Antioxidants, 11
Ant repellent
  Ant-Eliminating Lavender Neat Treatment, 338
  Peppermint Ant Killer, 339
  Peppermint–Tea Tree Ant Spray, 339
Anxiety
  Calming Temple Rub, 206
  Relaxing Lavender-Vetiver-Rose Bedtime Lotion, 207
  Yuzu–Ylang-Ylang Diffusion, 207

Apricot kernel oil, 22
Aromatherapy. *See also* Essential oils
  benefits of, 4–5
  reasons for using, 18
  science of, 10–11
Arousal
  Jasmine Linen Spray, 240
  Rose-Davana Perfume, 241
  Sensual Massage Oil, 241
Asthma
  Cajuput-Bergamot Diffusion, 132
  Relaxing Clary Sage–Lavender Chest Rub, 133
  Synergistic Asthma Inhaler, 133
Athlete's foot
  Clove Bud Spray, 294
  May Chang Foot Powder, 295
  Tea Tree Neat Treatment, 295

B

Backache
  Cedarwood Massage Oil, 156
  Cinnamon Leaf–Ginger Salve, 157
  Lavender-Benzoin Bath Salts, 157
Bathroom cleansers
  All-Purpose Disinfectant Spray, 322
  Daily Tea Tree–Eucalyptus Shower Spray, 323
  Lemon Scouring Powder, 323

Bee Sting Relief, Lavender-Eucalyptus, 353
Blisters
   Lavender Neat Treatment, 182
   Myrrh-Helichrysum Compress, 183
   Roman Chamomile–Tea Tree Balm, 183
Bloating
   Cinnamon Leaf–Fennel Seed Balm, 224
   Ginger–Black Pepper Digestive Massage, 225
   Minty Orange-Chamomile Lotion, 225
Blood-brain barrier, 11
Body odor
   Lavender Body Powder, 258
   Minty Rosemary-Patchouli Body Spray, 259
   Rosewood Deodorant, 259
Boils
   Chamomile-Helichrysum Gel, 184
   Synergistic Hot Compress, 185
   Tea Tree Steam Treatment, 185
Bowles, E. Joy, 13
Brittle Nails
   Frankincense Nail Balm, 296
   Lemon-Elemi Nail Soak, 297
   Synergistic Nail-Strengthening Blend, 297
Bronchitis
   Allspice–Sweet Orange Diffusion, 134
   Anise–Caraway Seed Vapor, 135
   Soothing Spearmint-Hyssop Gargle, 135
Bunions
   Copaiba-Peppermint Foot Cream, 298
   Frankincense Cold Compress, 299
   Tagetes Bunion Balm, 299

Burns
   Chamomile–Tea Tree Balm, 186
   Lavender-Geranium Compress, 187
   Lavender Neat Treatment, 187

C

Calluses
   Lavender-Myrrh Massage, 300
   Rose Geranium Sugar Scrub, 301
   Synergistic Callus Blend, 301
Canker sores
   Dill Seed Balm, 136
   Oregano Salve and Compress, 137
   Tea Tree Rinse, 137
Carrier oils, 21–22
Cellulite
   Anti-Cellulite Bath Salts, 260
   Synergistic Cellulite Massage Oil, 261
   Synergistic Skin-Firming Lotion, 261
Chapped lips
   Basic Lip Balm, 188
   Lavender-Peppermint Lip Salve, 189
   Lemon-Lavender Lip Balm, 189
The Chemistry of Aromatherapeutic Oils (Bowles), 13
Children, use of oils with, 31
CO_2 extraction, 12
Cold pressing, 12
Colds
   Bay Laurel–Lavender Diffusion, 138
   Caraway–Clove Bud Chest Rub, 139
   May Chang–Lemon Lotion, 139

Cold sores
- Melissa Neat Treatment, 190
- Soothing Niaouli-Hops Balm, 191
- Synergistic Cold Sore Ointment, 191

Colognes. *See also* Splashes
- Hungary Water, 314
- Winter Spice Cologne, 315

Concentration
- Basil, Rosemary, and Cypress Diffusion, 208
- Grapefruit-Spearmint Spritz, 209
- Rosemary-Lemon Hand Cream, 209

Congestion
- Caraway Seed–May Chang Shower Steam, 140
- Copaiba–Spanish Sage Vapor, 141
- Soothing Spruce-Yuzu Massage, 141

Conjunctivitis. *See* Pinkeye

Constipation
- Peppermint–Fennel Seed Lotion, 226
- Rosemary–Sweet Orange Compress, 227
- Synergistic Bath Blend, 227

Cracked heels
- Lemon-Lavender Foot Soak, 302
- Patchouli–Tea Tree Foot Balm, 303
- Synergistic Overnight Foot Cream, 303

Cuts and scrapes
- Lavender Neat Treatment, 158
- Patchouli-Myrrh Antiseptic Gel, 159
- Tagetes-Rosewood Balm, 159

D

Dandruff
- Peppermint-Rosemary Conditioner, 284
- Synergistic Dandruff Shampoo, 285
- Tea Tree–Orange Dandruff Treatment, 285

Diaper rash
- Frankincense-Myrrh Barrier Cream, 192
- Lavender-Neroli Baby Powder, 193
- Lavender–Roman Chamomile Cleansing Wipes, 193

Diarrhea
- Copaiba-Coriander Compress, 228
- Synergistic Abdominal Massage Blend, 229
- Triple-Spice Massage Blend, 229

Diffusions, 34

Dilutions, 35–37

Dry hair
- Clary Sage–Sandalwood Conditioner, 286
- Moisturizing Chamomile Hair Mask, 287
- Moisturizing Geranium-Myrrh Shampoo, 287

Dry hands
- Lavender-Rosewood Hand Cream, 304
- Skin-Softening Hand Soap, 305
- Soothing Hand Balm, 305

Dry skin
- Moisturizing Chamomile Body Wash, 262
- Soothing Benzoin-Myrrh Body Lotion, 263
- Sweet Orange–Rose Geranium Body Oil, 263

E

Eczema
   Cooling Oregano–Cucumber Seed Spray, 194
   Geranium-Lavender Balm, 195
   Soothing Palmarosa-Lavender Bath Salts, 195
Endogenous opioids, 10
Energy levels, boosting, 4
Enfleurage, 12
Equipment and tools, 23–24
Essential oils. *See also* Aromatherapy; Oils Index
   about, 6
   aroma categories, 20–21
   to avoid, 27
   chemistry of, 13–14
   contraindications, 31–34
   great-to-have, 35
   how they work, 5
   must-have, 35
   production of, 12–13
   safety guidelines, 26–34
   shopping for, 18–21
   storing, 25–26
   substituting, 38–39
Esters, 13
Exhaustion
   Basil-Geranium Shower Steam, 210
   Rosemary-Peppermint Temple Rub, 211
   Uplifting Citrus-Basil Diffusion, 211
Expression, 12
Extraction techniques, 12–13

F

Feelings and emotions, 4
Fever
   Aromatic Eucalyptus Sponge Bath, 142
   Cooling Peppermint Body Wrap, 143
   Cool Spearmint Compress, 143
Fibromyalgia
   Eucalyptus, Juniper, and Geranium Lotion, 144
   Minty Lemon-Lavender Temple Rub, 145
   Spicy Frankincense-Helichrysum Balm, 145
Fleas
   Indoor Flea Powder, 340
   Lavender Flea Powder, 341
   Synergistic Dog Flea-Collar Blend, 341
Floor cleaners
   Citrus Hardwood Floor Cleaner, 324
   Lavender-Eucalyptus Mop Solution, 325
   Mandarin-Neroli Carpet Powder, 325
Foot odor
   Grapefruit-Spearmint Foot Spray, 306
   Peppermint-Eucalyptus Pedicure Lotion, 307
   Rosemary-Lavender Foot Powder, 307
Fragrance oils, 7, 19
Free radicals, 11
Fungal infections, 5

G

Glass and mirror cleaners
   Heavy-Duty Window Cleaner, 326
   Lemon Window Cleaner, 327
   Streak-Free Glass and Mirror Cleaner, 327

Grapeseed oil, 21
Gut health, 224–237

H

Hair care, 284–291
Halitosis
   Citrus–Clove Bud Breath Drops, 146
   Lavender Mouthwash, 147
   Lavender-Spearmint Breath Spray, 147
Hangover
   Citrus-Mint Diffusion, 160
   Detoxifying Massage Oil, 161
   Restorative Shower Melts, 161
Hay fever
   Breathe-Easy Synergistic Blend, 350
   Melissa-Chamomile Diffusion, 351
   Niaouli Inhaler, 351
Headache
   Lavender, Marjoram, and Basil Balm for Tension Headaches, 162
   Rosemary, Basil, and Mint Shower Melts for General Headaches, 163
   Rosemary-Eucalyptus Vapor for Sinus Headaches, 163
Healing, 4, 129. *See also specific ailments*
Heartburn
   Minty Fennel Seed–Eucalyptus Lotion, 230
   Spearmint Compress, 231
   Synergistic Heartburn Blend, 231
Hemorrhoids
   Lemon-Cypress Compress, 232
   Neroli-Myrrh Wipes, 233
   Roman Chamomile Salve for Bleeding Hemorrhoids, 233
Hives
   Calming Ravintsara Balm, 196
   Roman Chamomile–Lavender Spritz, 197
   Soothing Myrrh Bath, 197
Household cleaners, 320–335
Hydrosols, 6

I

Identical oils, 19
Immunity, 4
Indigestion
   Cardamom Balm, 234
   Comforting Clove Bud Compress, 235
   Peppermint Massage, 235
Ingredients, 24
Ingrown hair
   Lavender Neat Treatment, 264
   Peppermint Sugar Scrub, 265
   Soothing Tea Tree Compress, 265
Ingrown toenails
   Healing Frankincense Balm, 308
   Lavender–Tea Tree Footbath, 309
   Lemon Eucalyptus–Clove Bud Compress, 309
Inhalation, 5
Insect bites and stings
   Chamomile-Lavender Gel, 352
   Lavender-Eucalyptus Bee Sting Relief, 353
   Lavender-Peppermint Anti-Itch Spray, 353

Insomnia
  Lavender-Chamomile Nighttime Shower Melts, 212
  Spikenard-Rose Bath Salts, 213
  Valerian-Cedarwood Bedtime Balm, 213

J

Joint pain
  Benzoin Balm, 164
  Peppermint-Pine Liniment, 165
  Spruce Compress, 165
Jojoba oil, 22
Journal of Alternative and Complementary Medicine, 5
Journal of Medical Microbiology, 5

K

Ketones, 13
Kitchen cleansers
  Microwave Disinfectant, 328
  Oven/Stovetop Gentle Scrubbing Soap, 329
  Quick Countertop Wipes, 329

L

Laryngitis/sore throat
  Lavender-Lemon Gargle, 149
  Lavender-Marjoram Sore Throat Spray, 148
  Soothing Bergamot-Lavender Neck Wrap, 149
Lawn and garden care
  Cinnamon Leaf Weedkiller, 354
  Slug and Snail Repellent, 355
  Tea Tree Antifungal Plant Treatment, 355

M

Maceration, 12
Memory enhancement, 4
Menopause
  Balancing Vitex Berry Lotion, 242
  Clary Sage Shower Melts, 243
  Peppermint–Rose Geranium Gel for Hot Flashes, 243
Menstrual symptoms
  Cypress–German Chamomile Compress for Menstrual Cramps, 244
  Fennel Seed–Grapefruit Massage for Bloating, 245
  Synergistic Blend for Irregular Cycles, 245
Mirror Cleaner, Streak-Free Glass and, 327
Moisturizers
  Basic Body Butter, 278
  Citrus-Flower Body Butter, 278
  Citrus Serum for Combination Skin, 279
  Easy Whipped Moisturizer, 279
  Frankincense and Commonsense Serum, 280
  Nourishing Nighttime Lotion, 281
  Sandalwood Serum, 281
Mold and mildew
  Mold and Mildew Prevention Spray, 330
  Tea Tree Mold Remover, 331
  Tea Tree Wall Mold Diffusion, 331
Monoterpenes, 13
Moodiness
  Lemon, Rosemary, and Chamomile Diffusion, 214
  Sandalwood-Vetiver Spray, 215
  Tangerine-Lavender Lotion, 215

Mosquitoes
    Mason Jar Luminaries, 342
    Mosquito Repellent Spray, 343
    Patchouli-Spearmint Repellent Lotion, 343
Moths
    Citronella-Lavender Mothballs, 344
    Pantry Moth Repellent, 345
    Patchouli–Palo Santo Potpourri, 345
Motion sickness
    Ginger Inhaler, 166
    Peppermint-Basil Travel Gel, 167
    Synergistic Traveler's Body Lotion, 167
Muscle cramps
    Lavender-Marjoram Compress, 168
    Minty Lavender-Cypress Gel, 169
    Soothing Massage Oil, 169
Muscle soreness
    Benzoin–Black Pepper Muscle Balm, 170
    Fir Needle Gel, 171
    Synergistic Pain-Relief Compress, 171

N

Nausea and vomiting
    Copaiba-Chamomile Compress, 236
    Melissa-Spearmint Bath Salts, 237
    Soothing Sandalwood Lotion, 237
Neat use of oils, 35–36
Neck pain
    Juniper-Peppermint Gel, 172
    Marjoram–Fir Needle Compress, 173
    Synergistic Pain-Relief Blend, 173

Nervousness
    Calming Chamomile-Neroli Steam, 216
    Clary Sage–Citrus Diffusion, 217
    Patchouli-Petitgrain Spritz, 217
Nosebleed
    Cypress Nasal Compress, 174
    Lavender Nasal Salve, 175
    Lemon-Lavender Nasal Compress, 175

O

Oily hair
    Dry Shampoo, 288
    Lavender–Tea Tree Conditioner, 289
    Rosemary-Peppermint Shampoo, 289
Oily skin
    Cooling Spearmint-Strawberry Mask, 266
    Deep-Cleansing Lavender-Lemon Steam, 267
    Refreshing Peppermint–Cucumber Seed Toner, 267
Olfactory system, 10–11
Organic oils, 20
Outdoor concerns, 350–359. *See also* Pests
Oxides, 14

P

Packaging of oils, 19
Pain relief, 5. *See also specific aches and pains*
Patch tests, 28
Perfume oils, 7, 19

Perfumes. *See also* Colognes
   Fleur Classique Parfum, 312
   Garden in the Woods Eau de Toilette, 313
   Lavender-Lemon Eau de Toilette, 313
   Luxurious Solid Perfume, 314
   types of, 310
Pests, 338–347
Pets
   Bodily Fluids and Pet Accident Cleaner, 334
   Indoor Flea Powder, 340
   Lavender Flea Powder, 341
   Synergistic Dog Flea-Collar Blend, 341
Phenols, 14
Pinkeye
   Cool Chamomile Compress, 150
   Lavender–Tea Tree Compress, 151
   Synergistic Pinkeye Blend, 151
Poison Ivy
   Lavender-Frankincense Bath, 356
   Peppermint-Myrrh Lotion, 357
   Synergistic Itch-Relief Spray, 357
Prediluted oils, 19
Pregnancy, use of oils during, 29–30
Psoriasis
   Cajuput–Cucumber Seed Gel, 198
   German Chamomile Bath Salts, 199
   Helichrysum Spray, 199
Puffy eyes
   Helichrysum–Cucumber Seed Compress, 268
   Lavender Eye Massage, 269
   Synergistic Eye Serum, 269
Purity of oils, 20

R

Razor bumps
   Honey-Lavender Mask, 270
   Lavender–Tea Tree Balm, 271
   Tea Tree Gel, 271
Refrigerator cleansers
   Lemon-Basil Sanitizing Spray, 332
   Minty Fresh Fridge, 333
   Quick Spot Cleaner, 333
Relaxation
   Everyday Citrus-Sandalwood Spritzer, 218
   Lavender-Basil Bath Salts for Restless Legs Syndrome, 219
   Synergistic Relaxation Diffusion, 219
Rosacea
   Rosacea Treatment for Mature Skin, 272
   Soothing Chamomile-Cypress Gel, 273
   Synergistic Rosacea Blend, 273
Rosehip oil, 22

S

Safety guidelines
   for children, 31
   contraindications, 31–34
   dosages, 26
   general, 28–29, 34
   oils to avoid, 27
   patch tests, 28
   for people with allergies, 29
   during pregnancy, 29–30
   for seniors, 31

Seniors, use of oils with, 31
Sensitization, 28, 34
Sesquiterpenes, 14
Sexual health, 240–249
Sinusitis
   Eucalyptus-Spearmint Vapor, 152
   Synergistic Sinusitis Inhaler, 153
   Synergistic Sinusitis Shower Melts, 153
Skin care and conditions, 4. *See also specific skin care needs and conditions*
Smell, sense of, 3, 10–11
Solvent extraction, 12–13
Sore throat. *See* Laryngitis/sore throat
Spiders
   Indoor Spider Repellent Spray, 346
   Lemon-Mint Spider Repellent Powder, 347
   Synergistic Spider Spray, 347
Splashes, 310
   Citrus and Spice Splash, 312
   Healing Aftershave Splash, 315
Split ends
   Sandalwood Split-End Gel, 290
   Synergistic Split-End Conditioner, 291
   Ultra-Rich Conditioning Mask, 291
Sprain
   Minty Helichrysum-Chamomile Compress, 176
   Synergistic First-Aid Gel and Sprain Compress, 177
   Synergistic Healing Balm, 177

Stain removers
   Bodily Fluids and Pet Accident Cleaner, 334
   Grass Stain Remover, 335
   Lemon Grease Treatment, 335
Steam distillation, 12
Storing oils, 25–26
Stress, 4–5
   Benzoin-Bergamot Lotion, 220
   Cardamom-Mandarin Temple Rub, 221
   Grapefruit–Ylang-Ylang Diffusion, 221
Stretch marks
   Galbanum Cream, 200
   Geranium-Neroli Cream, 201
   Post-Pregnancy Stretch Mark Slather, 201
Sunburn
   Geranium-Lavender Sunburn Gel, 358
   Helichrysum Milk Bath, 359
   Lavender–Cucumber Seed Spray, 359
Sweet almond oil, 22

T

Toner, Green Tea, 280
Tools and equipment, 23–24
Toothache
   Chamomile-Peppermint Compress, 178
   Clove Bud Neat Treatment, 179
   Synergistic Toothache Blend, 179
Topical application, 5, 11
Transdermal action, 11

U

Urinary tract infection (UTI)
    Lavender Rinse, 246
    Synergistic Antibacterial Massage Blend, 247
    Synergistic Antiseptic Bath Salts, 247

V

Vaginal yeast infection
    Lavender–Tea Tree Tampon, 248
    Lemon Salve, 249
    Synergistic Antifungal Douche, 249
Vomiting. *See* Nausea and vomiting

W

Warts
    Lavender Neat Treatment for Post-Wart Removal, 202
    Oregano Neat Treatment, 203
    Tea Tree Neat Treatment, 203
Wrinkles
    Rosewood-Patchouli Toner, 274
    Synergistic Firming Serum, 275
    Synergistic Smoothing Blend, 275